Foundations Interprofessional Collaborative Practice in Health Care

D1026646

Margaret M. Slusser, PhD, RN
Associate Professor of Health Science
Founding Program Coordinator
B.S. in Health Science Program (BSHS)
School of Health Sciences
Stockton University
Galloway, New Jersey

Luis I. García, PhD
Assistant Professor of Health Science
School of Health Sciences
Stockton University
Galloway, New Jersey

Carole-Rae Reed, PhD, RN, APN-BC
Associate Professor of Health Science
School of Health Sciences
Stockton University
Galloway, New Jersey

Patricia Quinn McGinnis, PT, MS, PhD
Professor of Physical Therapy
School of Health Sciences
Stockton University
Galloway, New Jersey

ELSEVIER

ELSEVIER

3251 Riverport Lane
St. Louis, Missouri 63043

FOUNDATIONS OF INTERPROFESSIONAL COLLABORATIVE
PRACTICE IN HEALTH CARE   ISBN: 978-0-323-46241-9

Copyright © 2019, Elsevier Inc. All rights reserved.

No part of this publication may be reproduced or transmitted in any form or by any means, electronic or mechanical, including photocopying, recording, or any information storage and retrieval system, without permission in writing from the publisher. Details on how to seek permission, further information about the Publisher's permissions policies and our arrangements with organizations such as the Copyright Clearance Center and the Copyright Licensing Agency, can be found at our website: www.elsevier.com/permissions.

This book and the individual contributions contained in it are protected under copyright by the Publisher (other than as may be noted herein).

Notices

Practitioners and researchers must always rely on their own experience and knowledge in evaluating and using any information, methods, compounds or experiments described herein. Because of rapid advances in the medical sciences, in particular, independent verification of diagnoses and drug dosages should be made. To the fullest extent of the law, no responsibility is assumed by Elsevier, authors, editors or contributors for any injury and/or damage to persons or property as a matter of products liability, negligence or otherwise, or from any use or operation of any methods, products, instructions, or ideas contained in the material herein.

Library of Congress Control Number: 2018938600

Executive Content Strategist: Lee Henderson
Senior Content Development Specialist: Laura Goodrich
Publishing Services Manager: Julie Eddy
Senior Project Manager: Tracey Schriefer
Design Direction: Amy Buxton

Printed in India

Last digit is the print number: 9   8   7   6   5   4

Working together to grow libraries in developing countries

www.elsevier.com • www.bookaid.org

This book is dedicated to all present and future healthcare professionals; we hope this book can assist them in mastering the Core Competencies for Interprofessional Collaborative Practice. We believe successful collaboration is essential to achieving safe, high-quality, and accessible patient- and population-centered care in all settings. Further, we dedicate this book to our patients and their significant others who are the most important members of the healthcare team, both as active participants, and recipients of care. Finally, we dedicate this work to all educators who, through teaching, mentoring, and role-modeling, inspired us to become effective healthcare professionals and collaborators.

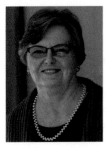

Margaret M. Slusser, PhD, RN

Margaret (Peg) Slusser received her diploma in nursing from Wilkes-Barre General Hospital School of Nursing, BSN from Wilkes University, and Master of Science (Psychiatric–Mental Health Nursing) and PhD in Nursing from the University of Pennsylvania. Her nursing career includes practicing as a staff nurse in critical care, serving as a staff development instructor, private practice as a Clinical Nurse Specialist in Psychiatric Mental Health, and ten years as a producer and writer for the Pennsylvania Public Television Network. Her career in nursing education includes tenured faculty positions at Wilkes University and Bloomsburg University of Pennsylvania, and a leadership position as Chairperson of the Department of Nursing and Health at DeSales University.

Dr. Slusser joined the faculty of Stockton University in 2012 as the Founding Program Coordinator of the Bachelor of Science in Health Science (BSHS) program. Established in 2012, the BSHS program uses the Core Competencies for Interprofessional Collaborative Practice (IPEC, 2011; 2016) as its conceptual framework. The mission of the BSHS program is to provide a quality, contemporary, pre–health professional education for undergraduate students who are preparing for graduate programs leading to healthcare careers or for other careers in the healthcare system. Dr. Slusser serves as an inaugural member of the School of Health Sciences Interprofessional Education (IPE) Committee, planning IPE programs for Stockton undergraduate and graduate students in Communication Disorders, Exercise Science, Health Science, Nursing, Occupational Therapy, Physical Therapy, and Public Health programs. She has presented nationally and internationally on the integration of the Core Competencies for Interprofessional Collaborative Practice into preprofessional and graduate health education programs through IPE.

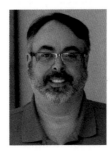

Luis I. García, PhD

Luis I. García is a tenured Assistant Professor of Health Science and the Program Coordinator of the Bachelor of Science in Health Science Program at Stockton University. Dr. García completed a Bachelor of Science in Psychology and a Master of Science in Community Counseling at the University of Wisconsin-Milwaukee. He completed a Doctor of Philosophy in Clinical Psychology with a concentration in Health Psychology at The George Washington University in Washington, DC. He completed a Postdoctoral Fellowship in HIV Prevention Research at the Center for AIDS Intervention Research (CAIR) at the Medical College of Wisconsin, in Milwaukee, WI. Dr. García's early university teaching focused on Human Development, Health Psychology, and Statistics; currently, his teaching focuses on Teamwork and Collaboration in Health Care and Research Methods for the Healthcare Professional.

Dr. García's expertise includes Interprofessional Education (IPE), HIV prevention research, community health, sexual identity, and Latino acculturation. His IPE research focuses on the impact of integrating the Core Competencies for Interprofessional Collaborative Practice in the education of undergraduate, preprofessional students. His HIV/AIDS research focuses on the influence of cultural and social factors in the decision of young Black men who have sex with men (MSM) to get tested for HIV. He has extensive experience conducting research in partnership with community-based organizations and in adapting and implementing evidence-based interventions in the community.

Dr. García has significant clinical experience as a health psychologist working with HIV-positive individuals, LGBT individuals, and Latinos, especially in the context of community-based health clinics. Currently, his clinical practice focuses on at-risk Latino youth and transgender teens.

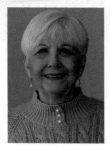

Carole-Rae Reed, PhD, RN, APN-C

Dr. Carole-Rae Reed received her Master of Science in Nursing and Doctor of Philosophy in Nursing from the University of Pennsylvania. Her commitment to interprofessional collaboration is evident throughout her long career. She engaged in postdoctoral study in Sleep and Chronobiology at the University of Pennsylvania School of Medicine, a truly interprofessional field. Dr. Reed has more than 40 years of clinical experience. As an Advanced Practice Nurse in mental health, Dr. Reed practiced collaboratively with a variety of healthcare professionals, community members, patients, and families to provide comprehensive mental health care. Her commitment to teamwork and patient-centered care led to a team award for an Access to Care project. Dr. Reed chaired an interdisciplinary task force on suicide prevention at a large urban medical center. Dr. Reed has an extensive background in research, holding positions as project manager and research coordinator at the University of Pennsylvania School of Nursing, Graduate Hospital, and Cooper University Hospital. She has numerous peer-reviewed publications and international presentations, many involving aspects of Interprofessional Education. She is a member of the Alpha Eta Society (Allied Health) and Sigma Theta Tau International Honor Society of Nursing. Dr. Reed is a tenured Associate Professor at Stockton University in the Bachelor of Science in Health Science (BSHS) program. This program is founded on the Core Competencies for Interprofessional Collaborative Practice. Her current research interests are in Interprofessional Education and Collaborative Practice, and Values and Ethics.

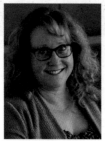

Patricia Quinn McGinnis, PT, MS, PhD, FNAP

Patricia Quinn McGinnis is Director and Professor in the Doctor of Physical Therapy Program at Stockton University in Galloway, NJ. She graduated from the University of Delaware with a Bachelor of Science in Physical Therapy. She earned a postprofessional Master of Science degree in Physical Therapy in the Neurologic Specialty area from the University of the Sciences in Philadelphia and a Doctor of Philosophy degree in Physical Therapy from Temple University. Dr. McGinnis teaches graduate courses in neuromuscular physical therapy, evidence-based practice, and professional issues. She has extensive clinical experience in the acute care and inpatient rehabilitation settings, providing patient-centered care as a member of healthcare team. Dr. McGinnis is an experienced qualitative researcher whose research endeavors include interprofessional education, clinical decision making, and development of professional core values. Her work includes peer-reviewed presentations at national and international conferences on outcomes of interprofessional education initiatives.

Her years in physical therapy education include a faculty position in the School of Health Professions at Rutgers–UMDNJ. She joined the faculty at Stockton in 1999 and later served as Associate Director of the postprofessional tDPT Program for practicing physical therapists. She was a founding member of the School of Health Sciences Interprofessional Education (IPE) Committee. Later she served as Chair of the IPE Committee and expanded participation in IPE activities across the university to include faculty and students from the Education, Psychology, Social Work, and Gerontology. Dr. McGinnis was the inaugural Interprofessional Education Fellow in the School of Health Sciences. In this role, she mentored faculty developing interprofessional learning activities across the university, as well as faculty looking to disseminate their efforts through professional presentations and publications.

In 2018, Dr. McGinnis was elected as a Distinguished Fellow of the National Academies of Practice (NAP) in Physical Therapy. She joins many outstanding healthcare leaders and practitioners of NAP, who are working collaboratively as an interprofessional community to influence and promote national health policy, legislation, quality health care, and research.

PROFESSIONAL CONSULTANT PANEL

Mark Adelung, MSN, RN
Assistant Professor of Nursing
Stockton University
School of Health Sciences
Galloway, New Jersey

Marc Baron, MSN, RN, CEN, PHRN
Children's Hospital of Philadelphia
Philadelphia, Pennsylvania

Felicita Calderon, RN (Retired)
Carolina, Puerto Rico

Jose J. Campos, DDS
Dentist
Private Practice
Bayamón, Puerto Rico

Victor I. Campos, MD
Occupational Medicine, Physician
Private Practice
Carolina, Puerto Rico

Reinaldo Colón, MS, RN
Neurosurgery Intensive Care Unit
Puerto Rico Medical Center
University of Puerto Rico–Medical Sciences Campus
Rio Piedras, Puerto Rico

Melissa Diener, MD
Gastroenterology, Physician
Private Practice
Egg Harbor Township, New Jersey

Anthony Dissen, MA, RDN
Instructor of Health Sciences
Stockton University
School of Health Sciences
Galloway, New Jersey

Kimberly A. Furphy, DHSc, OT
Program Director and Associate Professor
Master of Science in Occupational Therapy Program
Stockton University
Galloway, New Jersey

Priti Haria, PhD
Assistant Professor of Special Education
Stockton University
School of Education
Galloway, New Jersey

Jack B. Lewis, DSW, MSW, LCSW
Assistant Professor of Social Work
Stockton University
School of Social and Behavioral Sciences
Galloway, New Jersey

Joan M. Perks, PhD, RN, APN-C, CNE, CEN, CRNI
Associate Professor of Nursing
Stockton University
School of Health Sciences
Galloway, New Jersey

Barry Ransom, MS, RRT-NPS, RRT-ACCS
Visiting Assistant Professor of Health Sciences
Stockton University
School of Health Sciences
Galloway, New Jersey

Daisha Woodlin, RPhT
Registered Pharmacy Technician
Rite Aid Pharmacy
Vineland, New Jersey

INTERPROFESSIONAL EXPERT PANEL

Tracy A. Christopherson, MS, BAS, RRT
Doctoral Student
Rosalind Franklin University of Medicine and Science
North Chicago, Illinois

Lindsay Fox, MEd, RRT-NPS
Program Director
Respiratory Care
St. Louis Community College
St. Louis, Missouri

Victoria L. Gaffney, MSN, RN, CHSE
Associate Professor, Simulation Coordinator
Interprofessional Education Curriculum Coordinator of
    Nursing
Sinclair Community College
Dayton, Ohio

Barbara A. Ihrke, PhD, RN
Vice-President for Academic Affairs
School of Nursing
Indiana Wesleyan University
Marion, Indiana

Robert L. Joyner, Jr., PhD, RRT, RRT-ACCS, FAARC
Special Assistant to the Provost
Associate Dean, Richard A. Henson School of Science &
    Technology
Director, Respiratory Therapy Program
Department of Health Sciences
Salisbury University
Salisbury, Maryland

Jane Clifford O'Brien, PhD, OTR/L, FAOTA
Professor
Occupational Therapy
University of New England
Portland, Maine

Christine Patel, MA, RDH, BSDH,
Associate Professor
Dental Hygiene, Baccalaureate program
St. Petersburg College
St. Petersburg, Florida

Donald J. Raymond, MS, RRT
Respiratory Therapy Program Director Chippewa Valley
    Technical College
Respiratory Therapy
Chippewa Valley Technical College
Eau Claire, Wisconsin

Michelle R. Troseth, MSN, RN, FNAP, FAAN
President
National Academies of Practice (NAP)
Lexington, Kentucky

FOREWORD

The overall purpose of the Interprofessional Education Collaborative (IPEC) Expert Panel that produced the original *Core Competencies for Interprofessional Collaborative Practice* Report in 2011, and updated them in 2016 to be more inclusive of population health, was to define a broad framework for application to interprofessional education of future healthcare practitioners in the United States. Such preparation is believed to be fundamental to achieving the Triple Aim of improved patient experience of care, improved population health, and reduced costs of care. Building on existing work related to professional and interprofessional collaborative competencies both in and outside the United States, that Report and its update have spawned many organizational, educational, research, and evaluation responses, including translation into other languages. This book is one of those educational responses.

The authors thoughtfully and diligently apply the broad framework defined in the Report and its update to the fundamentals of interprofessional learning with application to practice. The first three chapters provide (1) an introduction to the concepts of Interprofessional Education (IPE) and Interprofessional Collaborative Practice (IPCP), (2) systems theory as the chosen theoretical framework for understanding IPCP, and (3) the concepts of wellness and patient-centered care. The systems theory chapter should be read, or reread as a concluding chapter, to deepen understanding of the theoretical bases that underlie the concept of IPCP in individual and population-based care because it is not directly linked to the content following this chapter.

Beginning with Chapter 4, each of the four domains of Interprofessional Collaboration, as defined and described in the 2011 Report and 2016 update, are considered and applied in a series of three chapters: Foundations, Competencies, and Case Studies. These foundational chapters contain descriptions of basic concepts related to each of the four domains, along with active learning exercises. These include "Caselets," brief cases with Discussion Questions. The foundational chapters integrate professional with interprofessional considerations, helping to foster the development of both professional and interprofessional identities.

The Competency chapters provide a detailed introduction to each of the four interprofessional collaboration competencies and their Sub-competencies. Case Studies with Discussion Questions provide for active learning around the Sub-competencies, along with a self-evaluation exercise for each of the Sub-competencies.

The Interprofessional Case Studies chapters provide a series of longer Case Studies, highlighting, for each case presented, which Sub-competencies are to be considered and applied. These case descriptions are followed by provocative, engaging, and often challenging Discussion Questions.

The Caselets and Case Studies are a treasure trove of application material. They are crafted carefully to emphasize the overall domain being addressed, while not excluding elements of other IPCP competency domains. Chapter 16, the concluding chapter, provides a series of collaborative Case Studies with an expectation to apply multiple aspects of the four competency domains of IPCP to each case situation.

All chapters begin with a list of Learning Outcomes. Each chapter ends with a summary of Key Points. Boxed content introduces limited global perspectives on each competency domain. Many of the chapters include, as well, a relevant "Research Highlight," which can be expanded for a more research-oriented IPE learning experience. The book content is not written from the perspective of any single profession but is truly written to orient many types of health professions students to the concept of IPCP. The Caselets and Case Studies incorporate many types of health (and other) professions. They emphasize, consistently, patient- or population-centered situations.

The book content can be used as a basic text for a course on understanding and applying the Core Competencies of Interprofessional Collaboration across the health professions. However, selected content also can be used to focus on one of the domains, such as Ethics and Values, for professional as well as interprofessional learning and practice. Active learning materials, such as the Caselets with Discussion Questions and the longer Case Studies, can stand on their own as ways to deepen understanding and application of basic concepts of IPCP by teachers and students.

This book is a practical realization of the hoped-for detailed application of the competencies for Interprofessional Collaborative Practice that was envisioned by IPEC and the original Expert Panel, strengthened substantially by the incorporated additions from the 2016 Report update.

Madeline H. Schmitt, PhD, RN, FAAN, FNAP
Professor Emerita
University of Rochester School of Nursing
Rochester, New York

Dr. Schmitt chaired the Expert Panel that wrote the 2011 *Core Competencies for Interprofessional Collaborative Practice* report for IPEC.

REFERENCES

Interprofessional Education Collaborative Expert Panel. (2011). Core competencies for interprofessional collaborative practice: Report of an expert panel. Washington, DC: Interprofessional Education Collaborative.

Interprofessional Education Collaborative. (2016). Core competencies for interprofessional collaborative practice: 2016 Update. Washington, DC: Interprofessional Education Collaborative.

TO THE INSTRUCTOR

This textbook represents an effort to provide a clear and illustrative guide for teaching students to understand and apply the Core Competencies for Interprofessional Collaborative Practice. Within this book, the four Core Competencies—Values/Ethics, Roles/Responsibilities, Interprofessional Communication, and Teams and Teamwork—along with their specific behavioral Sub-competency statements (IPEC, 2016) are explicated and supported by foundational theory and real-world case examples. Carefully constructed behavioral learning outcomes, provided as the Sub-competencies of each of the four Core Competencies, will serve as measurable student learning outcomes for use in curriculum development and in the construction of Interprofessional Education (IPE) learning experiences. Students can use the foundational chapters in the book to prepare for the successful accomplishment of identified learning outcomes.

Organization of the Text

- The book begins with a chapter titled **Interprofessional Education and Interprofessional Collaborative Practice,** which introduces the four Core Competencies and provides the national and international context that led to their development.
- The second chapter introduces readers to **systems theory** as an approach to Interprofessional Collaborative Practice. This theory serves as a backdrop to the four Core Competencies by illustrating how they affect health outcomes.
- The third chapter focuses on **wellness** as a paradigm for health care and explains the concepts of health and wellness at the individual and population levels. Instead of an illness-based approach, this chapter presents a comprehensive wellness paradigm within which to focus interprofessional collaboration.
- Chapters 4 through 15 focus on each of the four Core Competencies, each in a set of three chapters.
  - The first chapter in each set presents the **foundational concepts** and **knowledge** necessary to understand the basics of the specific Competency.

For example, Chapter 4 (Foundations of Values/Ethics) contains basic ethical theories and principles, provides a values-clarification exercise, and presents an ethical decision-making process designed for interprofessional collaboration.
  - The second chapter in each set presents the specific **Sub-competencies** related to the featured Core Competency. These Sub-competencies are the specific professional behaviors required to demonstrate mastery of the competency. These Sub-competency statements can serve as specific student learning outcomes that can be measured in a variety of ways. Each Sub-competency is explained with illustrative **Caselets** and unfolding **Case Studies** intended to clearly demonstrate the behavior required for mastery of each individual Sub-competency.
  - The final chapter in each set contains a collection of **Case Studies with Discussion Questions** that are specific to the featured Core Competency. The cases involve several different healthcare professions in a variety of settings and patient care or population health situations. The Case Studies can be customized as needed to meet discipline-specific needs by adding additional instructor-crafted **Discussion Questions** to meet specific student learning outcomes.
- Chapter 16 (**Interprofessional Collaborative Case Studies**) contains a collection of case studies designed to provide opportunities for interprofessional collaboration requiring integration of all four Core Competencies.

Chapter Features

Several features are provided throughout the text to stimulate learning and student self-assessment. **Active Learning** activities are designed to promote the learning of key points in the book; they can be completed independently in a very short time, assigned as homework, or integrated into the classroom as class activities. Additional features, such as **Global Perspectives** and **Research Highlights,** can serve as a basis for class discussions or for students to use to locate similar studies or identify global aspects of interprofessional collaboration. Information provided about **Additional Resources** is useful in broadening understanding of various aspects of interprofessional collaboration and the Core Competencies. **Key Points,** found at the end of all chapters (with the exception of the Case Study chapters) are summary points intended to assist students in their review of chapter content.

Case Studies and **Caselets** are provided throughout and are designed to be applicable to a wide variety of health professions. They may be used as presented by faculty in discipline-specific ways to enhance learning. Because each Case Study involves a variety of healthcare professions, students can divide into groups to work through each case, and each group member can play the role of a different professional. As an alternative, students can discuss the role of their specific profession in greater detail as it applies to the case. Case Studies can be used as individual student assignments, for which the student may be asked to respond to the associated Discussion Questions, or they can be used as a basis for class discussion. Some of the Case Studies and Caselets illustrate "missed opportunities" for interprofessional collaboration, to foster discussion and understanding of concepts. Instructors may choose to expand on a Case Study to suit their specific educational focus. Each Case Study and Caselet is followed by a set of related Discussion Questions; however, instructors may choose to develop their own questions to meet specific student learning outcomes. Questions are designed to provoke thought and discussion and to stimulate further learning and exploration of related concepts. No answers are provided because there is no single correct answer to these questions.

One **Exemplar Case Study** is provided to clearly illustrate each of the four Core Competencies. In these **exemplars,** students are provided with a clear illustration of successful implementation of each Competency and its related Sub-competencies; Sub-competencies are clearly identified for the student to reinforce the learning.

Instructor Resources provided on the companion Evolve website (http://evolve.elsevier.com/Slusser/ interprofessional/) include the following:

- An Image Collection containing all of the illustrations found in the book, for use in classroom or online presentations
- A selection of Case Studies and Caselets from the book

- A Grading Rubric that will assist instructors in scoring student responses in the Discussion Questions.

TO THE STUDENT

To provide safe, high-quality, accessible, patient- and population-centered care in today's complex healthcare climate, healthcare professionals must work collaboratively. As you prepare to work collaboratively with other health professionals, you need to know "what to do" and "how to do it." This book will present and illustrate essential behavioral competencies that you can incorporate into your own professional health education program or healthcare practice to serve in a truly interprofessional manner. The following are the four Core Competencies for Interprofessional Collaborative Practice:

- Values/Ethics for Interprofessional Practice
- Roles/Responsibilities
- Interprofessional Communication
- Teams and Teamwork (IPEC, 2011; 2016)

Practicing and incorporating these essential interprofessional collaboration competencies will help you to become "collaboration-ready." These competencies are the heart of this book.

Your instructor may identify specific learning outcomes for you to demonstrate that are based on these Core Competencies. This textbook will be helpful to you when you participate in Interprofessional Education (IPE) activities. It will provide you with basic information underlying the specific Sub-competencies of interprofessional collaboration that you will need to demonstrate.

Chapter Features

- **Learning Outcomes** and **chapter overviews** introduce each chapter and provide the lens through which you can view chapter content and evaluate your individual learning.
- **Active Learning Activities** are provided for you to complete independently. They are short activities designed to promote the learning of key chapter points. Your instructor may ask you to complete some of these activities as part of class activities or as homework.
- **Case Studies** are presented to provide you with clear examples of Sub-competencies or to illustrate how the application of specific professional behaviors could improve care to a patient or population. Some Case Studies will progressively unfold throughout a chapter to provide you with a continuity of focus.

- **Caselets** are short case studies used to illustrate specific points of learning.
- **Discussion Questions** follow each Case Study and Caselet to encourage you to focus on specific and significant aspects of related Sub-competencies.
- **Global Perspectives** boxes provide information to you about how the topic being discussed is viewed in contexts outside of the United States.
- **Research Highlights** are short discussions of high-quality research or systematic reviews supporting or illustrating the Core Competencies for Interprofessional Collaborative Practice or related concepts.
- **Exemplar Case Studies** provide a clear illustration of successful application of each of the four Core Competencies for Interprofessional Collaborative Practice. In these exemplars, Sub-competencies are clearly indicated to reinforce your learning.

- **Additional Resources** are listed and described to broaden your understanding of the various aspects of interprofessional collaboration and the Core Competencies.
- **Key Points** are summary points listed at the end of each chapter to reinforce the essential chapter content.

REFERENCES

Interprofessional Education Collaborative Expert Panel (IPEC). (2011). Core competencies for interprofessional collaborative practice. Washington, DC: Interprofessional Education Collaborative.

Interprofessional Education Collaborative (IPEC). (2016). Core competencies for interprofessional collaborative practice: 2016 update. Washington, DC: Interprofessional Education Collaborative.

ACKNOWLEDGMENTS

Because this book was truly a collaborative effort, it is difficult to identify and individually thank each person who helped and supported our author team. If you have inspired or supported us in any way, please know that you have our sincere appreciation even if you are not specifically named.

First, we offer our sincere admiration and gratitude to Dr. Madeline Schmitt and the Expert Panel that wrote the groundbreaking 2011 *Core Competencies for Interprofessional Collaborative Practice* report for IPEC. Their vision, identification, and framework for the Core Competencies enabled us to further this work by operationalizing the concepts and offering examples of their practical application.

Next, we recognize the support provided by the Elsevier team; in particular, we thank Lee Henderson, Executive Content Strategist, for believing in us and the concept for this text, and for promoting its publication from the very beginning. We are grateful to Laura Goodrich, Senior Content Development Specialist; Tracey Schriefer, Senior Project Manager; and others on the Elsevier staff for their guidance and patience during the process of making our vision a reality. We thank the reviewers from a variety of healthcare professions who made valuable suggestions that helped us to maintain our focus on Interprofessional Collaborative Practice.

We wish to express our appreciation to Stockton University, who supported us in the form of individual Research and Professional Development grants. We thank the university for its commitment to Interprofessional Education and valuing Interprofessional Collaborative Practice, its creation of an Interprofessional Education Fellowship, and its support of interprofessional activities for and by Stockton students and faculty. Special thanks go to School of Health Sciences and its Deans, faculty, and administrative staff for supporting us in our scholarship and research and facilitating our attendance and presentations at national and international conferences related to interprofessional education and collaborative practice.

Many thanks go to the patients with whom we practiced over the years. These patients and their families motivated us to provide a text that will help promote and develop the skills needed for interprofessional collaboration and patient-centered care. Patient experiences informed the Caselets and Case Studies in this book, either directly or indirectly. We appreciate what a privilege it is, as healthcare professionals, to work with and learn from patients and families.

Our colleagues throughout our careers significantly influenced the creation of this text. We learned the value of interprofessional collaboration from working with colleagues who recognized the importance of and need for collaboration to produce positive patient outcomes.

We called on our colleagues for input in various sections or to check our Case Studies, and they were more than willing to offer perspective. We experienced interprofessional collegiality in many ways that shaped our understanding of each of the four Core Competencies.

Our students inspired the creation of this text. Their eagerness to learn about interprofessional collaboration and teamwork led us to search for materials to assist them in developing the skills that would make them "collaboration ready." Because there were few such materials, we decided to create our own. Much of the content and many of the examples grew from learning activities we developed with our students. We thank them for their contribution to our own education.

The authors are grateful to each other. This text was the result of true collaboration. We wrestled with concepts and wording. We learned to appreciate each other's perspectives. We saw that the outcome was much better because of the team effort. We learned the true meaning and value of interprofessional collaboration.

Last, and certainly not least, we wish to thank our families and friends. The long hours, intense focus, and piles of papers that occupied our lives during the writing of this book required much patience and understanding from them. Your support sustained us throughout our journey and enabled this project to come to fruition. We are eternally grateful for your love, understanding, and constant support.

CONTENTS

1

Interprofessional Education and Interprofessional Collaborative Practice

LEARNING OUTCOMES

After studying this chapter, you will be able to:

1. Describe the evolution of professional health education in the United States.
2. Discuss the impetus for a new paradigm in the education of healthcare professionals.
3. Define Interprofessional Education (IPE).
4. Define Interprofessional Collaborative Practice (IPCP).
5. Describe the role of patients and their significant others in IPCP.
6. Describe the evolution of the Core Competencies for IPCP in the United States.
7. Differentiate between IPE and IPCP.
8. Provide examples of activities that could improve skills in interprofessional collaboration.
9. Discuss IPE and IPCP from a global perspective.

We are in the midst of an exciting evolution in health care. Healthcare professional education and healthcare practice are changing rapidly to increase the quality of both patient and population health. This transformation requires professionals, patients, and others involved in care to work collaboratively to improve patient and population outcomes. This chapter provides the backdrop for this change in the United States and globally.

In this chapter, you will begin a journey inspired by the vision that "interprofessional collaborative practice is the key to safe, high quality, accessible, patient-centered care desired by all" (IPEC, 2011, p. 1). To transform this vision into reality, healthcare professionals need to know what to "do"; therefore common behavioral competencies that can be incorporated into professional health education programs and healthcare practice have been identified. The goal of having common interprofessional collaboration competencies is to provide a foundation for consistency in heathcare provider education that will produce collaboration-ready graduates. The four identified Core Competencies for Interprofessional Collaborative Practice are (1) Values/Ethics for Interprofessional Practice, (2) Roles/Responsibilities, (3) Interprofessional Communication, and (4) Teams and Teamwork (IPEC, 2011; 2016). These competencies become the roadmap to Interprofessional Collaborative Practice (IPCP) and are the subject of this book. This chapter sets the stage for the chapters that follow.

HEALTHCARE PROFESSIONAL EDUCATION: A CALL FOR CHANGE

More than 100 years ago, a series of studies about the education of healthcare professionals, led by the 1910 Flexner Report, sparked groundbreaking educational reform. The Flexner Report transformed the nature and process of medical education in the United States with the establishment of the biomedical model of education as the gold standard. This model embraced the advancement of scientific knowledge as the essential characteristic of the modern physician (Duffy, 2011). This dramatic reform in education was not limited to physicians; it quickly spread to all areas of higher education in the healthcare professions. This educational transformation was recognized as contributing to the doubling of the life span during the 20th century (Frenk et al., 2010).

Over time, the Flexner model of professional education was not able to keep pace with 21st-century health challenges. Concerns about both the quality of health care and the quality of the educational programs preparing healthcare professionals in the United States were raised in a series of reports from the Institute of Medicine (IOM, 1972; 2000; 2001; 2003). Healthcare systems were struggling to cope with challenges brought on by advances in science and technology, new and changing sources of infection, inequities in health care delivery, and rising healthcare costs. Healthcare professionals educated within siloed, single-profession models tended to care for patients independently and rarely collaboratively. Healthcare professionals were poorly equipped to meet the healthcare needs of the future (IOM, 1972; Frenk et al., 2010). The IOM reports emphasized that to maximize the efficiency and effectiveness of the healthcare professional workforce, it would be necessary to redesign the system of healthcare professional education with interdependence between professions, rather than independence, as the goal. The intended outcome was for healthcare professionals to work collaboratively in providing care. The term used to define this interdependent group of healthcare professionals who would work collaboratively toward common goals was *team* (IOM, 1972; 2000; 2001; 2003). Educating students in the various healthcare professions to work collaboratively with other disciplines, in the context of interdisciplinary teams, required a change in educational methods. In posing a solution, the concept of what was then called *interdisciplinary education* was introduced (IOM, 1972).

Even after repeated IOM recommendations (IOM, 2000; 2001; 2003), a lack of teamwork, collaboration, and communication skills continued to be implicated in a wide range of adverse patient and healthcare outcomes (Brandt, 2015). The seminal report *Health Professionals for a New Century: Transforming Education to Strengthen Health Systems in an Interdependent World* (Frenk et al., 2010) echoed the IOM's call for educational reform. It became even clearer that negative outcomes were most likely to continue unless there was a significant shift in healthcare professionals' education that would enable and support quality, collaborative, team-based health care. Specifically, those educating health professionals were called upon to apply the power of interdependence, and not just role independence, in healthcare professional education. Many interdisciplinary educational endeavors began to be implemented over the years to meet this challenge, yet no significant changes in healthcare professionals' education were being realized (IPEC, 2011). The need for a new paradigm in the education of healthcare professionals persisted.

Educating healthcare professionals for interdependence, in addition to independence, required a significant shift in educational focus. Educational programs for healthcare professionals had been discipline-specific in nature. Students preparing for the same profession were educated exclusively with others preparing for the same professional scope of practice, in isolation from those preparing for other professions. For example, future nurses were educated in "nursing programs" and future physicians in "medical school." This isolated approach to preparing healthcare professionals is commonly referred to as a *silo approach* (Fig. 1.1). This approach worked well for teaching the scope and standards of each individual discipline, for demonstrating discipline-specific skills and practice, and for socialization into the individual professions. On the other hand, this approach did not provide intentional opportunities for educational experiences with students,

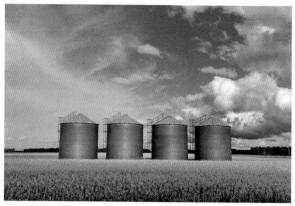

FIG. 1.1 Silos representing the traditional isolated teaching and learning model used in the discipline-specific education of healthcare professionals. (© libertygal/iStock/Thinkstock.)

or practitioners, from other professions that could be classified as interdisciplinary or interprofessional in nature. Graduates were practice-ready but not collaboration-ready. Although being practice-ready as independent practitioners is important, and discipline-specific curriculums remain an essential element of professional education, the need to enrich the current educational paradigm by adding an intentional element of an interdisciplinary education is essential if graduates are to become collaboration-ready as well. It was clear that new educational paradigms needed to include a focus on this interdependence between professions. To achieve this, it was widely agreed that educational approaches for healthcare professionals must include opportunities for students to engage in Interprofessional Education (IPE) as they prepare for IPCP (NLN, 2015).

THE INTERPROFESSIONAL COLLABORATIVE HEALTHCARE TEAM

The Team

There is a significant difference between what was traditionally called a *healthcare team* and what is now referred to as an *interprofessional collaborative healthcare team*. Healthcare providers traditionally identified themselves as members of "the healthcare team" without giving much thought to what that meant. Let's take a closer look at healthcare teams. It is important to be able to differentiate between the traditional, and often ineffective, multidisciplinary healthcare "team" and the desired interprofessional collaborative healthcare team. In most cases the traditional "team" is in fact a *group* of healthcare providers working independently of each other in the care of the same patient (i.e., parallel practice). These groups of healthcare personnel are called "teams" regardless of whether they actually collaborated in providing that care. A true team is defined as "a group with a specific task or tasks, the accomplishment of which requires the interdependent and collaborative efforts of its members" (Grumbach & Bodenheimer, 2004, p. 1247). The important difference between a *group* of providers, which more clearly describes what we traditionally called a healthcare team, and a true healthcare *team* is that the healthcare team works together and shares responsibility for making decisions to develop and deliver a plan of care (i.e., collaborative practice), whereas a *group* of providers does not. Team-based care is an approach to health care in which a group of people work together to accomplish a common goal, solve a problem, or achieve a specific result (IOM, 2015).

Interprofessional teamwork "engages members of two or more professions with complementary competencies in sustained collborative practice towards common goals" (CAIPE, 2013, p. 4). Interprofessional teamwork is essential in the delivery of safe, quality, patient-centered care, and it requires varying levels of cooperation, coordination, and collaboration between the professionals involved in the delivery of that care (IPEC, 2011). Interprofessional teamwork is a key element of IPCP. *Interprofessional collaborative practice* (IPCP) is specifically defined as, "When multiple health workers from different professional backgrounds work together with patients, families, carers [sic], and communities to deliver the highest quality of care" (WHO, 2010, p. 7).

The Role of the Recipient of Care in Interprofessional Collaborative Practice

It is important to intentionally define the role of the patient, or recipient of care, in IPCP. Collaborative, patient-centered care is a specific practice orientation in which healthcare professionals work in partnership with patients. Active participation of patients, their families, and/or their community as members of the healthcare team is clearly among the goals, values, and vision of interprofessional collaboration (IOM, 1972). The clear intent is that the care must be provided together with, rather than for, patients. Thus interprofessional collaboration requires participation of all stakeholders, nonprofessional ones included, on equal social grounds (Domanjnko, Ferfila, Kavcic, & Pahor, 2015).

This approach to care must be explicitly shared by all members of the team to avoid the traditional, more provider-centric interpretation of IPCP in which only the professionals collaborate to provide what they believe to be the best care for the patient. Unfortunately, patients, significant others, and sometimes whole communities are seen as being in less powerful positions than members of the healthcare team by virtue of having less professional healthcare education than the professionals on the team. This is unfortunate because although healthcare professionals are, in fact, experts by profession, patients and other nonprofessionals can and should be conceptualized as experts by experience. This conceptualization clearly acknowledges the importance of living with a certain condition, as well as the special kind of knowledge that is generated from it. The best way to include these experiential experts in collaborative health care is to let their voices be at the center of discussions related to their care. As healthcare professionals, we must empower and support the nonprofessional members of the collaborative team to actively collaborate in their own care (Domanjnko, Ferfila, Kavcic, & Pahor, 2015; Thistlethwaite, 2012). Shared decision making contributes to successful patient outcomes; the best treatment plan means very little if the patient or recipient of that care is not willing or able to engage in it.

The issue of what term to use when referring to the nonprofessional members of the collaborative team deserves some attention. Recipients of care are referred to by many different terms. In this text, for example, you will see terms such as *patient, client, recipient of care, consumer,* and *service user* used as deemed appropriate in specific discussions. We acknowledge that these terms are not universally accepted by all and are sometimes associated with specific power dynamics in healthcare relationships. The term *patient,* for example, is sometimes considered to indicate a passive recipient of care, one who is acted upon, whereas the term *client* has been said to imply more autonomy in a care relationship. The terms *consumer, customer,* and *service-user* reflect the growing commercialization of health care and, although they may infer a more active role in terms of self-determination and choice, these terms can seem somewhat cold and distant. Some terms have more positive associations with participation than others, but regardless of the term used, the nonprofessional members of the healthcare team must remain identified as valuable participants in their own care. The best way to avoid the imposition of an inappropriate term or label on the person or group receiving care is to empower them by asking them how they want to be referred to in the context of the collaborative team.

INTERPROFESSIONAL EDUCATION (IPE)

Traditional models used in the education of healthcare professionals emphasized the mastery of skills and roles within individual professions but gave relatively little attention to how those skills could be used collaboratively with other members of the healthcare teams. Widespread medical errors in hospitals were associated with substantial preventable mortality and morbidity; this clearly indicated inadequacies in health care delivery systems (IOM, 2001). One source of these inadequacies was attributed to a lack of teamwork, collaboration, and communication skills in the healthcare workforce, not to a lack of technical

skills (Brandt, 2015). A method of preparing healthcare professionals for IPCP was needed.

Interdisciplinary education, or interprofessional education (as it is now called), is the process of preparing students and professionals to engage fully in IPCP (CIHC, 2010; IPEC, 2011; 2016). To engage in interprofessional collaboration, all team members will need to understand the capabilities and limitations of the other team members, have a common language that promotes clear communication, and develop a set of skills to effectively coordinate and deliver team-based care. The goal of interprofessional learning is to intentionally prepare all students of the healthcare professions to work together through interprofessional collaboration with the common goal of building a US healthcare system that is focused on safer and better patient-centered and community/population-oriented care (IPEC, 2011).

One way to incorporate interprofessional learning experiences into healthcare professional education is through an educational strategy called *IPE. Interprofessional Education (IPE)* was first defined by the World Health Organization (2010) as the type of education that occurs when students or members of two or more professions learn with, from, and about each other to improve collaboration and the quality of care they can give to patients. The intention of IPE is to prepare healthcare professionals with the knowledge, skills, and attitudes needed for interprofessional collaboration and collaborative practice. IPE *is not* simply shared learning, such as that which occurs when students learn passively in an interprofessional student group assembled in the same room and exposed to the same content, as would be seen in a chemistry or anatomy course. The essential components of IPE are active ones; IPE activities provide opportunities for healthcare professionals to practice together as an interprofessional team and to demonstrate the core competencies that they will need to effectively deliver care as part of that interprofessional team. IPE, in its true form, is a specific and logical strategy for educating healthcare professional students about IPCP through the operationalization of the Core Competencies for IPCP (IPEC, 2016).

To more accurately reflect the intent of IPE, the National Center for Interprofessional Collaborative Practice and Education expanded the original meaning of the acronym (IPE) by intentionally including the word *practice* in the phrase. The "new" interpretation of the IPE acronym now indicates "interprofessional *practice* and education" and provides a way to create a shared

---

BOX 1.1   The National Center for Interprofessional Practice and Education

The National Center for Interprofessional Practice and Education (NEXUSIPE) is a public–private partnership formed in October 2012 through a cooperative agreement with the US Department of Health and Human Services, Health Resources, and Services Administration. The National Center is also funded in part by the Josiah Macy Jr. Foundation, the Robert Wood Johnson Foundation, the Gordon and Betty Moore Foundation, and the University of Minnesota. The National Center was charged by its funders to provide the leadership, evidence, and resources needed to guide the nation in the use of interprofessional education and collaborative practice as a way to enhance the experience of health care, improve population health, and reduce the overall cost of care.

Mission

The National Center offers and supports evaluation, research, data, and evidence that ignites the field of interprofessional practice and education and leads to better care, added value, and healthier communities.

Goal

The goal of the National Center Nexus is to provide the leadership, evidence, and resources needed to guide the nation on the use of interprofessional education and collaborative practice as a way to enhance the experience of health care, improve population health, and reduce the overall cost of care.

The Nexus

- A means of connecting healthcare professions' education, specifically interprofessional education, and transforming healthcare practice to create true partnerships and shared responsibility
- A place where clinical practices partner with healthcare professions' education programs in transforming health systems, serving as learning organizations that support continuous professional development while educating the next generation of healthcare professionals.
- Is present at sites across the country, where partners turn ideas into action and demonstrate how interprofessional practice and education are being used effectively in different clinical and learning environments.
- Pulls together vastly different stakeholders such as patients, families, and communities and incorporates students and residents into the interprofessional team to help achieve the Triple Aim of creating better experiences, improving health, and reducing costs. (NEXUSIPE, 2015)

---

space between interprofessional education, interprofessional practice, and collaborative practice. This expanded IPE includes specific goals related to improving health, creating support systems, and trying different models of practice. It intentionally supports people (including healthcare professionals, health workers, students, residents, patients, families, and communities) to learn together every day to enhance collaboration and improve health outcomes while reducing costs (NEXUSIPE, 2015). Box 1.1 provides more information about the National Center for Interprofessional Practice and Education.

Interprofessional Education Activities

Experiential learning, or learning from experience, is well suited to professional learning, in which the integration of theory and practice is needed. Participation in IPE activities promotes interprofessional collaboration as students and practitioners from different professions have the opportunity to learn about and reflect on the relationships they experience with the professionals involved, enhance their mutual understanding of each other's roles and responsibilities in a given care situation, and explore ways to combine their professional expertise to promote the delivery of quality health care (WHO, 2010). IPE activities are generally planned and intentional; we often think of IPE activities such as preplanned mock codes or community disaster simulations, but some of the most valuable IPE experiences *do* occur during everyday practice events, for example, during unit discussions, case conferences, patient rounds, or unplanned meetings with other healthcare professionals in the course of care provision (Fig. 1.2).

The key to identifying IPE experiences lies in one's own awareness of what IPE is, being able to recognize potential IPE experiences or the existing ones that one encounters. Consider whether you would identify the CarFit experience highlighted in Box 1.2 as a potential IPE activity.

The CarFit experience traditionally included only occupational therapy students and did not, at first, seem to be a suitable IPE activity. With further consideration and planning, it emerged as a prime example of an IPE activity that engaged students from nursing, occupational therapy, physical therapy, public health, and speech-language pathology in interprofessional learning. Students learned *with* each other in training for the event; they formed interprofessional teams to plan and collaborate about the assessment of each driver's fit to his or her own vehicle; they learned *from* each other as they participated in the assessment; and they learned *about* their varied professional perspectives, roles, and responsibilities in the assessment of individuals.

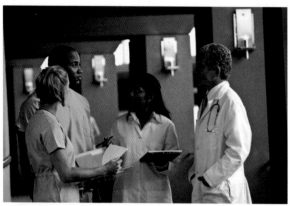

FIG. 1.2 Unplanned interprofessional education experiences occur in patient care interactions during a routine day. (© Comstock Images/Stockbyte/Thinkstock.)

Simulation-Enhanced Interprofessional Education

Simulation is a generic term used to refer to an artificial representation of real-world processes to achieve

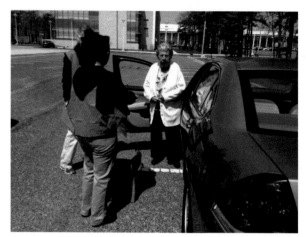

FIG. 1.3 Students interact with a CarFit participant. (From Ignatavicius D, Workman L, Rebar C: Medical-surgical nursing, 9e, St. Louis, 2018, Elsevier.)

BOX 1.2   Example of an Interprofessional Education Learning Activity: CarFit

Faculty in a School of Health Sciences were at an interprofessional education (IPE) planning session. Their goal was to identify and plan an IPE event that students from all programs could participate in. The occupational therapy (OT) faculty representative suggested CarFit as an IPE activity. One faculty member suggested that an upcoming "CarFit Day," usually participated in only by the OT students, could be used as the IPE activity for all programs in the school.

The professional programs in the school included undergraduate nursing and public health and graduate programs in communication disorders (CD), nursing, OT, and physical therapy (PT). Faculty on the committee were given the following information.

CarFit is an educational program created by the American Society on Aging and developed in collaboration with the American Automobile Association (AAA), AARP, and the American Occupational Therapy Association (AOTA). The program helps older drivers find out how well they fit into their own vehicle, highlights actions they can take to improve their fit, and promotes conversations about driver safety and community mobility.

To participate in CarFit Day all participating students would need to attend a CarFit Training Session. For the CarFit Day event, students would be assigned to participate as part of an interprofessional team (made up of one student from each of the school's professional programs) to evaluate the older drivers who would drive their own vehicles to the CarFit evaluation site (Fig. 1.3).

Activities

1. Watch the Introduction to CarFit video at http://www.car-fit.org/carfit/Videos.
2. Imagine that only you and others from your same profession will participate in the event; what might you assess in each driver?
3. Think of three other professional groups who might participate along with your own profession; what might they assess in each driver?

Discussion Questions

1. Do you think this activity could be made into an IPE activity for this School of Health Sciences?
2. Explain and support your answer using the definition of IPE.

educational goals through experiential learning (Al-Elq, 2010). Simulation-enhanced interprofessional education (Sim-IPE) is the overlap of the pedagogy of simulation and IPE (Decker et al., 2015). Sim-IPE empowers individuals to collaborate as a team in a controlled environment that replicates the healthcare setting. Participation in Sim-IPE has demonstrated improvement in the acquisition of knowledge, skills, attitudes, and behaviors of teamwork required to promote safe, quality patient care (Decker et al., 2015). Experiential learning often involves the use of case-based scenarios. Case-based simulations using low- to medium- to high-fidelity simulation provide the most common types of planned IPE experiences in educational and acute care settings. IPE simulation experiences are varied and are structured with specific learning outcomes in mind. There are different types and classifications of simulators; their costs vary according to the degree of their resemblance to the reality, or fidelity (Al-Elq, 2010). Simulation experiences offer the opportunity to participate in a patient or community care scenario as part of an interprofessional team. The simulated environment is designed to resemble the actual care environment as closely as possible. During the simulation experience participants practice and learn interprofessional communication, teamwork, and leadership, as well as about the roles and responsibilities of others. The simulation experience is often videotaped to measure learning outcomes and for immediate feedback to participants during a debriefing session.

Although many simulation scenarios are based on acute care situations, community-based simulated IPE experiences also provide experiences for interprofessional collaboration and practice. A common example of a community-based simulation is a simulated community disaster that may involve the collaborative efforts of public safety units, community agencies, first responders, acute care and community medical facilities, and educational institutions in coordinating their efforts to plan and practice a unified response. For example, communities host disaster drills focusing on events such as multivehicle accidents, chemical spills, plane crashes, fires, and floods. Community events do not always need to be on a large scale; small-scale simulations also offer multiple IPE opportunities.

High-fidelity simulations (Fig. 1.4) were shown to be educationally effective and complementary to medical education in patient care settings (Barry et al., 2005). An integrative review related to the use of simulation in

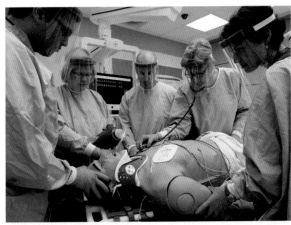

FIG. 1.4 Interprofessional education in an acute care setting using a high-fidelity patient simulator. (From Ignatavicius, D.; Workman, M. L.; Rebar, C. [2018]. *Medical-surgical nursing*, ed 9. St. Louis: Elsevier.)

nursing education concluded that simulation experiences are beneficial to nursing students in terms of knowledge, value, realism, and learner satisfaction (Weaver, 2011). Overall, simulation-based experiential learning is recognized as an effective way to promote teamwork (Decker et al., 2015).

Planning and Evaluating Interprofessional Education Activities

To be educationally sound, all IPE activities require planning, participant preparation, debriefing, and evaluation. The first step in **planning** is to identify measurable student learning outcomes to guide the development of the learning activity and to be used in the evaluation of the activity. Each of the Core Competencies that are presented throughout this book are accompanied by a set of behavioral Sub-competencies that can provide measurable student learning outcomes for the IPE activity being planned. An essential aspect in the planning phase is to be sure that all aspects of an IPE activity are present: participants must be able to learn *with*, *from*, and *about* each other as part of the activity.

The second step is **preparation** for the event. All participants should be fully aware of the identified learning outcomes and be prepared for active participation in the learning experience. For example, participants may prepare for the activity through the completion of standard curricular coursework, completion of required training, or attainment of some other background knowledge or experience. Participants may have assigned readings, role-specific preparation, or other written assignments (e.g., study questions) to complete before the simulation and evidence of their completion may be used as a student's admission ticket to the IPE activity.

The third step of an IPE activity is **participation.** Participation in all planned IPE activities begins with a formal overview or briefing related to the learning expectations conducted by the event facilitator(s). During this time, participants are oriented to the experience that will follow and may be given a specified amount of time to collaborate with team members in preparation for the actual event, if appropriate. Participation in the IPE event follows immediately. The IPE learning experience may be videotaped to measure learning outcomes and for immediate feedback to participants during a debriefing session after the event. A **formal evaluation** tool, designed to allow participants to evaluate their own achievement of the specified learning outcomes, should be completed by all participants immediately after the event.

Regardless of the type of IPE activity, **debriefing** is a key element of the experience because not everyone is naturally able to analyze, make sense of, and assimilate learning experiences on their own. *Debriefing* is a facilitator-led process that includes specific questions about the IPE experience just completed and guided reflection related to the details of that experience and the associated learning outcomes. The design of the debriefing session is tailored to the learning outcomes and to participant and team characteristics (Fanning & Gaba, 2007). Debriefing provides a structured forum for talking through the experiences of the activity and the opportunity to share emotions and perspectives related to them (Fig. 1.5). Debriefing bridges the gap between the experience of the IPE activity and the learning that the participant takes away from it. Studies suggest that gains in knowledge related to participating in simulation experiences are achieved only after debriefing and that the debriefing experience should be emphasized in all standardized simulation learning experiences (Shinnick, Woo, Horwich, & Steadman, 2011).

INTERPROFESSIONAL COLLABORATION COMPETENCIES

The Competency Approach

In response to the shared belief that healthcare educational programs must include opportunities for students to engage

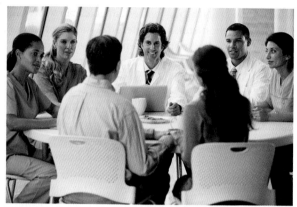

FIG. 1.5 Facilitator-led student debriefing following an IPE learning experience. (© monkeybusinessimages/iStock/Thinkstock.)

RESEARCH HIGHLIGHT

Simulation-Enhanced Interprofessional Simulation

Outcomes of simulation-enhanced interprofessional education (Sim-IPE) have been studied using both quantitative and qualitative methods.

Participants report perceived improvement in the following areas:
1. Knowledge, skills, attitudes, and behaviors related to teamwork
2. Appreciation of other professionals, their patient care roles, and skills
3. Awareness regarding the effective use of resources
4. Communication and collaboration
5. Self-confidence as it relates to teamwork
6. Clinical reasoning
7. Shared mental model
8. Understanding the importance of patient safety initiatives

Improvement has been observed and measured using reliable evaluation tools in the following areas:
1. Understanding professional healthcare roles
2. Identifying effective team performance supporting the best interest of patients and families
3. Improving team communications
4. Increasing awareness and acknowledgment of patients' needs and conditions
5. Improving patient outcomes and experiences (Decker et al., 2015, p. 294)

in IPE and practice interprofessional collaboration, curricular changes began to be seen in nursing, medicine, dentistry, pharmacy, and public health education. IPE was being identified by accreditation agencies and professional organizations as essential to achieving safe, quality patient-centered care. These early efforts demonstrated the intent of individual healthcare professions to include IPE and IPCP practice expectations for students in their own disciplines, but that was not enough. There was a need for a shared and unified approach that could be used by all disciplines in preparing students for interprofessional collaboration. There was a need to identify, agree upon, and strengthen core competencies for interprofessional collaboration across professions (IPEC, 2011).

A unifying concept that would enable the clear development of these core competencies across all professions was identified. That concept was *interprofessionality* (IPEC, 2011). *Interprofessionality* was defined by D'Amour & Oandasan (2005, p. 9) as:

> [T]he process by which professionals reflect on and develop ways of practicing that provides an integrated and cohesive answer to the needs of the client/family/population…[I]t involves continuous interaction and knowledge sharing between professionals, organized to solve or explore a variety of education and care issues all while seeking to optimize the patient's participation…Interprofessionality requires a paradigm shift, since interprofessional practice has unique characteristics in terms of values, codes of conduct, and ways of working. These characteristics must be elucidated.

The concept of *interprofessionality* became foundational to the identification of the mutually agreed upon core interprofessional competency domains and associated specific competencies. A framework within which to deliver this essential content was still needed, and three frameworks were identified that captured the interdependency between healthcare professions' education competency development for collaborative practice and practice needs (D'Amour & Oandasan, 2005; Frenk et al., 2010; WHO, 2010). Developers of these three frameworks identified IPE as "a means of improving patient-centered and community-/population-oriented care" (IPEC, 2011, p. 11).

The application of an interprofessional competency framework in the education of healthcare professionals was suggested by Barr (1998) to distinguish between three

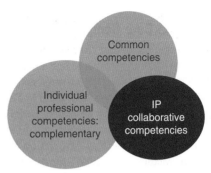

FIG. 1.6 Barr's three types of professional competencies. (From Interprofessional Education Collaborative Expert Panel [IPEC]. [2011]. *Core competencies for interprofessional collaborative practice: Report of an expert panel.* Washington, DC: Interprofessional Education Collaborative.)

types of competence from an interprofessional perspective: common, complementary, and collaborative competencies (IPEC, 2011; Fig. 1.6). The common or overlapping competencies are those expected of all healthcare professionals. These are competencies that are common or shared by more than one profession but not necessarily all professionals (Barr, 1998). For example, nurses, physicians, physicians' assistants, pharmacists, and others may all share the common competency of administering an immunization, whereas others, such as occupational therapists, probably do not.

Complementary competencies are unique competencies that distinguish one profession from another; for example, the care of a patient who has had a stroke with resultant disabilities may involve a physician, demonstrating competency in prescribing the appropriate diet to meet metabolic needs; a dietician, demonstrating a complementary competency in designing a meal plan that meets the specific nutritional and consistency requirements; the complementary competency of a speech therapist to evaluate swallowing; and the complementary competencies of a professional nurse to actually feed the patient safely and efficiently while maintaining as much independence as possible. The third type of competencies, interprofessional collaborative competencies, are those in which each profession needs to work together with others, such as other specialties within a profession, between professions, with patients and families, with nonprofessionals and volunteers, within and between organizations, within communities, and at a broader policy level (Barr, 1998; IPEC, 2011).

Identifying the Core Competencies

The IPCP competencies and the specific competencies associated with each of them were first identified in the document, *Core Competencies for Interprofessional Practice: Report of an Expert Panel* (IPEC, 2011). This report concluded 1 year of work by an expert panel that was sponsored by the American Association of Colleges of Nursing (AACN), the American Association of Colleges of Osteopathic Medicine (AACOM), the American Dental Education Association (ADEA), the Association of American Medical Colleges (AAMC), and the Association of Schools and Programs of Public Health (ASPPH). The panel found convergence in interprofessional competency content themes between the national literature and the global literature, among healthcare professional organizations in the United States, and across American educational institutions (IPEC, 2011). The work of this panel resulted in the identification of four Core Competencies: Values/Ethics, Roles/Responsibilities, Interprofessional Communication, and Teams and Teamwork (IPEC, 2011). Each of these interprofessional competencies was presented with the more specific Sub-competencies associated with them, each written as a measurable behavioral objective. The completed work reflected the vision of the panel that IPCP is key to safe, high-quality, accessible, patient-centered care. These Competencies were intentionally made general enough to allow flexible application within the professions and at the institutional level. As such, they allow "faculty and administrators to develop a program of study for their profession or institution that is aligned with the general competency statements but in a context appropriate to particular professional, clinical, practitioner, or institutional circumstances" (IPEC, 2016, p. 3). The response to this work is historic and resulted in both the redesigning of healthcare professions' education and new accreditation standards linked to the IPEC Competencies (Brandt, 2015).

The original document was updated in 2016. Although it maintained the original vision, the revision was responsive to two prominent changes that occurred in the healthcare system in the 5 years since its completion. These changes included an increased focus on the Institute for Healthcare Improvement's (IHI) Triple Aim (IHI, 2017) and the implementation of the Patient Protection and Affordable Care Act in 2010 (Rosenbaum, 2011). The *IHI Triple Aim* is a framework developed by the IHI that describes an approach to optimizing health system

The IHI Triple Aim

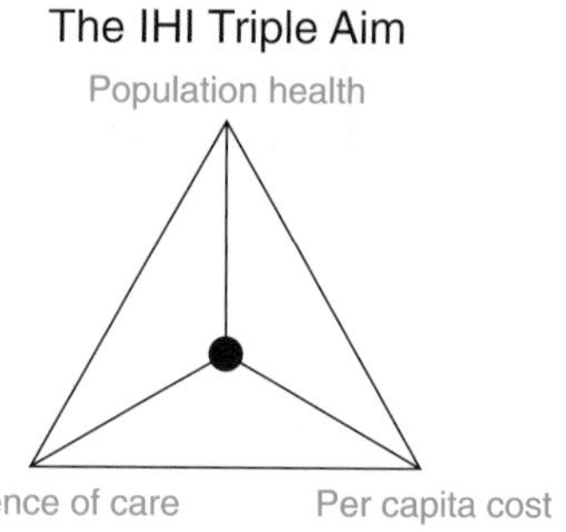

FIG. 1.7 The Institute for Healthcare Improvement Triple Aim. The Triple Aim framework was developed by the Institute for Healthcare Improvement in Cambridge, Massachusetts (www.ihi.org). Reprinted with permission.

performance. It is IHI's belief that new designs must be developed to simultaneously pursue three dimensions, referred to as the "Triple Aim": (1) improving the patient experience of care (including quality and satisfaction); (2) improving the health of populations; and (3) reducing the per capita cost of health care (IHI, 2017; Fig. 1.7). The Patient Protection and Affordable Care Act established the basic legal protections that had been absent and a near-universal guarantee of access to affordable health insurance coverage, from birth through retirement (Rosenbaum, 2011). In light of these two changes in health care, the IPEC Board recognized that population health approaches needed to be explicitly incorporated in the present model. The 2016 update integrated explicit considerations for population health with individual Sub-competencies to create an expanded competency model appropriate for use in achieving the current health system goals (IPEC, 2016). This updated model provides a broader and stronger framework that enables clinical care providers, public health practitioners, and professions from other fields to collaborate more efficiently and effectively across disciplines to optimize health care and advance population health (IPEC, 2016).

In addition to revisions integrating population health emphasis, the updated version reframed Interprofessional Collaboration as the document's central domain. Responsive to the work of Englander et al. (2013), instead of depicting the four Core Competencies (i.e., Values/Ethics, Roles/Responsibilities, Interprofessional Communication, and Teams and Teamwork) as individual domains within IPCP, Interprofessional Collaboration is now prominent as the central domain with the four general Competencies and related Sub-competencies presented as they relate

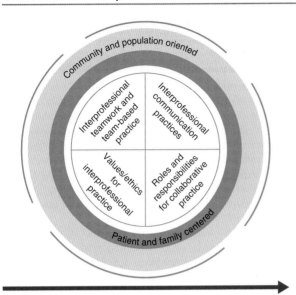

The learning continuum pre-licensure through practice trajectory

FIG. 1.8 Interprofessional Collaboration as Central Competency Domain. (From Interprofessional Education Collaborative Expert Panel [IPEC]. [2016]. *Core competencies for interprofessional collaborative practice: 2016 update.* Washington, DC: Interprofessional Education Collaborative.)

to Interprofessional Collaboration (IPEC, 2016). This chapter sets the stage for the presentation and operationalization of each of the four Core Competencies. Fig. 1.8 illustrates the Competencies within the domain of Interprofessional Collaboration.

GLOBAL FOCUS ON INTERPROFESSIONAL EDUCATION AND INTERPROFESSIONAL COLLABORATIVE PRACTICE

In response to two significant reports, *Health Professionals for a New Century: Transforming Education to Strengthen Health Systems in an Interdependent World* (Frenk et al., 2010) and *The Future of Nursing: Leading Change, Advancing Health (IOM, 2011),* the IOM created the Global Forum on Health Professions Education in 2012. The Global Forum is an ongoing, convening activity of the National Academies of Sciences, Engineering and Medicine; it brings together stakeholders from multiple nations and professions to network, discuss, and illuminate issues within healthcare professional education. The Forum

routinely convenes organizations focused on IPE and IPCP to accelerate national change as part of ongoing worldwide initiatives. Currently there are 60 appointed members to the Forum who are academic experts and healthcare professionals representing 19 different disciplines from eight countries (National Academies of Sciences, Engineering, and Medicine, 2018). The Global Forum uses guiding principles to direct its work; these principles emphasize engaging students, being patient- and person-centered, and creating an environment of learning with and from partners outside of the United States. In March 2016, the division of the National Academies of Sciences, Engineering, and Medicine (the National Academies) that focuses on health and medicine was renamed the Health and Medicine Division (HMD) instead of using the name Institute of Medicine (IOM). The Health and Medicine Division continues the consensus studies and convening activities previously undertaken by the IOM (National Academies of Sciences, Engineering, and Medicine, 2015).

IPE has been acknowledged internationally as being an essential component of educating healthcare professionals for IPCP. The number of competency domains and their categorization vary internationally; however, it is important to note that the expert panel did report finding "convergence in interprofessional competency content between national literature and global literature, among health professions organizations in the United States, and across American educational institutions" (IPEC, 2011, p. 15).

Both national and international efforts have been forged to create partnerships in both the creation and dissemination of a body of knowledge on IPE. In the United States, between the 1970s and early 2000, various professional conferences focused on cross-professional practice and education were held. International efforts in IPE progressed during the late 1980s and throughout the 1990s to include the establishment of national centers and collaboratives. See information on the Centre for the Advancement of Interprofessional Education in the United Kingdom and the Canadian Interprofessional Health Collaborative (CIHC) in the Global Perspective boxes.

In the United States, the need for a reenvisioned IPE presence emerged during 2003 when it became clear that previously held national meetings around IPE had been discontinued and there was increased international attention in this area. In the absence of a national organization, individuals in the United States collaborated

GLOBAL PERSPECTIVES ON INTERPROFESSIONAL EDUCATION IN THE UNITED KINGDOM

The Centre for the Advancement of Interprofessional Education (CAIPE) was established in the United Kingdom in 1987 as a membership organization and as a UK-based charity. CAIPE supports students, academics, practitioners, researchers, and others who seek to promote health and well-being and to improve the health and social care of the public by advancing interprofessional education.

The aims of CAIPE include the following:

- The promotion and development of IPE, learning, practice and research through the active involvement of all members
- Collaboration with like-minded individuals and organizations nationally and globally in IPE, research, learning, and practice
- Collaboration with national stakeholders and statutory, professional, and regulatory bodies in the promotion and development of IPE through research and practice
- Acting as an independent "think tank" to improve collaborative practice and thereby the quality of service provision by the professions learning and working together
- Being a national and international authoritative voice on IPE in both academia and the workplace
- Providing information and advice through national and internationsal activities and publications, corporate forums and workshops
- Facilitating the development of a workforce fit for practice
- Making an impact on quality of service

From Centre for the Advancement of Interprofessional Education (CAIPE). (2017). Retrieved from https://www.caipe.org/.

GLOBAL PERSPECTIVES ON INTERPROFESSIONAL EDUCATION IN CANADA

The Canadian Interprofessional Health Collaborative (CIHC) is made up of health organizations, health educators, researchers, healthcare professionals, and students from across Canada. CIHC believes interprofessional education and collaborative patient-centered practice are key to building effective healthcare teams and improving the experience and outcomes of patients. The CIHC identifies and shares best practices and its extensive and growing knowledge in interprofessional education and collaborative practice.

The CIHC National Interprofessional Competency Framework was developed for integration into education and practice. Six competency domains were identified to highlight the knowledge, skills, attitudes, and values that are believed to shape judgments essential for interprofessional collaborative practice:

1. Interprofessional communication
2. Patient-/client-/family-/community-centered care
3. Role clarification
4. Team functioning
5. Collaborative leadership
6. Interprofessional conflict resolution

From Canadian Interprofessional Health Collaborative (CIHC). (2010). *A national competency framework*. Vancouver, BC: CIHC.

with CIHC to develop the first Collaborating Across Borders Conference (CAB I): An American-Canadian Dialogue on Interprofessional Health Education. Today Collaborating Across Borders (CAB) is the premier Canada–United States joint conference focused on IPE and collaborative practice. The conference offers a venue where educators, clinicians, researchers, policy makers, and students from both sides of the border can engage in rich, productive dialogue. The conference series continues to be held biennially and, in keeping with the theme, alternates across the border between Canada and the United States.

From the CAB effort, American institutional leaders emerged with an interest to establish a US-based interprofessional organization, now known as the American Interprofessional Health Collaborative (AIHC, 2015). Box 1.3 contains more information about AIHC.

IPE is receiving growing attention throughout Europe. The challenges for European institutions to implement IPE are great because of the varied countries there, each with their own legislation on education and health care. During the past 30 years, many initiatives have been seen in the form of journals, such as the *Journal of Interprofessional Care,* and international meetings, such as the biennial All Together Better Health (ATBH) Conferences (see www.atbh.org). IPE has become a global movement (Vyt, Pahor, & Tervaskanto-Maentausta, 2015).

BOX 1.3 **The American Interprofessional Health Collaborative**

The American Interprofessional Health Collaborative (AIHC) was incorporated in 2011 to improve health outcomes by fostering a learning community with a shared commitment to collaboration across healthcare professions. Acknowledging that in many respects, healthcare professions education remained isolated from practice realities, and profession-specific learning did not prepare future and current healthcare professionals for working together, AIHC aimed to transcend boundaries to connect "traditional" healthcare professions, educators, new and emerging health and care providers, care coordinators, administrators of health care delivery and payment systems, and policy makers in partnership with patients, communities, and populations.

The AIHC transcends the following boundaries to transform learning, policies, practices, and scholarship toward an improved system of health and wellness for individual patients, communities, and populations:

• Professional boundaries
• Organizational boundaries
• Various perspectives and philosophies of interprofessional teamwork and collaboration
• Stages of professional development
• Boundaries around education, practice, and research

• Boundaries around professionals and individuals, communities, and populations
• Geographic and national boundaries

The AIHC believes educating those entrusted with the health of individuals, communities, and populations to value and respect each other's unique expertise and skills and to work together is fundamental to care that is effective, safe, of high quality, and efficient in terms of cost, resources, and time.

The American Interprofessional Health Collaborative is committed to the preparation and deployment of a workforce that exemplifies ethics and values for interprofessional collaboration; that understands the breadth and complexity of roles and responsibilities for collaborative practice; that has the foundational skills for effective interprofessional communication; and has the requisite competencies for interprofessional teamwork and provision of team-based care of individuals, communities, and populations.

The American Interprofessional Health Collaborative promotes the scholarship and leadership necessary to develop interprofessional education and transform healthcare professions education across the learning continuum, for students, practitioners, and educators.

(AIHC, 2015)

ADDITIONAL RESOURCES

The resources in this section include organizations working on IPE and IPCP, foundational documents in IPE and IPCP, and other resources for interprofessional education.

Organizations Focusing on IPE and IPCP
This subsection lists organizations with significant IPE and IPCP work and resources. Included are direct links to these organizations. Further resources can be found within the organizations listed here.

Interprofessional Education Collaborative (IPEC)
https://www.ipecollaborative.org/resources.html

This is a compilation of Interprofessional Education (IPE) and Interprofessional Collaborative Practice (IPCP) resources including direct links to foundational IPEC documents and the MedEdPortal.

The Interprofessional PORTAL (MedEdPORTAL) https://www.mededportal.org/

The MedEdPORTAL is a program of the Association of American Medical Colleges that provides access to high quality, peer-reviewed, competency-based learning modules

for interprofessional education (IPE). The mission of the MedEdPORTAL is to promote educational scholarship and collaboration by facilitating the open exchange of peer-reviewed health education teaching and assessment resources.

National Center for Interprofessional Practice and Education (NCIPE) https://nexusipe.org/informing/resource-center

The National Center for Interprofessional Practice and Education is charged to provide leadership, evidence, and resources to promote interprofessional practice and education. The National Center facilitates networking among professionals interested in IPE and IPCP and it is a repository of evaluations, research, data and evidence about interprofessional practice and education.

The American Interprofessional Health Collaborative (AIHC) https://aihc-us.org/what-is-aihc

The AIHC transcends boundaries to transform learning, policies, practices, and scholarship toward an improved system of health and wellness for individual patients,

Continued

communities, and populations. AIHC is composed of individuals and organizations that are committed to influencing a more positive future.

The Canadian Interprofessional Health Collaborative (CIHC) https://www.cihc.ca/about/overview

CIHC is the national Canadian organization promoting interprofessional and patient-centered education and practice. CIHC is the Canadian counterpart of the Interprofessional Education Collaborative (IPEC) in the United States.

The Global Forum on Innovation in Health Professional Education (Global Forum) http://nationalacademies.org/hmd/activities/global/innovationhealthprofeducation.aspx

The Global Forum is an ongoing, convening activity of the Health and Medicine Division (HMD) of the National Academies of Sciences, Engineering and Medicine (previously the Institute of Medicine [IOM] program unit of the National Academies), that brings together stakeholders from multiple nations and professions to network, discuss, and illuminate issues within health professional education.

Foundational Documents in IPE and IPCP

This subsection lists foundational documents in IPE and IPCP. Many of these documents are associated with the organizations listed above; however, direct links to the documents are provided here.

The Core Competencies for Interprofessional Collaborative Practice: 2016 Update Interprofessional Education Collaborative. (2016). Retrieved from https://nebula.wsimg.com/2f68a39520b03336b41038c370497473?AccessKeyId=DC06780E69ED19E2B3A5&disposition=0&alloworigin=1

The Core Competencies for Interprofessional Collaborative Practice: 2011 Original Interprofessional Education Collaborative. (2011). Retrieved from https://nebula.wsimg.com/3ee8a4b5b5f7ab794c742b14601d5f23?AccessKeyId=DC06780E69ED19E2B3A5&disposition=0&alloworigin=1

Team-Based Competencies: Building a Shared Foundation for Education and Clinical Practice. Interprofessional Education Collaborative [IPEC] (2011). Author. Retrieved from https://nebula.wsimg.com/191adb6df3208c643f339a83d47a3f28?AccessKeyId=DC06780E69ED19E2B3A5&disposition=0&alloworigin=1

The Health Resources and Services Administration (HRSA), the Josiah Macy Jr. Foundation, the Robert Wood Johnson Foundation (RWJF), and the ABIM Foundation, in collaboration with the Interprofessional Education Collaborative (IPEC), sponsored this two-day conference. This conference brought together more than 80 invited participants, including chief executive officers, deans, policy makers, and other opinion leaders from the diverse fields of nursing, medicine, pharmacy, public health, dentistry, and osteopathic medicine. Building on the work of the IPEC expert panel, this leadership conference reviewed the IPEC draft of Core Competencies and created the groundwork for an action plan for using the competencies to transform health professional education and health care delivery in the United States.

A National Interprofessional Competency Framework. Canadian Interprofessional Health Collaborative (CIHC). (2010). Retrieved from http://www.cihc.ca/files/CIHC_IPCompetencies_Feb1210r.pdf

This is the seminal document of the Canadian Interprofessional Health Collaborative (CIHC) and provides a framework for interprofessional practice and education in Canada. This report is analog to the 2011 IPEC report, *The Core Competencies for Interprofessional Collaborative Practice*.

Resources for IPE Courses, Curriculum Development and Related Guidelines

This subsection offers resources to develop curricula for the teaching of Interprofessional Collaborative Practice (IPCP), including a full course. Guidelines to transform clinical simulations into an Interprofessional Education (IPE) experience are also offered.

INACSL Standards of Best Practice: Simulation[SM] https://www.inacsl.org/i4a/pages/index.cfm?pageid=3407

Best Practice Guidelines to achieve optimal outcomes in simulation-enhanced interprofessional education (Sim-IPE) have been developed based on evidence in the literature. INACSL developed *Best Practice Guidelines for Simulation-enhanced Interprofessional Education (Sim-IPE): The INACSL Standards of Best Practice: Simulation*[SM] to advance the science of simulation, share best practices, and provide evidence-based guidelines for implementation and training. INACSL offers a detailed process for evaluating and improving simulation operating procedures and delivery methods

Advancing Interprofessional Clinical Prevention and Population Health Education: Curriculum Development Guide for Health Professions Faculty. Meyer, S. M., Garr, D. R., Evans, C., & Maeshiro, R. (2015). https://nexusipe.org/http://www.teachpopulationhealth.org/uploads/2/1/9/6/21964692/ipe_crosswalk_2016_update.pdf

This curriculum guide links the Clinical Prevention and Population Health Curriculum Framework with the Core

📄 **ADDITIONAL RESOURCES—cont'd**

Competencies for Interprofessional Collaborative Practice. It is intended for faculty members educating healthcare professionals who want to design and implement interprofessional learning activities related to clinical prevention and population health. The Healthy People Curriculum Task Force prepared this guide to inform curriculum development focused on students' abilities to participate effectively as members of interprofessional health care teams delivering clinical prevention and population health services.

Curriculum for an Interprofessional Seminar on Integrated Primary Care (IS-IPC) http://www.apa.org/education/grad/curriculum-seminar.aspx

This curricular resource is designed to develop educational experiences for an interprofessional group of learners about the competencies needed to work together in an integrated healthcare team. It is designed for use with learners early in their health professions training; however, the content is adaptable for learners at other levels. The IS-IPC contains eight modules that can be used individually or combined for a more extensive educational experience and can easily be customized for specific educational needs. Topics include: an introduction to interprofessional education and collaborative practice, integrated primary care, population health, ethics, leadership, quality improvement, healthcare financing, and health policy and advocacy.

The Toronto Model for Interprofessional Education and Practice. Information can be found in Nelson, S., Tassone, M., & Hodges, B. D. (2014). *Creating the Health Care Team of the Future: The Toronto Model for Interprofessional Education and Practice.* Cornell University Press.

This book is based on the Toronto Model of interprofessional education and care (IPE/C). The authors describe the history and evolution of University of Toronto's Program and share "lessons learned." Written in workbook format, the book is geared toward health professional educators and clinical faculty. The emphasis is on "how to" develop and implement IPE programs.

KEY POINTS

- The Flexner model of professional education did not meet 21st-century health challenges. There were concerns about both the quality of health care and the quality of the educational programs preparing healthcare professionals. Healthcare systems were struggling to cope with advances in science and technology, new and changing infections, high rates of medical errors, inequities in health care delivery, and rising healthcare costs.

- To maximize the efficiency and effectiveness of the healthcare professional workforce, it was necessary to redesign the system of healthcare professional education with interdependence among professions, rather than independence, of practice as the goal. Healthcare professionals need to work together collaboratively, not individually, in providing care.

- Interprofessional teamwork is essential in the delivery of safe, quality, patient-centered care. It is the key element of interprofessional collaborative practice.

- Interprofessional collaborative practice is defined as, "when multiple health workers from different professional backgrounds work together with patients, families, [carers], and communities to deliver the highest quality of care" (WHO, 2010, p. 7). In addition, interprofessional teamwork includes working in partnerships between professions or between organizations with individuals, families, groups, and communities (CAIPE, 2013, p. 3).

- IPE is a strategy used to incorporate interprofessional learning experiences into healthcare professional education.

- *IPE* is defined by the World Health Organization (2010) as the type of education that occurs when students or members of two or more professions *learn with, from,* and *about* each other to improve collaboration and the quality of care they can give to patients.

- To more accurately reflect the intent of IPE, the original meaning of the acronym was intentionally expanded to include the word *practice* in the phrase. The "new" IPE acronym indicates "interprofessional *practice* and education." It provides a way to create a shared space among IPE, interprofessional practice, and collaborative practice.

- IPE can occur in formal planned activities such as in high-fidelity simulation or in informal interactions of interdisciplinary team members in routine patient care activities related to a given recipient of care.

- Educationally sound IPE activities require planning, participant preparation, debriefing, and evaluation.
- An interprofessional competency framework was suggested by Barr (1998) to distinguish between three types of competencies from an interprofessional perspective: common, complementary, and collaborative competencies.
- Core Competencies for IPCP were identified by an expert panel (IPEC, 2011) and were updated in 2016.
- The Core Competencies for Interprofessional Practice are Values/Ethics for Interprofessional Practice, Roles/Responsibilities, Interprofessional Communication, and Teams and Teamwork.
- The 2016 update of the IPEC *Core Competencies for Interprofessional Collaborative Practice* integrated explicit considerations for population health with individual Sub-competencies to create an expanded competency model appropriate for use in achieving the current health system goals. The updated model provides a broader and stronger framework for clinical care providers, public health practitioners, and professions from other fields to collaborate efficiently and effectively across disciplines to optimize health care and advance population health.
- The 2016 update of the IPEC *Core Competencies for Interprofessional Collaborative Practice* identified interprofessional collaboration as the central domain with the four general Competencies and related Sub-competencies discussed in this chapter arrayed below. This replaced the former depiction of the four Core Competencies as individual domains within interprofessional collaborative practice.
- The 2106 update did not change the names of the IPEC Core Competencies.
- IPE has been acknowledged internationally as being an essential component of educating healthcare professionals for interprofessional collaborative practice.

REFERENCES

Al-Elq, A. H. (2010). Simulation-based medical teaching and learning. *Journal of Family and Community Medicine, 17*(1), 35–40.

American Interprofessional Health Collaborative (AIHC). (2015). Retrieved from https://aihc-us.org/what-is-aihc.

Barr, H. (1998). Competent to collaborate: Towards a competency-based model for interprofessional education. *Journal of Interprofessional Care, 12*(2), 181–187.

Barry Issenberg, S., Mcgaghie, W. C., Petrusa, E. R., et al. (2005). Features and uses of high-fidelity medical simulations that lead to effective learning: A BEME systematic review. *Medical Teacher, 27*(1), 10–28.

Brandt, B. F. (2015). *Interprofessional education and collaborative practice: Welcome to the "new" forty-year old field.* The Advisor, 9-17. Retrieved from http://www.naahp.org/Portals/2/OtherImages/TheAdvisor/Articles/35-1-02.pdf.

Canadian Interprofessional Health Collaborative (CIHC). (2010). *A National Competency Framework.* Vancouver, BC: CIHC.

Centre for the Advancement of Interprofessional Education (CAIPE). (2013). *Introducing interprofessional education.* Fareham, UK: CAIPE CarFit retrieved from http://www.car-fit.org.

Centre for the Advancement of Interprofessional Education (CAIPE). (2017). Retrieved from https://www.caipe.org/.

D'Amour, D., & Oandasan, I. (2005). Interprofessionality as the field of interprofessional practice and interprofessional education: An emerging concept. *Journal of Interprofessional Care, 19*(Suppl. 1), 8–20.

Decker, S. I., Anderson, M., Boese, T., et al. (2015). Standards of best practice: Simulation standard VIII: Simulation-enhanced interprofessional education (Sim-IPE). *Clinical Simulation in Nursing, 11*(6), 293–297.

Domanjnko, B., Ferfila, N., Kavcic, M., et al. (2015). Beyond Interprofessionalism: Caring *together with* rather than *for* people. In A. Vyt, M. Pahor, & T. Tervaskanto-Maentausta (Eds.), *Interprofessional Education in Europe: Policy and Practice.* Antwerpen-Apeldoorn: Garant.

Duffy, T. P. (2011). The Flexner Report—100 years later. *The Yale Journal of Biology and Medicine, 84*(3), 269–276.

Englander, R., Cameron, T., Ballard, A. J., et al. (2013). Toward a common taxonomy of competency domains for the health professions and competencies for physicians. *Academic Medicine, 88*(8), 1088–1094.

Fanning, R. M., & Gaba, D. M. (2007). The role of debriefing in simulation-based learning. *Simulation in Healthcare, 2*(2), 115–125.

Frenk, J., Chen, L., Bhutta, Z., et al. (2010). Health professionals for a new century: Transforming education to strengthen health systems in an interdependent world. *The Lancet, 376*(9756), 1923–1958.

Grumbach, K., & Bodenheimer, T. (2004). Can health care teams improve primary care practice? *Journal of the American Medical Association (JAMA)*, *291*, 1246–1251.

Institute for Healthcare Improvement (IHI). (2017). *Initiatives: The Triple Aim Initiative*. Retrieved from http://www.ihi.org/Engage/Initiatives/TripleAim/Pages/default.aspx.

Institute of Medicine (IOM). (1972). *Educating for the health team*. Washington, DC: National Academy of Science.

Institute of Medicine (IOM). (2000). *To err is human: Building a safer health system*. Washington, DC: National Academy of Science.

Institute of Medicine (IOM). (2001). *Crossing the quality chasm*. Washington, DC: National Academy of Science.

Institute of Medicine (IOM). (2003). *Health professions education: A bridge to quality*. Washington, DC: National Academy of Science.

Institute of Medicine (IOM). (2011). *The future of nursing: Leading change, advancing health*. Washington, DC: National Academies Press.

Institute of Medicine (IOM). (2015). *Measuring the impact of interprofessional education on collaborative practice and patient outcomes*. Washington, DC: National Academy of Science.

Interprofessional Education Collaborative Expert Panel (IPEC). (2011). *Core competencies for interprofessional collaborative practice: Report of an expert panel*. Washington, DC: Interprofessional Education Collaborative.

Interprofessional Education Collaborative Expert Panel (IPEC). (2016). *Core competencies for interprofessional collaborative practice: 2016 update*. Washington, DC: Interprofessional Education Collaborative.

National League for Nursing (NLN) Board of Governors. (2015). *Interprofessional collaboration in education and practice: A living document from the National League for Nursing*. Retrieved from http://www.nln.org/docs/default-source/default-document-library/ipe-ipp-vision.pdf?sfvrsn=14.

Rosenbaum, S. (2011). The Patient Protection and Affordable Care Act: Implications for public health policy and practice. *Public Health Reports*, *126*(1), 130–135.

Shinnick, M. A., Woo, M., Horwich, T. B., et al. (2011). Debriefing: The most important component in simulation? *Clinical Simulation in Nursing*, *7*(3), e105–e111.

The National Academies of Sciences, Engineering, and Medicine, Health and Medicine Division. (2015). *Institute of Medicine to Become National Academy of Medicine*. Retrieved from http://www8.nationalacademies.org/onpinews/newsitem.aspx?recordid=04282015&_ga=2.3138356.504490429.1522779166-560925224.1522779166.

The National Academies of Sciences, Engineering, and Medicine. (2018). *Global Forum on Innovation in Health Professional Education*. Retrieved from http://nationalacademies.org/hmd/Activities/Global/InnovationHealthProfEducation.aspx.

The National Center for Interprofessional Practice and Education (NEXUSIPE). (2015). *About IPE*. Retrieved from https://nexusipe.org/informing/about-ipe.

Thistlethwaite, J. E. (2012). *Values-based interprofessional collaborative practice working together in health care*. Cambridge, UK: Cambridge University Press.

Vyt, A., Pahor, M., & Tervaskanto-Maentausta, T. (Eds.). (2015). *Interprofessional education in Europe: Policy and practice*. Antwerpen-Apeldoorn: Garant.

Weaver, A. (2011). High fidelity patient simulation in nursing education: An integrative review. *Nursing Education Perspectives*, *32*(1), 37–40.

World Health Organization (WHO). (2010). *Framework for action on interprofessional education & collaborative practice*. Geneva: WHO. Retrieved from http://www.who.int/hrh/nursing_midwifery/en/.

Systems Theory: An Approach to Interprofessional Collaborative Practice

LEARNING OUTCOMES

After studying this chapter, you will be able to:

1. Discuss the importance of a theoretical framework in guiding Interprofessional Collaborative Practice (IPCP) and Interprofessional Education (IPE).
2. Define a system and the components of a system.
3. Explain the General Systems Theory.
4. Differentiate between simple and complex systems.
5. Explain the application of the General Systems Theory to understanding problems in the healthcare system.
6. Identify six primary components of all healthcare systems.
7. Define systems thinking.

This chapter focuses on systems theory as framework to understand Interprofessional Collaborative Practice (IPCP). It begins with a description of the scope of theories available for use in understanding IPCP and then focuses on the general systems theory. The chapter provides an introductory discussion related to systems in general, including a definition and the basic components of a system. A more in-depth discussion about the general systems theory follows, including newer associated concepts and offshoot theories such as complex systems theory, complex-adaptive systems theory, and chaos theory. The bioecological model is then discussed to provide the perspective needed to understand the patient as the center of care. The chapter ends with an application of the general systems theory to Interprofessional Collaborative Practice (IPCP) and healthcare teams, using systems thinking as the main tool for the application.

A FRAMEWORK FOR INTERPROFESSIONAL EDUCATION AND COLLABORATIVE PRACTICE

Interprofessional collaboration among healthcare professionals usually takes place within a healthcare or educational system. To better understand the context in which professionals collaborate, an understanding of systems is useful. We chose the General Systems Theory (GST) (von Bertalanffy, 1968) as a framework with which to understand how systems function; GST was developed to be used by multiple disciplines and to apply universally to all systems.

Theories are useful in helping to describe, understand, and predict many phenomena; they also can explain the underlying mechanisms of the phenomenon of interest. Interprofessional collaboration has been identified as the construct that, when operationalized through Interprofessional Collaborative Practice (IPCP), results in safe, high-quality, accessible, patient- and population-centered care (IPEC, 2011; 2016). In this case the "phenomenon" we need to describe, understand, and predict is IPCP. The identification of a theoretical framework for IPCP can help to predict the impact that IPCP will have on patient and population health outcomes. In short, having a theoretical framework to engage in IPCP is not just desirable, it is necessary.

A significant number of theories have been identified as suitable for application to IPE and IPCP; some already have been applied to IPCP (Reeves et al., 2007). These theories come from at least eight different perspectives (Box 2.1). Each of these approaches have pros and cons, and some may be more appropriate than others in addressing different aspects of IPCP in specific contexts. In choosing a theory to frame IPCP within this book,

BOX 2.1	**Theories Identified as Suitable for Application to Interprofessional Education and Interprofessional Collaborative Practice**		
Perspective	**Theory/Theorist**	**Perspective**	**Theory/Theorist**
Theories That Have Been Applied to Interprofessional Education (IPE) and Interprofessional Collaborative Practice (IPCP)		Organizational	Organizational learning (Argyris & Schön)
			Punctuated equilibrium (Gersick)
Social psychology	Contact theory (Allport)		Institutional theory (DiMaggio & Powell)
	Groupthink (Janis)	**Theories Identified as Appropriate for Application to IPE and IPCP but Not Applied Yet**	
	Group development (Tuckman & Jensen)		
	Social exchange theory (Challis et al.)	Individual	Action-centered leadership
			Active learning
	Cooperation theory (Axelrod)		Attribution theory of leadership
	Relational awareness theory (Drinka et al.)		Discovery learning
			Leadership grid
	Team reflexivity (West)		Mind mapping
	Realistic conflict theory (Brown et al.)		Situational leadership theory
			Valence–instrumentality– expectancy theory
	Social identity theory (Ellemers et al.)		Vroom–Yetton leadership model
	Social learning theory (Bandura & Cervone)	Team/group	Abilene paradox
			Action learning
	Self-categorization theory (Turner)		Autonomous work groups
	Transformation/transactional leadership (Bass)		Case-based learning
			Collaborative/cooperative learning
Sociology	Discourse theory (Foucault)		Collective effort model
	Surveillance theory (Foucault)		Existence relatedness growth theory
	Self-presentation theory (Goffman)		
	Negotiated order perspective (Strauss)		Field theory
			Inquiry-based learning
	Professionalization theory (Freidson)		Sensitivity training
			Synchronous learning
	Practice theory (Almas)		T-groups
	Power and influence theory (French & Raven)		Team learning
		Organization/ system	Behavioral theory of the firm
Adult learning	Reflective learning (Schön)		Contingency theory
	Problem-based learning (Barrows & Tamblyn)		Differentiation-integration theory
			Diffusion of innovation theory
	Experiential learning (Kolb)		Implementation theory
	Situated learning (Lave & Wenger)		Leavitt's diamond
Systems	General systems theory (von Bertalanffy)		Organizational theory
			Stakeholder theory
	Presage-process-product (Biggs)		Sociotechnical theory
	Chaos (Krippner)		Unfreeze–change–refreeze
	Complexity (Cooper)		Virtual learning community
	Activity theory (Engestrom)		

From Reeves, S., Suter, E., Goldman, J., Martimianakis, T., Chatalalsingh, C., & Dematteo, D. (2007). *A scoping review to identify organizational and education theories relevant for interprofessional practice and education.* Vancouver, BC: Canadian Interprofessional Health Consortium (CIHC). Retrieved from http://www.cihc.ca/files/publications/ScopingReview_IP_Theories_Dec07.pdf

we sought a theory that demonstrated the robustness needed to describe the components of the myriad of healthcare systems found throughout the United States and globally, and their complex interactions. A theory that provides a holistic approach to understanding IPCP and is compatible with a person-centered perspective is also required. A review of the literature suggests the general systems theory as the theory that best meets these criteria.

Although GST was selected to illustrate the impact of IPCP and its Core Competencies within the healthcare system, other theories associated with GST are described here because of their frequent use in the literature to understand certain aspects of the healthcare system. For example, the bioecological model is commonly used in public health to understand the impact several hierarchies of systems (e.g., family, city, culture) have on the health of individuals or populations. Similarly, two other theories born from GST, complex-adaptive systems theory (also known as *complexity theory*) and chaos theory, are discussed because they have been useful in explaining some of the unexpected behaviors of the healthcare system.

INTRODUCTION TO SYSTEMS THEORY

A significant number of definitions for a *system* are available; however, there is no universal agreement (Adams et al., 2013). In general, most definitions of a system describe (1) a group of elements, (2) interacting with each other and their environment, (3) making a larger whole, and (4) having a purpose defined by the purpose and function of the elements (Cordon, 2013). In this text, *system* is defined as "a set of related parts that work together in a particular environment to perform whatever functions are required to achieve the system's objectives" (Carr, 2016, p. 14).

Systems theory appeared in the early part of the 20th century as a reaction to the 300-year-old reductionist approach of science (Cordon, 2013; Sexton & Stanton, 2016); reductionism is an approach to science that attempts to understand a larger whole by studying its parts (Cordon, 2013). In contrast, systems theory is a holistic approach to science (Cordon, 2013), an approach that tries to understand the emergent properties of a complex system by studying the totality of the system. An *emergent property* is a characteristic of a larger entity that appears as a consequence of the interactions among the smaller entities that make the larger entity, but the

characteristic is not present in the smaller entities. Consciousness is an emergent property of the brain. It emerges when billions of neurons interact with each other, but individual neurons do not display consciousness.

GENERAL SYSTEMS THEORY

The GST was developed by Ludwig von Bertalanffy to define the general principles underlying all systems, regardless of the nature of the system (von Bertalanffy, 1968). *GST* can be defined as a set of models, principles, and laws that apply to all systems or their subclasses, irrespective of their particular kind, the nature of their component elements, and the relationships or "forces" among them (von Bertalanffy, 1968). GST is useful in understanding the healthcare system and the impact of the Core Competencies on IPCP within that system.

In GST, systems are characterized by their "wholeness," "organization," "dynamics," "primary activity," and "equifinality" (Meir, 1969). *Wholeness* means the system is a unit in itself, distinct from its parts, and with its own properties (Meir, 1969). *Organization* refers to the structure of the system and the function of the organization (Meir, 1969). The organization of each system's components is particular to the system and necessary for the system to function (von Bertalanffy, 1968). For example, the location of the cell membrane, cytoplasm, and nucleus in a cell is not random, but intrinsic to the functioning of the cell. Systems are made of smaller systems *(subsystems),* and they are part of larger systems *(suprasystems). Dynamics* refers to the interactions of the system with those subsystems and suprasystems. These dynamics develop and make the system function (Meir, 1969). Systems are also characterized by their primary activity. This consists of inherent behaviors of the system that are independent of external stimuli (Meir, 1969). For example, a single pharmaceutical company can be considered a system, in which its several departments (e.g., research and development, accounting, marketing) can be considered subsystems. Any given subsystem (i.e., department) in the larger system (i.e., pharmaceutical company) has a primary activity that is independent from another subsystem: Research and development conducts biomedical research and develops new and better medications, accounting keeps track of the earnings and payments, and marketing is in charge of making the product attractive to the public (Fig. 2.1). Finally, systems have equifinality. This means that the goals of the system can

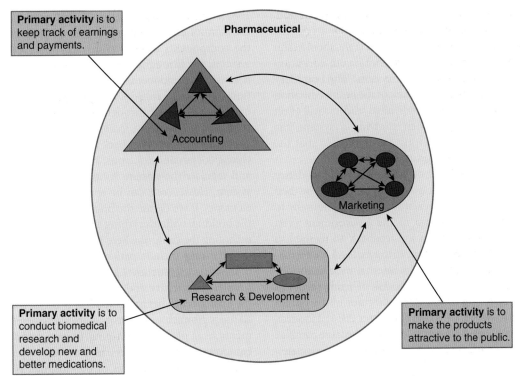

Primary activity is to keep track of earnings and payments.

Pharmaceutical

Accounting

Marketing

Research & Development

Primary activity is to conduct biomedical research and develop new and better medications.

Primary activity is to make the products attractive to the public.

FIG. 2.1 Representation of the primary activity of subsystems within a larger system.

be achieved in many different ways; however, the path the system takes to achieve its goals depends on the conditions of the environment (Meir, 1969).

GST applies to two types of systems: closed and open systems. Closed systems are systems with limited or no exchanges with their environments (von Bertalanffy, 1968); in the natural sciences, closed systems do not have exchanges of matter with the environment, and isolated systems have no exchanges of matter or energy. Because systems require energy, material, or information to achieve their goals (Carr, 2016), closed systems tend to lose organization and deteriorate (*entropy*) because of the lack of energy, material, or information (Sexton & Stanton, 2016). There are no good examples of closed systems in health care because, as stated previously, they tend to deteriorate until they cannot function anymore and dissipate. However, let's imagine a scenario in which a medical military unit in the battlefield assisting wounded soldiers is cut off from the rest of the troops. This medical unit can be considered a closed system because it cannot get more supplies and it cannot send or receive more wounded soldiers. If these conditions persist, the medical

unit will eventually run out of wounded soldiers to treat or medical supplies to treat wounded soldiers. Because of the lack of exchanges with the environment, this system will deteriorate and eventually will not be able to perform its function.

On the other hand, open systems are systems that interact with their environments (von Bertalanffy, 1968). These systems exchange energy, material, or information with their environment, so they are better able to adapt (*negentropy*) to external stimuli (Sexton & Stanton, 2016). Negentropy, or negative entropy, refers to a tendency in the system to become more and better organized. Examples of open systems are humans, an interprofessional collaborative team, and a hospital.

Closed and open systems are separated from their environment by their boundaries. The *boundary* of a system is the line or point at which the system can be distinguished from its environment (Gillies, 1982). In open systems, the boundary is permeable, so exchanges between the system and the environment can take place (Gillies, 1982). In closed systems, the boundary is easier to identify—for example, the walls of a thermos. The boundaries of an open system may be difficult to find. For example, it is easy to tell whether a hospital is inside the healthcare system, but what about a high school health education teacher? Is the high school health education teacher a part of the healthcare system? The boundary is not easily apparent, but the work of the health education teacher toward the health of individual students will affect the healthcare system. When studying a system, the boundaries of the system must be defined so that the components of the system can be determined.

Another characteristic of systems is their tendency toward *equilibrium.* When systems are stimulated by their environment, they must react by changing internally to compensate for the change in the environment (von Bertalanffy, 1968). Systems use feedback to reestablish equilibrium (Sexton & Stanton, 2016); *feedback* is information the system draws from its internal process to self-regulate (Gillies, 1982). The process of using feedback to self-regulate and maintain equilibrium in the system was called *homeostasis* (Sexton & Stanton, 2016). However, this term has been replaced by *adaptation* because complex systems have the ability to learn, be proactive (anticipate), and produce novel responses (creativity) to the environment, which is beyond merely responding to changes in the environment using feedback (Cordon, 2013; Gillies, 1982; Sexton & Stanton, 2016).

Basic Components of Systems

It is possible to reduce a system to four basic elements: input, throughput (process), output, and feedback (Fig. 2.2). *Input* is the energy, material, or information that enters the system (Gillies, 1982). *Throughput* is the process the system uses to convert the energy, material, or information into the product produced by the system (Gillies,

1982). Understanding the throughput requires knowing the components of the system and understanding how the components interact with each other. In complex systems, the throughput may be difficult to understand because the components of the system and/or its interactions may not be fully known. *Output* is the product, or outcome, obtained through the process of the system (Gillies, 1982). Finally, *feedback* is the process in which part of the output is fed back into the system (Martínez-García & Hernández-Lemus, 2013) to monitor, evaluate, and regulate the system. A hospital is a fairly complex system. However, it can be reduced to these four basic elements. If we define the boundaries of the hospital as the building with everything and everyone that is inside, including the campus where it sits, then the input of this hospital may include patients, the friends and families of the patients, supplies (e.g., medication, medical devices, needles), electricity and water, and money (to finance the operation). The throughput (or process) may include all the personnel (e.g., doctors, nurses, engineers), departments (e.g., pharmacy, imaging, human resources), and equipment (e.g., computers, mops, stethoscopes) needed to carry out the functions of the hospital. Notice that any element of the throughput is also a system itself and could be reduced to the same four basic elements. The output of the hospital may include healthier patients, health education, waste, and money (e.g., salaries). The feedback of this system may include the infection rates, patient falls, overall mortality, and patient census (i.e., daily number of patients). These same principles apply to even more complex systems, although determining what constitutes the system, the input, the throughput, the output, and the feedback may be difficult.

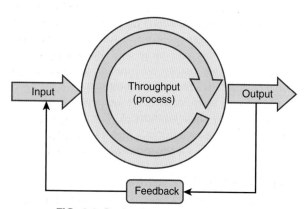

FIG. 2.2 Basic elements of a system.

✳ ACTIVE LEARNING

Answer the following questions about the healthcare system, keeping in mind that input, throughput, output, and feedback may change depending on how one draws the boundaries of the system:

1. What are five things that serve as input for the healthcare system?
2. What are five components of the throughput of healthcare system?
3. What are five things the healthcare system produces (output)?
4. What are five pieces of information the healthcare system uses as feedback?

BOX 2.2   Basic Principles of a Systems Approach

1. A system is greater than the sum of its parts.
2. The portion of the world studied (the system) must exhibit some predictability.
3. Though each subsystem is a self-contained unit, it is part of a wider and higher-order entity.
4. The central objective of a system can be identified by the fact that other objectives will be sacrificed to attain the central objective.
5. Every system, living or mechanical, is an information system.
6. An open system and its environment are highly interrelated.
7. A highly complex system may have to be broken into subsystems so each can be analyzed and understood before being reassembled into a whole.
8. A system consists of a set of objectives and their relationships.
9. A system is a dynamic network of interconnecting elements. A change in only one of the elements must produce change in all the others.
10. When subsystems are arranged in a series, the output of one is the input for another; therefore, process alterations in one requires alterations in other subsystems.
11. All systems tend toward equilibrium, which is a balance of various forces within and outside of a system.
12. The boundary of a system can be redrawn at will by a system analyst.
13. To be viable, a system must be strongly goal-directed, be governed by feedback, and have the ability to adapt to changing circumstances.

From Gillies, D. A. (1982). *Nursing management: A systems approach.* Philadelphia: WB Saunders.

Principles of the General Systems Theory

Thirteen basic principles of a systems approach were drawn from GST (Gillies, 1982; Box 2.2). These principles provide an approach to understanding the healthcare system and are applicable to IPCP.

These principles facilitate understanding a complex system like the healthcare system. For example, because the healthcare system is an open system, it is highly interrelated with its environment (principle 6). This explains why it is difficult to draw the boundaries of the healthcare system. Although some elements like a hospital are clearly inside the system, as discussed previously, a high school health education teacher could be thought of as being part of the healthcare system or part of its environment. As part of the environment, a health education teacher supplies healthier individuals to the healthcare system (input). As a component of the healthcare system, the teacher can be seen as a subsystem whose primary activity is to promote health among individuals inside the healthcare system (throughput).

Complex Systems

Systems such as living organisms, culture, or the healthcare system are complex systems. *Complex systems* are systems that produce unpredictable behavior as a result of the synergy of nonlinear interactions (*nonlinearity*) of multiple inputs (Martínez-García & Hernández-Lemus, 2013). The output of complex systems is produced by *multiple causalities* (inputs). Multiple causalities often get reinforced by *circular causality*; this is a phenomenon in which information flows between different hierarchies of the system, creating complicated feedback loops (Martínez-García & Hernández-Lemus, 2013). Complex systems have positive and negative feedbacks. Positive feedback increases the dynamics of the system, whereas negative feedback reduces those dynamics (Martínez-García & Hernández-Lemus, 2013). Another characteristic of complex systems is *asymmetry*. This is related to differences in the contributions of different components of the system (Martínez-García & Hernández-Lemus, 2013); this means that the same interaction on one part of the system may have a small impact, but it may have a big impact on a different part of the system. Complex systems also have *memory* (hysteresis). This means that the same input can have a different output in subsequent iterations because of the history of the system (Majdandzic et al., 2014). Finally, complex systems have complex structures that include the nesting of subsystems and networking (Bronfenbrenner, 1979; Cohen & Havlin, 2010). *Nesting* means that systems are organized in multiple hierarchical structures in which subsystems are fully contained by suprasystems (Bronfenbrenner, 1979). Complex systems also tend to be organized into highly interacting local *networks* with fewer interactions observed between local networks (Cohen & Havlin, 2010); this simplifies the system and makes it more efficient.

Complex-Adaptive Systems

A complex-adaptive system is a system with nonlinear interacting components that have the capacity for learning and can produce reactive or proactive adaptive behavior (Cordon, 2013). This means that learning is an emergent property of this kind of complex system. Another emergent property of complex-adaptive systems is the ability to *adapt*, which is the ability to self-organize in response to demands from the environment (Cordon, 2013).

Because the healthcare system is a complex-adaptive system, introducing Interprofessional Collaborative Practice (IPCP) into it can produce unpredictable outcomes. However, as a complex-adaptive system, the healthcare system also has the ability to learn and adapt to changes. This means that, although it is not possible to fully predict all the outcomes associated with introducing IPCP, we can be fairly certain the system will adapt to this new way of practicing. Introducing changes to complex systems can produce unpredictable results, but a significant number of national and international experts agree that IPCP should help reduce human error and produce an overall positive effect on health care (CAIPE, 2013; CIHC, 2010; IPEC, 2011; WHO, 2010).

IPCP happens in the context of healthcare teams, which are complex-adaptive subsystems within a larger complex-adaptive system (e.g., healthcare workforce). Understanding the environment in which it operates (e.g., hospital) is important when implementing an Interprofessional Education (IPE) program to promote IPCP (Sargeant, 2009); IPCP and IPE are subsystems of the healthcare system, and these subsystems are interrelated (Sargeant, 2009). In short, the subsystems IPCP, IPE, and healthcare teams interact with each other and with other subsystems in the healthcare system. However, through learning and adaptation, healthcare teams should be able to adapt to IPCP and IPE programs. This is especially true if the program is tailored to the environment in which the healthcare team operates and the program changes in response to the changes in the practice of the healthcare team.

Intervening in complex systems may seem overwhelming and dangerous, given it can produce unpredictable results. However, it is worth noting that another theory born from GST, chaos theory, suggests that order and chaos are related; order emerges from chaos. Further, systems that seem to be in chaos may still be contained within ordered boundaries (Cordon, 2013), and because of *adaptation*, the system may be self-organizing and be moving toward order. Systems seek order and will try to adapt to changes (Cordon, 2013). This means that we should not hesitate to introduce thoughtful interventions

in the healthcare system. A well-thought-out intervention will force the system to change and produce some positive outcomes.

The Bioecological Model

The bioecological model is a systems theory that is particularly useful to understand patient-centered care (PCC), which is discussed in Chapter 3. This theory was developed by Urie Bronfenbrenner as a model of human development using principles from systems theory. This model also borrowed ideas from other disciplines such as ecology. In this model, adaptation to changes in the environment are seen as *goodness of fit*, that is, adaptation is the balance between the individual and its environment (Pardeck, 1988). The bioecological model conceptualizes the individual as a system nested in a hierarchy of five suprasystems, each one nested inside another (Fig. 2.3). This model is a person-centered, holistic approach to understanding the health of the individual. The six nested systems are the person, microsystem, mesosystem, exosystem, macrosystem, and chronosystem (Tacón, 2008). PCC is an approach to healthcare practice that puts the patient at the center. This means the treatment of the patient is planned considering the totality of the individual, and it includes the patient and his or her loved ones in the process (a formal definition and an explanation of PCC is offered in Chapter 3). To engage in PCC, healthcare teams need to understand the factors interacting with the patient up and down the hierarchy of systems.

The *person* is the system at the center of the hierarchy of systems. The individual brings his or her unique characteristics to the overall system; these include things like genetics, age, life experiences, and temperament. Healthcare teams tend to be more aware of the factors within the person system (e.g., age, diagnosis, genetic risk, vital signs) than with the factors in any other system in the hierarchy.

The *microsystem* is the setting in which the person lives. It includes institutions like the family, peers, school, church, hospitals, and the neighborhood (Bronfenbrenner, 1979). Healthcare teams, as part of a health institution (e.g., hospital), exist in the microsystem of the patient. If the patient is seen in a hospital that has not adopted IPCP and PCC, the patient may be at an increased risk of medical errors and reduced quality of care. Similarly, the patient may live in a food desert (an area without access to fresh fruit, vegetables, and other healthful whole foods) or in a rural community that lacks an outpatient

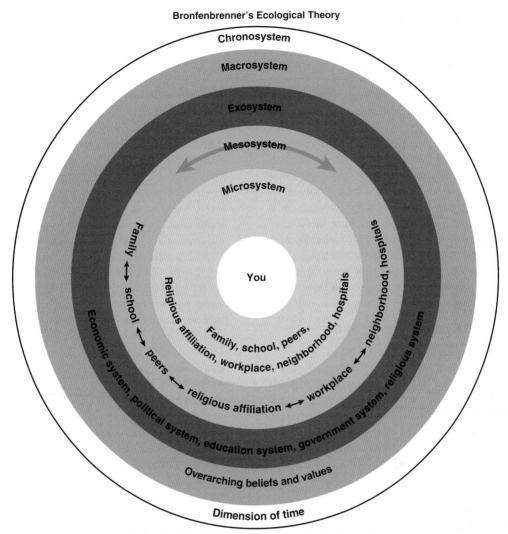

Bronfenbrenner's Ecological Theory

FIG. 2.3 Bronfenbrenner's bioecological model.

service necessary for her recovery; these are examples of how factors in the microsystem of the patient may affect the work of the healthcare team.

Mesosystem refers to the interactions among the components of the microsystem. A health-related example of the mesosystem is the intersection of health and religious institutions—for example, a patient who is part of a religious community that objects to blood transfusion or to abortions even to save the life of the mother. Because the patient becomes part of the healthcare team, PCC is an excellent way to determine these kinds of factors in the mesosystem of the patient.

The *exosystem* includes the interactions among large aspects of the social context of the person and their immediate context (Bronfenbrenner, 1979). For example, the economy of the country exists in the exosystem. A downturn in the economy may result in job loss, and therefore problems accessing health care. Other examples include shortages of the flu vaccine or being displaced by a natural disaster. Usually, patients have little to no control over the factors in the exosystem; nonetheless, they affect their health.

Macrosystem refers to the overall cultural context of the person. The boundaries of this system are defined by the laws and norms of the country (Bronfenbrenner, 1979). An example of the effect of the macrosystem on the health of a person is the social norms that discourage males from seeking health care. Another example is changes in healthcare policy. Changes in the macrosystem of the patient tend to come slowly (evolving), although sometimes they can come suddenly, such as in the case of revolutions.

Chronosystem refers to time patterns that emerge over the course of a lifetime. Chronosystem refers to a cohort effect or the sociohistorical context of the person. This system was not part of the original model created by Bronfenbrenner (Tacón, 2008). Conditions being equal in all the lower systems, two individuals from two different generations will experience different outcomes because of the specific time patterns of their respective generations. For example, a young adult today may have a healthier old age than his or her parents because of the current focus on wellness in today's generation.

Application of Systems Theory to the Healthcare System

The healthcare system is a complex system (Swanson et al., 2012) with a large number of subsystems. Analysis of problems, the development of interventions, and the deployment of those interventions require a theoretical framework that can manage the complexity of the healthcare system. Systems thinking can provide the tools to make thoughtful changes to the healthcare system that will translate into better health outcomes to patients.

Components of the Healthcare System

The World Health Organization (2010) identified six primary components of any healthcare system: leadership and governance, health information systems, human resources for health care, health financing, service delivery, and healthcare products. As components of any healthcare system around the world, each of these components is in itself a complex system.

1. *Leadership and governance* refers to those pieces of the healthcare system that can only be handled by governments. It includes things like producing health policy; providing a vision, strategy, and planning to improve the system; addressing unanticipated problems; preparing for disasters; and enacting effective regulations (Shi & Singh, 2017; WHO, 2010).
2. *Health information systems* include technologies and processes to gather, manage, and disseminate information. At a national level, it includes processes to collect, evaluate, and monitor information about health trends. At a local level, it includes technologies that facilitate health care delivery, such as electronic medical records (Shi & Singh, 2017; WHO, 2010).
3. *Human resources for health care* refers to the professionals who work in the healthcare system, including professionals from medicine, nursing, dentistry, and pharmacy; nonphysician practitioners (e.g., physician assistant, nurse practitioner); allied healthcare professionals (e.g., occupational therapists, physical therapists); technicians and assistants (e.g., phlebotomists, dental hygienists); public health professionals (e.g., health educators); healthcare administrators; and a multitude of support staff such as receptionists, environmental service workers, and dietary aides. This component also includes the institutions that train those professionals, professional organizations, and public policies focused on ensuring that sufficient professionals are available to meet the needs of the country (Shi & Singh, 2017; WHO, 2010).
4. *Health financing* includes several strategies to finance health care, including governments levying taxes to pay for healthcare services (e.g., single payer), governments providing the health care (e.g., Veteran Health Administration, and the National Health Service in the United Kingdom), private (e.g., Blue Cross) and public (e.g., Medicare) health insurance, reimbursement methods to pay healthcare professionals (e.g., fee-for-service, salary), and managed care, which is both a type of service delivery and a type of health financing (Shi & Singh, 2017; WHO, 2010).
5. *Service delivery* refers to the ways in which health care is delivered to patients. It includes several settings and levels. The *common settings* include outpatient services, hospitals, managed care, and long-term care. *Levels of care* refers to primary care (i.e., basic and routine services); secondary care (i.e., short-term, sporadic consultation, and interventions beyond primary care); and tertiary care, which involves complex, highly specialized, institution-based interventions (e.g., hospitalization) (Shi & Singh, 2017; WHO, 2010).
6. *Healthcare products* include the diagnostic and treatment equipment and supplies necessary for the healthcare system to function well, pharmaceutical products such as medications and vaccines, regulation of the use of those healthcare products such as prescription drug regulation, and policies to ensure the

production and availability of such products (WHO, 2010).

Although these six subsystems of the healthcare system may appear more cohesive than a country's healthcare system as a whole, they are also large and complex, with many subsystems of their own. Stimulating any one of these subsystems can produce significant changes in the subsystem being stimulated, in other subsystems, and in the healthcare system as a whole. Because small disturbances can produce massive changes in complex systems (Cordon, 2013), a thoughtful method to transform the healthcare system is necessary if one wants to improve it.

System Thinking

System thinking is a holistic approach to thinking and solving problems in which issues are construed as complex systems and the thinker focuses on the interrelatedness and interactions of the components of the system, rather than in the components of the system (Behl & Ferreira, 2014). System thinking is a system in and of itself, and it can be defined as "a set of synergistic analytic skills used to improve the capability of identifying and understanding systems, predicting their behaviors, and devising modifications to them in order to produce desired effects" (Arnold & Wade, 2015, p. 675). It is logical that a system is required to analyze and transform another system in a thoughtful way. System thinking is a thoughtful approach to making improvements to the healthcare system (Swanson et al., 2012). Several skills to intervene in the healthcare system have been defined (Box 2.3). System thinking suggests that when addressing a problem, it should be framed as a "pattern of behaviors," so understanding the problem means understanding the interactions driving the behavior. In complex systems, many behaviors of the system are native to the system; this means the behavior is a response to internal dynamics. When addressing a problem, one should look for the "internal actors" involved and understand how they interact with the problem. It may also require "understanding the context" in which those interactions take place. Because the problem is the result of the interactions between subsystems (e.g., internal actors), it is not necessary to understand how each subsystem works; one can concentrate on what "causes" or "generates" the problem.

Finally, complex systems have "feedback loops." This means that whatever caused the behavior, the behavior feeds back to the source of the problem, to make the

---

> **BOX 2.3 Skills of the System Thinking Approach**
>
> 1. *Dynamic thinking* means framing a problem in terms of a pattern of behavior over time.
> 2. *System-as-cause thinking* refers to placing responsibility for a behavior on internal actors who manage the policies and "plumbing" of the system.
> 3. *Forest thinking* is believing that to know something requires understanding the context of relationships.
> 4. *Operational thinking* means concentrating on causality and understanding how a behavior in the system is generated.
> 5. *Loop thinking* involves viewing causality as an ongoing process, not a one-time event, with effect feeding back to influence the causes and the causes affecting each other.

World Health Organization (WHO). (2009). *System thinking for health systems strengthening*. Geneva, Switzerland: Author. Retrieved from http://apps.who.int/iris/bitstream/10665/44204/1/9789241563895_eng.pdf.

---

behavior ongoing. Similarly, the solution to the problem will have to be ongoing because the feedback loop will create resistance to change. Three strategies rooted in system thinking have been defined for transformational interventions to healthcare practice (Swanson et al., 2012): "collaboration across disciplines, sectors, and organizations," "ongoing, iterative learning," and "transformational leadership." *Collaboration across disciplines, sectors, and organizations* means that solutions to problems in the healthcare system will require solutions that involve the collaboration of the "actors" involved in the problem; no one professional, administrator, or organization can solve the problem by themselves. *Ongoing, iterative learning* indicates that as solutions are being applied, the context of the problem changes, so the "actors" must continuously adapt, learn, and apply the new knowledge to the solution. *Transformational leadership* means that interventions to change the practice of healthcare professionals require leaders willing to challenge the prevailing paradigm and sacrifice personal and organizational interest for systemic benefits.

The Outcomes of Interprofessional Education and Interprofessional Collaborative Practice

Making improvements to the healthcare system requires addressing health practice, health education, health research, and health policy (Swanson et al., 2012). This

BOX 2.4   **Areas of Improvement Associated With Interprofessional Education**

1. Diabetes care
2. Emergency department culture and patient satisfaction
3. Collaborative team behavior and reduction of clinical error rates for emergency department teams
4. Collaborative team behavior in operating rooms
5. Management of care delivered in cases of domestic violence
6. Mental health practitioner competencies related to the delivery of patient care

From Andrews, L. (2016). Cochrane review summary-interprofessional education: Effects on professional practice and healthcare outcomes. *Singapore Nursing Journal, 43*(3), 25–26.

text focuses on improving health outcomes through IPE and IPCP. The infusion of IPE and IPCP into the healthcare system is expected to result in safer, high-quality, accessible, patient- and population-centered care (IPEC 2011; 2016). Although research on the effects of IPE and IPCP on health outcomes is sparse, a literature review by Andrews (2016) found evidence of improvements in several areas (Box 2.4).

System thinking is the correct approach to implement IPE and IPCP in the healthcare system. It focuses on the interactions among healthcare professionals, rather than focusing on each healthcare professional. Swanson et al. (2012) proposed that collaboration across disciplines is one of the "methods and strategies" of system thinking. This means that the health outcomes of patients can be improved by teaching healthcare professionals how to collaborate (i.e., Interprofessional Collaborative Practice [IPCP]), which is the goal of Interprofessional Education (IPE).

IPE/IPCP IN HEALTHCARE TEAMS: A SYSTEMS CASE STUDY

Consider the following exemplar case of a community HIV clinic where every patient is assigned to (1) a nurse practitioner who acts as the primary health provider, (2) an infectious disease physician who manages the HIV treatment, (3) a mental health counselor who evaluates new patients and thereafter meets them if referred by

another healthcare professional in the clinic or by request of the patient, and (4) a social worker who manages referrals to ancillary services for the patient, such as housing, health insurance, and transportation. These professionals used a consultation model of care in which they communicate with each other to obtain feedback when making decisions about the patient. For example, the infectious disease doctor may consult with the social worker about where is best to refer the patient for an outpatient procedure, given the particular circumstances of the patient: insurance, transportation, etc. In this case study, let's assume the model of care they used works fine for stable, well-established patients, but it may not be very efficient for new patients or patients with significant needs—for example, homeless patients or patients with medical complications. To improve the quality of care in the clinic, the medical director and the chief executive officer of the clinic decide to introduce IPCP to the clinic and move the practice from a consultation model to an integrated practice model. To achieve this, they hire a consultant who restructures the clinic's workforce and establishes an IPE program. The consultant arranges the healthcare professionals into teams consisting of a nurse practitioner, an infectious disease physician, a mental health counselor, and a social worker, and instead of assigning patients to healthcare professionals, patients are assigned to a team. As the physical space allows, the offices of the healthcare professionals were moved closer to each other. As an integrated practice unit, each healthcare team member is equally involved in the care of the patient, has access to the resources necessary to practice, and constantly interacts to exchange necessary patient information. Furthermore, to increase communication, teams meet on Friday afternoons to develop or review the single plan for the cases scheduled for the following week, especially difficult cases. Teams are encouraged to use a semiformal format for these meetings, at which some socialization can happen; for example, it is common for team members to bring refreshments to the meeting. In these meetings, for example, the team may decide to bring another healthcare professional to consult in a particularly difficult case. As part of the IPE program, teams are sent together to trainings and participate in in-services as a unit. The continuing education director of the clinic has also introduced several educational activities to the teams to promote learning together. For example, each team member is responsible to present and lead a discussion about a professional article about a pertinent topic. Teams are also encouraged to bring professionals from other specialties to the Friday meetings. The team can learn about specialties they do not interface frequently with and therefore be prepared whenever that specialty is needed. This also builds relationships with other healthcare professionals and improves consultation with and referrals to specialties outside of the team. Occasionally, the patient is invited to portions of the meetings to discuss the treatment plan; otherwise, the social worker tends to be the spokesperson for the patient's point of view.

SYSTEM ANALYSIS OF THE CASE STUDY

In the previous configuration (i.e., consultation-based practice), for every patient, a "temporary healthcare team" is formed to treat the patient. Because of the small number of healthcare professionals in the clinic, the same configuration of professional is repeated for several patients; however, these "temporary teams" did not interact long enough around the same purpose (e.g., a patient) to develop a significant group identity (this is discussed in more detail in Chapter 13). In this configuration, each healthcare professional is a subsystem of the complex-adaptive system "temporary team." The boundaries of this system are very vague.

In this case study, the short-lived interaction may not allow sufficient time and intensity of interaction for the system to learn and adapt. Because of this model of practice, these "temporary teams" may be missing out on one of the benefits of complex-adaptive systems: the ability to anticipate and produce novel responses. These emergent properties appear when the system is allowed to learn and adapt. In an integrated practice unit, the healthcare team is a complex-adaptive system, and its boundaries are better defined than in the consultation-based model. The clinic is the immediate environment of this system.

In the integrated practice unit model, each healthcare professional, and the patient, are complex-adaptive subsystems of the system "healthcare team." Because of the prolonged interactions between the subsystems of the healthcare team (i.e., healthcare professionals and patients), the system is continuously learning and adapting, and therefore improving its functioning. Because the healthcare professionals know each other better (e.g., personalities, strength and weaknesses), they are able to anticipate how team members may react, making interactions smoother. They know who is better at performing a specific task, they know how to communicate with each other efficiently, and they are likely to recover from disturbances in the team (e.g., disagreements) quicker. Notice that in this case study, little attention was put on changing the individual subsystems (e.g., healthcare professionals), but it focused on the interactions of the subsystems; for example, increasing interactions by forming permanent teams, promoting collaboration by having a single plan to which every team member contributes, promoting team cohesion by requiring everyone to take responsibility for the education of the team, and having weekly meetings that include socializing.

✳ ACTIVE LEARNING

Think about a productive team you have been part of, perhaps for a class project, in a club, or at work. Answer the following questions:

1. What kind of interactions between the team members (subsystems) made the team work more efficiently?
2. What kind of interactions made the team less efficient?
3. What kind of conditions could have made the team function more efficiently?

 ADDITIONAL RESOURCES

This chapter introduced you to the concept of system theory, including the GTS and more advanced system theories. The purpose of introducing these theories is to help you understand the interrelatedness of the health care system and the potential outcome of adopting the

Core Competencies of Interprofessional Collaborative Practice (IPCP) in the healthcare system. The resources in this section were selected to help you deepen your understanding of system theory, and therefore, the impact of the Core Competencies in the healthcare system.

Continued

📄 **ADDITIONAL RESOURCES—cont'd**

Foundational Books in Systems Theory

General System Theory: Foundations, Development, Applications. von Bertalanffy, L. (1968). George Braziller: New York, NY.

In the book, *General System Theory: Foundations, Development, Applications,* von Bertalanffy launched the field of systems by introducing the general systems theory. It was quickly applied to many fields such as computer sciences, business, and biology.

Living Systems. Miller, J. G. (1978). New York, NY: McGraw-Hill.

Bronfenbrenner, U., & Morris, P. A. (1998). The ecology of developmental processes. In *Handbook of Child Psychology.* Vol. 1. New York: John Wiley & Sons. pp. 993–1023.

Miller and Bronfenbrenner expanded the field of systems with their books on living systems and human development, respectively. They conceptualized living beings are complex systems.

Videos Explaining Aspects of Systems

The Interrelatedness of Complex Systems

https://youtu.be/17BP9n6g1F0

This video from Sustainability Illustrated, explains how the interrelatedness of components of a complex system can produce unintended consequences, when we don't understand how the components of the system interact with each other.

System Thinking

Access this program, including the curriculum, at http://evaluationforleaders.org/. Access the video at https://youtu.be/2vojPksdbtl

This video explains system thinking in the context of an intervention for obesity. The video is provided thanks to the University of British Columbia, Mobile Learning in Evaluation for Health Leaders. This program teaches health administrators to evaluate health programs in the context of complex systems.

Complex Systems

https://youtu.be/vp8v2Udd_PM

This video from Complexity Labs, explains the basic principles of complex systems. Complexity Labs is a platform for the exchange of information, research, and educational media related to complex system theory. More resources about complex systems can be found on their website: http://complexitylabs.io/about/.

KEY POINTS

- GST is useful in understanding the context in which IPCP occurs and in identifying potential effects of the interprofessional team's actions. Theories are useful in helping to describe, understand, and predict many phenomena; they also can explain the underlying mechanisms of the phenomena of interest.

- Interprofessional collaboration, when operationalized through IPCP, results in safe, high-quality, accessible, patient- and population-centered care (IPEC 2011; 2016).

- In general, systems have the following four common components (Cordon, 2013): It consists of a group of elements (e.g., objects, forces), the elements that make up the system interact with each other and with their environment, the elements form a larger whole, and the function or purpose of the elements within the system affect the function or purpose of the system.

- Systems are characterized by their wholeness, organization, dynamics, primary activity, and equifinality (Meir, 1969).

- Systems are made of smaller systems (subsystems), and they are part of larger systems (suprasystems).

- Systems can be characterized by their primary activity; these are inherent behaviors of the system that are independent of external stimuli (Meir, 1969).

- Systems have four basic elements: input, throughput (process), output, and feedback. Input is the energy, material, or information that enters the system to be transformed (Gillies, 1982).

- Throughput is the process the system uses to convert the energy, material, or information into the product produced by the system (Gillies, 1982).

- Output is the product obtained through the process of the system (Gillies, 1982).

- Feedback is the process in which part of the output is fed back into the system (Martínez-García & Hernández-Lemus, 2013) to monitor, evaluate, and regulate the system.

- GST is a set of models, principles, and laws that apply to all systems or their subclasses, regardless of their kind; the nature of their component elements; and the relationships or "forces" between them (von Bertalanffy, 1968).

- Thirteen basic principles of a systems approach were drawn from the GST (Gillies, 1982). These principles provide an approach to understanding the healthcare system and are applicable to both IPE and IPCP.
- Complex systems display emergent properties; systems such as a living organism, culture, or the healthcare system are complex systems.
- An emergent property is a characteristic of a larger entity that appears as a consequence of the interactions among the smaller entities that make the larger entity, but the characteristic is not present in the smaller entities.
- The bioecological model was developed by Urie Bronfenbrenner as a model of human development using principles from systems theory and ecology (Pardeck, 1988).
- The bioecological model conceptualizes the individual as a system nested in a hierarchy of five systems, each one nested inside another. It is a person-centered, holistic approach to understand the health of the individual.
- The six nested systems of the bioecological model are the person, microsystem, mesosystem, exosystem, macrosystem, and chronosystem (Tacón, 2008).
- The World Health Organization (2010) identified six primary components of any healthcare system: leadership and governance, health information systems, human resources for health care, health financing, service delivery, and healthcare products.
- *System thinking* is defined as "a set of synergistic analytic skills used to improve the capability of identifying and understanding systems, predicting their behaviors, and devising modifications to them in order to produce desired effects" (Arnold & Wade, 2015, p. 675).
- The systems thinking approach has the following skills: dynamic thinking, system-as-cause thinking, forest thinking, operational thinking, and loop thinking.

REFERENCES

Adams, K. M., Hester, P. T., & Bradley, J. M. (2013). A historical perspective of systems theory. *Proceedings of the 2013 Industrial and Systems Engineering Research Conference.* Retrieved from https://www.researchgate.net/publication/288782223_A_historical_perspective_of_systems_theory.

Andrews, L. (2016). Cochrane review summary—Interprofessional Education: Effects on professional practice and healthcare outcomes. *Singapore Nursing Journal, 43*(3), 25–26.

Arnold, R. D., & Wade, J. P. (2015). A definition of systems thinking: A system approach. *Procedia Computer Science, 44,* 669–678.

Behl, D. V., & Ferreira, S. (2014). Systems thinking: An analysis of key factors and relationships. *Procedia Computer Science, 36,* 104–109.

Bronfenbrenner, U. (1979). *The ecology of human development.* Cambridge, MA: Harvard University Press.

Canadian Interprofessional Health Collaborative (CIHC). (2010). *A national competency framework.* Vancouver, BC: CIHC.

Carr, A. (2016). The evolution of systems theory. In T. L. Sexton & J. Lebow (Eds.), *Handbook of family therapy* (pp. 13–29). New York, NY: Routledge.

Centre for the Advancement of Interprofessional Education (CAIPE). (2013). *Introducing interprofessional education.* Fareham, UK: CAIPE.

Cohen, R., & Havlin, S. (2010). Complex networks: Structure, robustness and function. Cambridge, MA: Cambridge University Press.

Cordon, C. P. (2013). System theories: An overview of various system theories and its application to healthcare. *American Journal of Systems Science, 2*(1), 13–22.

Gillies, D. A. (1982). *Nursing management: A systems approach.* Philadelphia, PA: WB Saunders.

Interprofessional Education Collaborative Expert Panel (IPEC). (2011). *Core competencies for Interprofessional Collaborative Practice: Report of an expert panel.* Washington, DC: Interprofessional Education Collaborative.

Interprofessional Education Collaborative Expert Panel (IPEC). (2016). *Core competencies for Interprofessional Collaborative Practice: 2016 update.* Washington, DC: Interprofessional Education Collaborative.

Majdandzic, A., Podobnik, B., Buldyrev, S. V., et al. (2014). Spontaneous recovery in dynamical networks. *Nature Physics, 10,* 34–38.

Martínez-García, M., & Hernández-Lemus, E. (2013). Health systems as complex systems. *American Journal of Operations Research, 3,* 113–126.

Meir, A. Z. (1969). General systems theory: Developments and perspectives for medicine and psychiatry. *Archives of General Psychiatry, 21*(3), 302–310.

Pardeck, J. T. (1988). An ecological approach for social work practice. *The Journal of Sociology and Social Welfare, 15*(2), 133–142.

Reeves, S., Suter, E., Goldman, J., et al. (2007). *A scoping review to identify organizational and education theories relevant for interprofessional practice and education.* Vancouver, BC: Canadian Interprofessional Health Consortium (CIHC). Retrieved from http://www.cihc.ca/files/publications/ScopingReview_IP_Theories_Dec07.pdf.

Sargeant, J. (2009). Theories to aid understanding and implementation of Interprofessional Education. *Journal of Continuing Education in the Health Professions, 29*(3), 178–184.

Sexton, T. L., & Stanton, M. (2016). Systems theories. In J. C. Norcross, G. R. VandenBos, & D. K. Freedheim (Eds.), *APA handbook of clinical psychology: Theory and research* (Vol. 2, pp. 213–239). Washington, DC: APA.

Shi, L., & Singh, D. A. (2017). *Essentials of the U.S. health care system* (4th ed.). Burlington, MA: Jones & Bartlett Learning.

Swanson, R. C., Cattaneo, A., Bradley, E., et al. (2012). Rethinking health systems strengthening: Key systems thinking tools and strategies for transformational change. *Health Policy and Planning, 27*, iv54–iv61.

Tacón, A. M. (2008). Approaches to chronic disease and chronic care: From oxymoron to modern Zeitgeist. *Disease Management and Health Outcomes, 16*(5), 285–288.

von Bertalanffy, L. (1968). *General system theory: Foundations, development, applications.* New York, NY: George Braziller.

World Health Organization (WHO). (2009). *System thinking for health systems strengthening.* Geneva, Switzerland: Author. Retrieved from http://apps.who.int/iris/bitstream/10665/44204/1/9789241563895_eng.pdf.

World Health Organization (WHO). (2010). *Framework for action on interprofessional education & collaborative practice.* Geneva, Switzerland: Author. Retrieved from http://apps.who.int/iris/bitstream/10665/70185/1/WHO_HRH_HPN_10.3_eng.pdf?ua=1.

Adopting the Frameworks of Wellness and Patient-Centered Care

LEARNING OUTCOMES

After studying this chapter, you will be able to:

1. Describe the historical development of wellness as a concept.
2. Define *wellness*.
3. Describe the illness–wellness continuum and positive health.
4. Define *salutogenesis*.
5. Describe eight dimensions of wellness.
6. Compare and contrast disease prevention and health promotion.
7. Explain the concept of social determinants of health and its relationship to wellness.
8. Define *patient-centered care*.
9. Describe several elements necessary for effective patient-centered care.
10. Describe barriers to patient-centered care.
11. Define *health literacy* and *patient education*.

This chapter offers two models that are useful in understanding health and health care in relation to Interprofessional Collaborative Practice (IPCP): *wellness* and *patient-centered care*. The chapter describes the historical development of wellness and provides a definition of this approach to health. A discussion of wellness-related concepts such as the illness–wellness continuum, salutogenesis, and dimensions of wellness is provided. The chapter contextualizes wellness with discussions about disease prevention, health promotion, and social determinants of health.

Patient-centered care is defined, and several elements to engage effectively in patient-centered care are described. Barriers to patient-centered care are presented. Finally, the chapter addresses the need for health literacy and patient education to ensure the participation of the patient in the healthcare team. Several strategies and resources to address low health literacy in patients are listed.

WELLNESS

Health and Wellness in the 19th Century

In the 19th century, nutrition, hygiene, the health of the home and work environment, global travel, and access to health care were identified as the main health and wellness concerns (Brunton, 2014). Most of the treatments that we take for granted today had not been developed (e.g., penicillin), and the approach to health and wellness focused simply on preventing infections, accidents, and diseases related to malnutrition. The 19th century saw an increase in safety regulations that affected the safety of food, water, and the workplace (Brunton, 2014).

In the 19th century, most people around the world still lived in rural communities and fed themselves by growing their own food, grazing animals, and collecting seasonal fruits and vegetables. This food supply system presented two main problems. First, people had access to only a limited range of foods. This sometimes contributed to malnutrition because the available food (e.g., potatoes, rice, wheat) could not always provide all the necessary nutrients. Second, famines related to natural disasters (e.g., droughts) were common and could devastate the crops that families or communities depended on for an entire year (Brunton, 2014). The industrialization of farming and advances in transportation (e.g., trains) improved the variety and reliability of the food supply in the 20th century.

One of the most important health developments seen in the 19th century was the identification of hygiene as a health intervention. The medical recommendation of the time was to bathe, wash one's clothes, and clean the house with clean water as a way of avoiding infections. However, access to clean water soon became a significant issue as people moved from rural areas to the cities and the bodies of water close to the urban areas became contaminated. Some important hygiene developments in the 20th century were the construction of water reservoirs, piping water directly to cities (for those who could afford it), the availability of public baths, the ventilation of buildings, and hygiene education in public schools (Brunton, 2014).

The focus of personal hygiene was extended to the environment, especially in cities. The rapid growth of cities produced a large amount of waste that was difficult to deal with. Most of the waste generated would end up in the streets and rivers, and the city government would pick it up only infrequently. Because living in cities became a health hazard, the 19th century saw the development of waste management systems and regulations meant to make life in the city healthier. For example, the width of streets and the size of rooms in dwelling buildings were regulated to increase ventilation and reduce disease (Brunton, 2014).

The advances in transportation in the 19th century allowed for the easy movement of people around the country and around the world. However, this ease of movement came with a high cost: With easy movement came the spread of new diseases. People were now exposed to climates they were not use to, for example, tropics or deserts. In some instances, people did not know how to cope with new climates, and in other cases they had difficulties physically adapting to them (Brunton, 2014).

Access to health care was dependent on the seriousness of the ailment and the resources of the family. Most people had enough knowledge of healing practices to take care of common health problems with home remedies or popular medicine. For more serious ailments, people sought the assistance of community healers (e.g., herbalists, bloodletters, bonesetters). Families with more resources had access to medical doctors (Brunton, 2014).

From Reductionism to the Emergent Property of Complex Systems

By the beginning of the 20th century, science had contributed great advances to medicine, such as the discovery of penicillin (1928) and the development of vaccines, including ones for influenza (1918), tuberculosis (1921), and polio (1955). Until the beginning of the 20th century, science had successfully used a *reductionist* approach, one in which the universe can be understood by studying its parts and how they interact with each other (Brunton, 2014). However, in the past 100 years, science moved from the reductionistic approach toward the study of the emergent properties of complex systems. For example, understanding how neurons function does not explain the emergence of consciousness. Wellness may also be an emergent property of the complex system "human body"; a series of scientific discoveries, including the discovery of the flight-or-fight response, the placebo effect, and the existence of specific neuropeptides and receptors the brain uses to communicate with body systems, have demonstrated the brain can affect a person's state of wellness (mind–body connection).

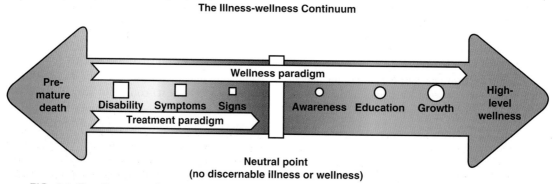

The Illness-wellness Continuum

FIG. 3.1 The illness–wellness continuum. (From Travis, J., & Ryan, R. S. [2004]. *The wellness workbook: How to achieve enduring health and vitality* [3rd ed.]. Berkeley, CA: Celestial Arts.)

The History of the Concept of Wellness

The idea that the body, and therefore health, is influenced not just by *physical* factors (e.g., infections) but also by *mental* factors (e.g., the placebo effect) received serious consideration during the second half of the 20th century. A comprehensive idea about wellness was first proposed in 1961 by Dunn, based on 3 decades of work at the National Office of Vital Statistics (Jordan, 2016); Dunn is widely regarded as the father of the wellness movement.

A decade after Dunn proposed the idea of high-level wellness, Travis proposed the wellness paradigm, conceptualizing illness and wellness as a continuum (Fig. 3.1) that ranges from high-level wellness to premature death (Travis & Ryan, 2004). Soon after, Hettler develop the concept of *Dimensions of Wellness* (Fig. 3.2); the original model had six dimensions of wellness. The model has been expanded since then to include additional dimensions (Becker & McPeck, 2013). Antonovsky (1979) proposed the concept of salutogenesis (i.e., the origin of health) as a counterpart to pathogenesis (i.e., the origin of disease); he proposed that health should be studied in the same way that disease is studied. Using the concept of salutogenesis, Becker added a positive health dimension to the illness–wellness continuum, producing the positive health model (Fig. 3.3) (Becker & McPeck, 2013).

A comprehensive history of the development of wellness is outside the scope of this book, but it is worth mentioning some early attempts to shift the focus of the healthcare system from disease to wellness. Robbins and Hall (1970) proposed a system that could be used to predict population health problems and take steps to prevent them. Lalonde (1974), Canada's Minister of National Health and Welfare, released the landmark report, *A New Perspective on the Health of Canadians: A Working Document*. In it, he stated that most premature death and disability was related to lifestyle choices; therefore health care should focus on prevention. Around the same time, Ardell (1977) proposed shifting US national health planning from building more hospitals to promoting a healthy lifestyle.

Wellness as a Framework for Health Care
What Is Wellness?

Wellness is the conscious and deliberate process of making choices to improve one's health (Johnson, 1986; Swarbrick, 2006; 2013). It is "an integrated method of functioning which is oriented toward maximizing the potential of which the individual is capable" (Dunn, 1977, p. 4). Wellness assumes that the levels of health that a person can

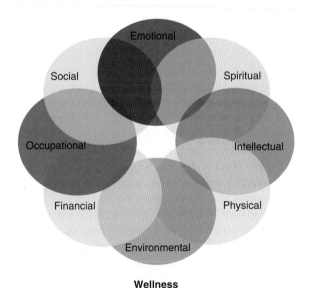

FIG. 3.2 The eight dimensions of wellness. (From Substance Abuse and Mental Health Services Administration [SAMHSA]. [2016]. Eight dimensions of wellness. Retrieved from https://www.samhsa.gov/wellness-initiative/eight-dimensions-wellness.)

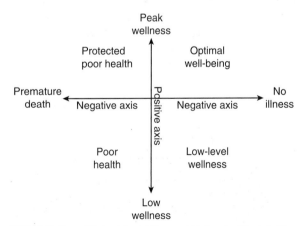

FIG. 3.3 Two-Dimensional Illness-Wellness Model: The Positive Health Model. (From Becker, C., & McPeck, W. [2013]. *Creating positive health: It's more than risk reduction* (white paper). Retrieved from http://www.nationalwellness.org/resource/resmgr/WhitePapers/NWIWhitePaper_BeckerMcPeck20.pdf.)

achieve aren't limited by the presence or absence of disease. The logical implication of this paradigm for healthcare professionals is that our roles and responsibilities extend beyond just healing our patients; we should work with people at all levels and dimensions of wellness.

Wellness assumes that humans are an integrated system with interdependent subsystems (Dunn, 1977). This means that it is illogical to treat one component of wellness (i.e., physical health) while ignoring the rest. Wellness is a holistic approach to health, so when we are treating a person for a physical condition (e.g., hip replacement), we are also concerned about other physical subsystems that might be affected, as well as other dimensions of health, such as how their mood is being affected, the quality of their social support, their employment and financial situation, their understanding of the situation, and more. For example, a patient recovering from an injury who needs to, but cannot afford to, take time off from work may require assistance in identifying other financial resources that could minimize the impact of missing work while recovering.

Wellness involves maximizing and maintaining an individual's health potential (Dunn, 1977). Wellness is not a destination, but a lifelong process involving day-to-day decisions and behaviors meant to achieve and maintain a maximum level of functioning. However, the wellness model assumes that individuals are capable of fully engaging in that process (Box 3.1), which is not always true (Chambers-Clark, 1996). Nonetheless, as healthcare professionals, our professional roles and responsibilities are to assist those we serve in achieving and maintaining their maximum levels of functioning.

BOX 3.1   Assumptions of the Wellness Model About Individuals' Capabilities

To effectively engage in wellness behavior, individuals must be able to do the following:
- Self-assess their own wellness needs
- Take action to meet their wellness goals
- Evaluate their progress toward wellness
- Be in the process of moving toward wellness
- Learn how to move to a higher level of wellness
- Learn from modeling, use clearly structured goals, and have the means to meet those goals and the necessary peer support

From Chambers-Clark, C. (1996). *Wellness practitioner: concepts, research, and strategies.* New York: Springer.

From the Illness–Wellness Continuum to Positive Health

As mentioned previously, early on, wellness was conceptualized as an illness–wellness continuum (Hafen, 2016; Travis and Ryan, 2004), by which one's state of health was illustrated on a continuum from premature death to high levels of wellness (see Fig. 3.1). In this perspective, gains on one pole (e.g., wellness) are at the expense of the other (e.g., illness), so that by maximizing one's health one could prevent disease and early death. High levels of health can and do have an effect on illness (Seligman, 2008); however, health and illness are not opposites (Becker & McPeck, 2013).

Today, illness and wellness are conceptualized as two-dimensional (see Fig. 3.3), with one dimension representing levels of wellness (i.e., positive health axis) and the other dimension representing levels of illness (i.e., negative health axis). The negative health axis extends from *no illness* to *premature death* and the positive health axis from *peak wellness* to *low wellness* (Becker & McPeck, 2013). In this model, the goal of the healthcare system and healthcare professionals should be to maintain optimal well-being (first quadrant of Fig. 3.3) (Lane, 2016). This expanded model is the positive health model (Becker & McPeck, 2013).

Salutogenesis: A New Prescription for Health Care

Salutogenesis is the study of the origin of health. As discussed previously, the concept of salutogenesis can best be understood in contrast to its opposite, pathogenesis, which is the study of the origin of disease. Wellness, and associated concepts such as positive health, are underpinned by the concept of salutogenesis. Traditionally, health researchers have focused on the etiology of disease (Becker & Rhynders, 2013) and healthcare professionals have focused "on symptom reduction, rapid stabilization, and interventions focused on deficiencies and incapacity" (Swarbrick, 2006, p. 312). Historically, society has poured tremendous amounts of resources into understanding what causes disease and how to fight it, rather than focusing resources on understanding the origins of health.

Salutogenesis, in contrast to pathogenesis, seeks to identify the factors that support and increase health. Salutogenesis explains health as a "reservoir of resources." From this perspective, illness arises when the demands of a particular event (e.g., infection, injury) exceed the available health resources in reserve (Antonovsky, 1979).

It is important to keep in mind that the size of each person's "reservoir" varies according to many different factors. For example, genetic makeup will allow for the potential of a larger reservoir in some people and a smaller reservoir in others; however, within that potential, the individuals can increase or decrease the reserves with their health behaviors (e.g., disease prevention, health promotion). Salutogenesis requires healthcare professionals to assist patients to increase their own health reserves as well as to treat their diseases.

The concept of salutogenesis can be used to explain, at least in part, why two individuals may be exposed to the same pathogen, but only one becomes ill; why recovery from the same disease may be longer in one individual than another; or why an infection may kill one patient, but not another. Individuals with larger health reserves may better weather an infection or injury than individuals with smaller health reserves. The concept of wellness means focusing on the positive health axis, so the individual can better combat the events on the negative health axis. Salutogenesis does not focus on solving a problem; it focuses on achieving optimal health (Becker & Rhynders, 2013).

Dimensions of Wellness

For thousands of years, philosophers discussed the "dual nature" of humans (i.e., the mind–body problem) and the interaction between these two aspects of humanity (Crane & Patterson, 2000; Massey, 2015). The recent focus on wellness recognizes this multidimensional nature of human beings and its relationship to health.

Dunn (1977) described *body, mind, and spirit* as distinct but blended aspects of human beings, and he argued that because of this interrelatedness, not being well in one aspect negatively affects the others. In the context of wellness, treating individuals as whole persons requires attention to the unique intersections of their physical, mental, and emotional aspects (Jonas, 2005). To maintain optimal health (first quadrant of Fig. 3.3), attention must be paid to all aspects of the human being.

The Six Dimensions of Wellness model addressed this multidimensional concept of health. It included the aspects of occupational, physical, social, intellectual, spiritual, and emotional wellness (Hettler, 1980). Subsequently, environmental (Foster & Keller, 2007) and financial wellness (Swarbrick, 2006) were added. The expanded model was adopted by the Substance Abuse and Mental Health Services Administration (SAMHSA) (2016) as the Eight Dimensions of Wellness model. Although other dimensions, such as creative wellness (i.e., participating in arts and cultural activities), have been proposed (Davis, Saltzburg, Wellman, & Clyburn, 2014), this chapter focuses on the Eight Dimensions of Wellness model (see Fig. 3.2).

The Eight Dimensions of Wellness

The presentation of the eight dimensions of wellness that follows is from the perspective of the patient. However, it is important to keep in mind that these dimensions also influence the healthcare professional, on a personal and professional level.

Intellectual Wellness

Intellectual wellness involves the development of problem-solving skills, creativity, and learning. Individuals with intellectual wellness seek to expand their level of knowledge and skills to their full potential. Intellectually well individuals prefer to stretch and challenge their minds rather than become self-satisfied; they identify potential problems and actively seek a solution rather than wait, worry, and procrastinate (Hettler, 1980; National Wellness Institute [NWI], n.d.). Intellectually well patients are active partners in their own health care; these individuals strive to understand their healthcare needs, identify problems, seek solutions, and ask questions.

Emotional Wellness

Individuals with high levels of emotional wellness are aware of and accepting of their own feelings; they are enthusiastic about their lives and maintain a positive outlook. Those with emotional wellness realistically assess their limitations, but instead of letting that knowledge defeat them, they are motivated to achieve their full potential. They tend to control and cope well with their own feelings and associated behaviors. Emotionally well individuals maintain satisfying, interdependent relationships with others based on mutual commitment, trust, and respect (Hettler, 1980; NWI, n.d.). Emotionally well individuals tend to have healthy relationships and appropriate support systems. The implication to practice of emotional wellness is having patients who are optimistic about their treatment and who have emotional resources to face difficult times.

Physical Wellness

Individuals with high levels of physical wellness recognize the need for regular exercise and well-balanced nutrition. They avoid the use of tobacco, drugs, and excessive alcohol consumption; they seek medical attention when needed. Physically well individuals appreciate the relationship between engaging in the health behaviors described previously and the way their bodies perform. They work to build physical strength, flexibility, and endurance while being safe (e.g., wearing a seatbelt or helmet) (Hettler, 1980; NWI, n.d.). The implication to practice of physical wellness is that patients with physical wellness have a high potential to resist disease, and when ill are more likely to recover quickly.

Social Wellness

Social wellness is focused on the ability to recognize one's importance in society and one's influence on multiple environments (Hettler, 1980; NWI, n.d.). Socially well individuals "make willful choices to enhance personal relationships and important friendships, and build a better living space and community" (NWI, n.d., p. 1). Social wellness also includes good communication skills, the capacity for intimacy, accepting each other's differences, and cultivating a supportive social network (e.g., family, friends) (Hales, 2005). The implications to practice of social wellness includes good relationships between healthcare professionals, patients, and their social networks. Patients who are aware of how their actions affect their environment may be less likely to miss or cancel appointments, communicate better, and may try to ensure the optimal functioning of the healthcare services they receive. Similarly, healthcare professionals with high levels of social wellness may be more effective healthcare workers.

Occupational Wellness

The basic tenant of occupational wellness is satisfaction with one's work and enrichment in one's life through work (Hettler, 1980; NWI, n.d.). Individuals with a high level of occupational wellness find it rewarding to contribute their "unique gifts, skills, and talents" (NWI, n.d., p. 1) and find purpose through work; occupational wellness includes balancing work and leisure time (Hales, 2005). The implication of occupational wellness to the practice of healthcare professionals may include, especially in countries in which health insurance is tied to employment (e.g., United States), patients who are not worried about being unable to access or afford health care. High levels of

occupational wellness may reduce work-related stress and result in a happier life, which in turn may promote faster healing. It is worth noting that patients will benefit from healthcare professionals having high levels of occupational wellness; healthcare professionals who derive meaning from their work may be more effective and less likely to experience burnout.

Financial Wellness

Financial wellness is not part of the original six dimensions described by Hettler (1980). However, it was added because, although it is possible to participate in work that is personally rewarding (e.g., student, actor), the work may not result in financial security. The Center for the Study of Student Life (2015) defines *financial wellness* as a state in which a person is "fully aware of his/her own financial state and budgets, saves, and manages his/her finances in order to achieve realistic financial goals" (p. 17). Financial wellness means having sufficient resources and managing them effectively, meeting one's needs, and achieving one's goals. The implication of this dimension to practice is that patients who have and manage their resources effectively will be able to have access to and afford health care.

Spiritual Wellness

Individuals who are spiritually well find meaning and purpose in human existence; their internal and external worlds live in harmony, and their values, beliefs, and actions are consistent (Hettler, 1980; NWI, n.d.). Individuals with high levels of spiritual wellness focus on pondering the meaning of life and are tolerant of the beliefs of others. The implication to practice of spiritual wellness is similar to occupational wellness. Individuals with high levels of spiritual wellness may be happier and have more congruence between what they think and do. This may facilitate the patient–professional relationship and give them resilience to endure difficult treatments.

Environmental Wellness

Environmental wellness was one of the first new dimensions to be added to the original model. It recognizes the importance of one's surroundings to the health of the individual (Foster & Keller, 2007). An environmentally well person "recognizes the responsibility to preserve, protect, and improve the environment and appreciates the interconnectedness of nature and the individual" (Center for the Study of Student Life, 2015, p. 17). Individuals with high levels of environmental wellness seek to make their environment healthier by protecting the food and water supply, reducing infectious disease and violence in society, and protecting the air from pollution. They may also promote measures to improve the environment, standard of living, and quality of health of the population (Wellness Center, n.d.). The implication of this dimension to healthcare practice may include healthcare professionals and patients advocating for policies that protect and promote environmental wellness as well as reduce disease.

CASE STUDY

Wellness

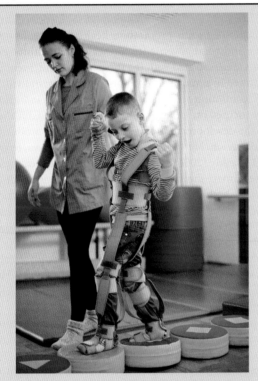

(© olesiabilkei/iStock/Thinkstock.)

Karen is a twenty-something young woman who recently graduated top of her class with a master in occupational therapy; she always wanted to work with children, so she interned in an early childhood treatment center near her parent's home. After graduation, she was quickly hired by the treatment center where she interned and was able to move back with her parents. She loves her new job, it pays her well, and she has good relationships with her coworkers. Karen is also excited about her new job sending her to learn sign language, so she can better communicate with some of her young patients. In her senior year, Karen took an elective course in ornithology, which helped her to develop an appreciation of birds. She recently joined the local chapter of the Audubon Society and joins them several times a year to watch migrating birds.

This year Karen also became engaged to her boyfriend, who graduated from college a year ago and secured a job in a nearby town. She and her boyfriend have been spending weekends looking for houses in the area. Karen also started planning her wedding with her mother, her sister, and her best friend. Since Karen came back home, she has been having difficulties with her younger sister. However, Karen feels that including her younger sister in the wedding planning can help their relationship. They spend many afternoons showing each other samples of wedding dresses, invitations, and cakes. She smiles to herself every time she thinks about having her family, and high school and college friends at her wedding.

Karen likes to practice what she preaches, so even though she is not a morning person, she wakes up early in the morning to go to the gym before she goes to work. She also eats balanced meals and does not smoke. This helps her to manage better her type I diabetes. Even when she is very healthy, she visits her doctor regularly to manage her diabetes and tries to take her medication as indicated.

Anyone who looks at Karen's life would think that she is happy and well. However, inside, a part of her does not feel fulfilled. Karen feels her life lacks some kind of purpose or meaning she can't quite pinpoint and that she has not been able to find in her job, relationships, and hobbies.

Discussion Questions

1. Evaluate Karen's wellness on each of the eight dimensions of wellness described in this chapter. Rate each dimension as "well" for those dimensions that do not need an intervention, "needs improvement" for those that could use some attention, and "not well" for those dimensions that need a formal intervention.

2. Propose an intervention for dimensions rated as "needs improvement" or "not well." Note: dimensions rated "not well" may require greater effort than dimensions rated "needs improvement."

3. Which dimension seems to be troubling Karen the most? Speculate how the lack of wellness in that dimension could affect her overall health.

Disease Prevention and Health Promotion

Although disease prevention and health promotion share many goals (WHO, n.d.), disease prevention is more closely associated with the negative axis (pathogenesis) and health promotion with the positive axis (salutogenesis) of the positive health model (see Fig. 3.3) (Breslow, 2000). For instance, disease prevention focuses on disease, even when disease is not present; for example, improving hygiene practices to prevent infection. This focus, while necessary, is limited and can result in missed opportunities to improve health (Duxbury, 2000). In contrast, health promotion is concerned with increasing the health resources of the individual (Leddy, 2006) and pays less attention to the disease. For example, health promotion applied to a patient with a swallowing disorder will most likely focus on educating the patient about how to manage his or her condition and where and how to access services. This suggests that both disease prevention and health promotion are necessary to have a comprehensive approach to health care.

What Is Disease Prevention?

The World Health Organization (n.d.) defines *disease prevention* as interventions aimed to reduce the impact of disease and associated risk factors. In other words, disease prevention involves actions taken to avoid the occurrence or development of a health problem (WONCA, 2016). These actions may include mitigating or removing certain determinants of poor health and encouraging health behaviors such as practicing oral hygiene and regularly monitoring blood pressure in the presence of hypertension (AFMC, n.d.).

Disease prevention is a model used to classify and understand healthcare interventions based on the "health status" of the individual. Currently, five categories of disease prevention have been articulated (Box 3.2); however, most health-related governmental and nongovernmental organizations (e.g., NIH, WHO) aim their efforts toward primary, secondary, and tertiary prevention.

What Is Health Promotion?

Health promotion is the "process of empowering people to increase control over their health and its determinants through health literacy efforts and multisectoral action to increase healthy behaviors" (WHO, n.d., par. 5). Good health promotion interventions not only educate individuals to take control of their own health, but also serve to increase the skills of the individual and provide a social infrastructure to increase the chances of success (AFMC, n.d.). For example, promoting biking as a way of exercise may be insufficient if the city does not provide safe bike trails. Similarly, smoking cessation programs benefit from decreasing places where smoking is allowed and raising the cost of cigarettes through taxation. Health promotion is closely related to wellness because it focuses on increasing the health resources of an individual, rather than remedying an existing health problem.

The World Health Organization (2016) identified three elements of health promotion: health literacy, healthy cities, and good governance for health. These three elements are associated with the three levels of intervention identified in some health promotion models: individual level, community level, and political level. The *individual level* focuses on behavioral change through education and the development of skills and self-efficacy producing the behavior (Nutbeam, Padmadas, Maslovskaya, & Wu, 2013). Leddy (2006) suggests that at this level healthcare professionals should focus on making sure individuals "gain the health-related knowledge, attitudes, and practices associated with achieving specific health-related behaviors" (p. 11). Examples of health promotion at the individual level include quitting smoking, improving nutrition, exercising, and having regular medical checkups. Health literacy is central to this level of health promotion (WHO, 2016); that topic is covered in more detail under Patient-Centered Care.

Individual-level health promotion has been studied more than the other two approaches. This may be because it is easily accessible to healthcare professionals. For example, assisting patients to quit smoking, lose weight, or begin to exercise is easier than mobilizing the community to clean a toxic landfill or changing national public policy. A significant number of models explain health promotion behavior at the individual level—for example, the human potential for change, health belief model, theory of reasoned action/planned behavior, self-efficacy and social cognitive theory, transtheoretical model, Pender's health promotion model, and many more (Pender, Murdaugh, & Parsons, 2015). Most health promotion interventions focus on changing individual behavior and neglect to address changes to the environment (Stokols, 2000).

Community-level health promotion involves changes in the environment and the recognition that lifestyle and environment are interrelated (Leddy, 2006). For Nutbeam et al. (2013) it means "community mobilization" to

---

BOX 3.2 Categories of Disease Prevention

Primordial prevention refers to "actions to minimize future hazards to health and hence inhibit the establishment of factors (environmental, economic, social, behavioral, cultural) known to increase the risk of disease" (AFMC, n.d., p. 44). This category of prevention focuses on removal or mitigation of broad social determinants of health, for example, improving sanitation or promoting green sources of energy (AFMC, n.d.).

Primary prevention tries to "prevent the onset of specific diseases via risk reduction: by altering behaviors or exposures that can lead to disease, or by enhancing resistance to the effects of exposure to a disease agent" (AFMC, n.d., p. 45). Primary prevention is the closest prevention category to wellness because it focuses on trying to enhance resistance to disease and injury. Some examples include smoking cessation, vaccination, good nutrition, and exercise.

Secondary prevention includes "procedures that detect and treat pre-clinical pathological changes and thereby control disease progression" (AFMC, n.d., p. 45). The focus of secondary prevention is early detection of disease (e.g., breast cancer) and the management of controlled diseases (e.g., hypertension). Screening activities such as mammography to detect breast cancer before symptoms of the disease appear or regularly measuring blood pressure for a person with hypertension are examples of secondary prevention.

Tertiary prevention focuses on reversing or mitigating the effect of an existing disease. This category of prevention seeks to prevent complications related to a symptomatic disease (Duxbury, 2000). In the case of breast cancer, removing the tumor is a tertiary preventive measure because the removal of the tumor may

"reverse" the condition. However, "where the condition is not reversible, tertiary prevention focuses on rehabilitation, assisting the patient to accommodate to his or her disability" (AFMC, n.d., p. 45). For example, someone with hypertension may need to make changes to accommodate the disability such as taking medication, regularly monitoring blood pressure, and avoiding salt.

Quaternary prevention includes "actions taken to identify patients at risk of over-medicalization, to protect them from new medical invasion, and to suggest to them interventions ethically acceptable" (Jamoulle & Roland, 1995, p. 3). This category of intervention may also include debriefing, quality assurance, and improvement processes (Gofrit et al., 2000). The focus of quaternary prevention is to prevent damage by removing excessive treatment or replacing current treatment with a treatment that has fewer or milder side effects. Gofrit et al. (2000) suggest that quaternary prevention may be the most interprofessional type of intervention because it requires "collecting information about the process, multidisciplinary analysis of the data, deriving conclusions, and distributing them to all the involved bodies" (p. 499). This means that for quaternary prevention to work, interprofessional collaboration is essential. An example of quaternary prevention is a patient whose back pain is being managed with narcotics. This person could be weaned from the narcotic and moved to a combination of nonopiate analgesics and exercise. Nonopiate pain relievers may have fewer side effects and less risk for falls and drug dependence. Exercise is effective at reducing some types of back pain and provides other benefits to the overall health of the person.

---

provide support. Cities are essential in the promotion of health by creating infrastructure, both physical (e.g., primary healthcare facilities) and social (e.g., preventive measures), that can support the community (WHO, 2016). An example is creating fitness trails within community parks to promote physical activity as a way of promoting health and wellness in the community.

Probably the most important feature of community-level health promotion is the existence of structures that support individual-level health promotion. Analysis of factors associated with "blue zones" have found several structural factors supporting the health and longevity of the individuals living in those societies. *Blue zones* are "parts of the world where people live the longest … areas

where we have a demographically confirmed, geographically defined, area where people are either reaching age 100 at extraordinary rates, have the highest life expectancy, or the lowest rate of middle age mortality" (Worrall, 2015, par. 3). For example, Pes et al. (2013) found that the inclination of the terrain where people lived in a town in Sardinia was associated with male longevity; it was noted that most males worked as shepherds, so their work involved moderate but continuous physical activity. In this case people did not have to decide or remember to exercise; it was built into their lifestyle. Another structural factor associated with blue zones is social support. A study with centenarians in Okinawa found "that people take care of each other, forming more coherent and supportive links than in the western world" (Mishra, 2009, p. 274). Communities can be structured in a way that remove barriers and facilitate individual efforts to become healthier.

Political-level health promotion involves the creation and maintenance of an environment conducive to adopting and maintaining a healthy personal lifestyle (Leddy, 2006). In this approach, the government may have the most responsibility; governments "must factor health implications into all the decisions they make, and prioritize policies that prevent people from becoming ill and protect them from injury" (WHO, 2016, p. 1). Examples of political-level promotion are taxing tobacco, alcohol, and products high in sugar and salt, and developing policies for residential areas so they are walkable and free of pollution (WHO, 2016). However, it may also require individuals to exert personal leadership to bring about social change that promotes health; a good example is Mothers Against Drunk Driving, which influenced changes in state and federal policy around drunk driving and consequently has saved many lives and prevented many injuries.

Social Determinants of Health and Wellness

Wellness, as a health model, can be very empowering and optimistic. For example, the idea that individuals can increase their health and avoid injury and disease by engaging in some behaviors (e.g., exercising, eating well, meditating) and avoiding others (e.g., smoking, riding motorcycles without helmets) may give the impression that we have more control over our health than we actually do. *Health behaviors* are "any activity undertaken by an individual, regardless of actual or perceived health status, for the purpose of promoting, protecting or maintaining health, whether or not such behavior is objectively effective towards that end" (WHO, 1998, p. 8). However, our behavior is not the only factor that determines our health.

Determinants of health "are the range of personal, social, economic, and environmental factors that determine the health status of individuals or populations. They are embedded in our social and physical environments" (Healthy People 2020, 2008, p. 21). Five broad categories of determinants of health are commonly cited: biology and genetics, individual behavior (health behaviors), social environment, physical environment, and health services (CDC, 2014). A wellness approach to health will probably have a greater impact on individual behaviors, but less so on the rest. Actually, determinants of health in the biology and genetics category are extremely difficult or impossible to change—for example, age, gender, genetic disorders, or missing a limb. The other three determinants of health (i.e., social environment, physical environment, and access to health services) are often known as social determinants of health.

Social determinants of health are "the complex, integrated, and overlapping social structures and economic systems that are responsible for most health inequities. These social structures and economic systems include the social environment, physical environment, health services, and structural and societal factors" (CDC, 2014, par. 14). It is possible, although not easy, to influence social determinants of health. For example, a problem in the physical environment of an individual, such as living near a polluting factory, may require the individual to (1) move away from the contamination, (2) mobilize the community to force the factory to control the pollution, or (3) lobby the government to change state or national pollution standards. Access to health care is heavily influenced by public policy; public policy affects the availability and quality of health care an individual can access and the cost of health care. For example, people living in rural areas may have to drive long distances to access some health services if the government does not incentivize healthcare providers to service those areas. Finally, the social environment can also affect the health of an individual. De Maio et al. (2017) found that low birth weight in Black and Latino babies is related to the experience of discrimination of their parents.

PATIENT-CENTERED CARE: A NEW FRAMEWORK FOR HEALTH CARE

In the past, the confidence a patient placed on the advice of a doctor was based on the character and behavior of the doctor (Silverman, 2012); patients trusted their doctor because they looked and sounded like they knew what they were doing. Sir William Osler, the father of modern medicine, changed the way physicians and patients related to each other; he believed that doctors should behave like "Victorian gentlemen," whose place is superior in rank to others (Silverman, 2012). This way of relating with patients, and other healthcare professionals, left little room to question the actions and decisions of the physician. However, this model has changed significantly in the past 50 years because of a substantial number of factors. For example, the dramatic increase in the number of healthcare professions has required an increase in interprofessional collaboration (Marr, 2014). In addition, the increased complexity of care, the growing demands on physicians, and the development of new models of health care delivery have also contributed to a shift to an interprofessional framework (M. Schmitt, personal communication, March 5, 2018). These and other factors have also transformed the traditional relationship between patients and their healthcare professionals. Palmer (2016) notes that "patients now self-diagnose, research their conditions, consult online support groups, and visit multiple specialists to learn about their diagnoses" (p. 48). Now, many patients have the expectation they will be active participants in their own health care. (The author makes the point that patients are in the best position to determine how providers can best meet their needs, which is a basic tenant of Patient-Centered Care.)

What Is Patient-Centered Care?

Patient-centered care means different things to different people. Tanenbaum (2015) analyzed a significant number of models and grouped them into four types: whole patient versus their parts, patients versus providers, patients/providers/states versus the system, and person-centered medicine. *Whole patient versus their parts* refers to definitions of patient-centered care that focus on a holistic view of the patient (Tanenbaum, 2015). These definitions are particularly useful in the context of primary care. *Patients versus providers* focuses on the view of the patient as a consumer. These types of definition tend to equalize the power between the patient and the provider (Tanenbaum, 2015). *Patients/providers/states versus the system* definitions of patient-centered care focus on the "incentives—economic, legal and professional—that motivate the providers to act in their own interest" (Tanenbaum, 2015, p. 279). Finally, person-centered medicine combined several humanistic approaches and has emerged, in part, as a response to evidence-based medicine (Tanenbaum, 2015). Miles & Mezzich (2011) proposed the following definition of person-centered medicine: It is medicine of the person, for the person, by the person, and with the person. This definition captures the spirit of the official definition of patient-centered care provided by the Institute of Medicine: care that is "respectful of and responsive to individual patient preferences, needs, and values, and ensuring that patient values guide all clinical decisions" (IOM, 2001, p. 6). This is the definition of patient-centered care adopted in this book.

Patient-centered care is so important to IPCP that the Canadian Interprofessional Health Collaborative (2010) included it as one of their Core Competencies: "Learners/practitioners seek out, integrate and value, as a partner, the input and the engagement of the patient/client/family/community in designing and implementing care/services" (p. 13). Although not a separate competency, patient-center care is woven within the Core Competencies for IPCP that are discussed throughout this book. For example, the Interprofessional Education Collaborative (IPEC, 2016) described four Sub-competencies in terms of patient-centered care: "VE1. Place interests of patients and populations at center of interprofessional health care delivery and population health programs and policies, with the goal of promoting health and health equity across the lifespan" (p. 11), "VE8. Manage ethical dilemmas specific to interprofessional patient/population centered care situations" (p. 11), "CC8. Communicate the importance of teamwork in patient-centered care and population health programs and policies" (p. 13), and "TT3. Engage health and other professionals in shared patient-centered and population-focused problem-solving" (p. 14). In other words, to practice patient-centered care is to practice collaboratively and vice versa.

Elements of Patient-Centered Care

Research conducted with healthcare professionals has identified several elements pertaining to effective patient-centered care. Sidani et al. (2014) identified collaborative care as one of the main elements of effective patient-centered care. This means that patients must be full members of the healthcare team and fully participate in the care decision making, in the carrying out of treatment, and in the management of the disease. *Collaborative care* requires increasing the autonomy of the patient by shifting power from the healthcare professionals to the patient (Lusk & Fater, 2013). For example, the autonomy of the patient can be increased by having shared decision making (SDM; Gallo et al., 2016). SDM and collaborative care require that patients and their families have access to information so their participation in the healthcare team is real (Gallo et al., 2016).

Another element of effective patient-centered care is the provision of *individualized care* (Lusk & Fater, 2013; Sidani et al., 2014). This means that care must be adapted to the needs of the patient or family—for example, considering the patient's and family's preferences and needs (Gallo et al., 2016). Individualized care also requires the healthcare professional to be culturally competent, which entails tailoring "care to patients with diverse values, beliefs, and behaviors" (Johnson, 2015, p. 87). It is worth noting that consideration of the patient's values, beliefs, and behaviors is closely related to the Core Competencies of Values/Ethics (e.g., "VE3. Embrace the cultural diversity and individual differences that characterize patients, populations, and the health team") and Interprofessional Communication (e.g., "CC2. Communicate information with patients, families, community members, and health team members in a form that is understandable, avoiding discipline-specific terminology when possible").

Patient-centered care requires *patient/family education and patient-to-provider information sharing* (Gallo et al., 2016). For patients and their families to be effective members of the healthcare team, it is necessary to educate them about relevant issues such as the disease process, treatment options, and self-care actions. Similarly, patient-centered care requires patients and families to share relevant information about the patient, the disease, and the preferences and needs of both (Gallo et al., 2016). This exchange of information increases the relationship between healthcare professionals, patients, and their families and improves the effectiveness of the healthcare team.

A less frequently cited element of patient-centered care is *holistic care*. This involves paying attention to the whole person (Sidani et al., 2014). This element of patient-centered care is closely associated to wellness. Just paying attention to the physical complaint of the patient is not enough to provide good patient-centered care. Buist (2016) suggests that healthcare professionals are trained to selectively listen for confirmation of their diagnosis when interviewing the patient, thus missing many important details that may be important to the patient's total wellness. By really listening to the patient, the professional can better understand the preferences and needs of the patient and family, and may learn about other issues not directly related to the physical complaint, but that can impact the treatment.

Finally, having a caring attitude was identified as another element of good patient-centered care (Lusk et al., 2013). A *caring attitude* may involve intentions, commitments, attitudes, and actions that convey the idea that one cares for the well-being of the patient. It may also include facilitating social–emotional support (Gallo et al., 2016)—for example, providing support structures such as support groups, respite care for caretakers, and networking opportunities for the patient and their loved ones.

The Picker Institute's (n.d.) eight principles of patient-centered care (Box 3.3) were developed through qualitative research involving patients, families, and healthcare professionals; a review of the literature; and original research. These principles include most of the elements discussed in this section.

The Josie King story is an excellent case study on how things can go wrong when patients and their families are not involved in the health care of the patient. This case study is an excellent resource for classroom discussion. You can find more information about the Josie King Story at the end of this chapter in the Additional Resources box.

Barriers to Patient-Centered Care

Several barriers to effective patient-centered care have been identified. An overarching barrier is the *lack of evidence* about the efficacy of the patient-centered care approach (Frampton & Guastello, 2014). This lack of concrete evidence makes skeptics of practitioners and administrators alike. At a personal level, *lack of motivation* and a *lack of holistic view* have been identified as barriers for healthcare professionals to engage in patient-centered care (Esmaeili et al., 2013). For the healthcare professionals to engage effectively in patient-centered care, they must believe in the model and they must be interested in the whole person, not just on the health concern related to their own professional role and responsibilities.

Some institution-level barriers include lack of teamwork coordination and lack of understanding about the role of the patient in the team, lack of resources such as a shortage of personnel, lack of time, workload pressures (Esmaeili et al., 2013), and leadership in each professional silo impeding change (Rubenstein et al., 2014).

Health Education, Patient Education, and Health Literacy
Health Education

For patients and their families to be effective members of the healthcare team, they must possess the appropriate knowledge, that is, information (e.g., about the disease, treatment) and skills (e.g., navigating the healthcare system). *Health education* comprises "consciously constructed opportunities for learning involving some form of communication designed to improve health literacy, including improving knowledge, and developing life skills which are conducive to individual and community health" (WHO, 1998, p. 4). Health education involves providing information and assisting patients to develop skills that will help them to improve their health behaviors. Although effective health education requires a concerted effort at

---

BOX 3.3   Principles of Patient-Centered Care

1. **Respect for patients' values, preferences, and expressed needs.** Patients want to be kept informed regarding their medical condition and involved in decision-making. Patients want hospital staff to recognize and treat them in an atmosphere that is focused on the patient as an individual with a presenting medical condition. This principle means that (1) illness and medical treatment may affect quality of life, so care should be provided in an atmosphere that is respectful of the individual patient and focused on quality-of-life issues; (2) informed and shared decision-making is a central component of patient-centered care; and (3) healthcare professionals should provide the patient with dignity, respect, and sensitivity to his/her cultural values.

2. **Coordination and integration of care.** Patients may feel vulnerable and powerless in the face of illness. Proper coordination of care can ease those feelings. Three specific areas of coordination may be able to reduce feelings of vulnerability through cooperation and integration of (1) clinical care; (2) ancillary and support services; and (3) front-line patient care.

3. **Information, communication, and education.** Patients often express the fear that information is being withheld from them and that they are not being completely informed about their condition or prognosis. This fear can be alleviated by providing information about (1) the clinical status, progress, and prognosis of the disease; (2) describing the processes of the treatment; and (3) by stimulating autonomy, self-care, and health promotion with information and patient education.

4. **Physical comfort.** Physical care that comforts patients, especially when they are acutely ill, is one of the most elemental services that caregivers can provide. Three areas seem to be particularly important to patients: (1) pain management; (2) assistance with activities and daily living needs; and (3) the hospital surroundings and environment, which should be kept clean and accessible to family and friends for visits while preserving the privacy of the patient.

5. **Emotional support and alleviation of fear and anxiety.** Fear and anxiety associated with illness can be as debilitating as the physical effects. Caregivers should pay particular attention to (1) anxiety over clinical status, treatment, and prognosis; (2) anxiety over the impact of the illness on themselves and their family; and (3) anxiety over the financial implications of illness.

6. **Involvement of family and friends.** Patients become concerned with the role of family and friends in the patient care, including being concerned with the effects of their illness on their loved ones. These concerns can be addressed with (1) accommodations to allow for family and friends to provide social and emotional support; (2) respect for and recognition of the patient "advocate's" role in decision-making; (3) support for family members as caregivers; and (4) recognition of the needs of family and friends.

7. **Continuity and transition.** Patients often express considerable anxiety about their ability to care for themselves after discharge. Meeting patient needs in this area requires staff to (1) provide understandable, detailed information regarding medications, physical limitations, dietary needs, and other important data; (2) coordinate and plan ongoing treatment and services after discharge and ensure that patients and family understand this information; and (3) provide information regarding access to clinical, social, physical, and financial support on a continuing basis.

8. **Access to care.** Patients need to know they can access care when it is needed. Attention must also be given to time spent waiting for admission or time between admission and allocation to a bed in a ward. Focusing mainly on ambulatory care, the following areas may be important to the patient: (1) access to the location of hospitals, clinics, and physician offices; (2) availability of transportation; (3) ease of scheduling appointments; (4) availability of appointments when needed; (5) accessibility to specialists or specialty services when a referral is made; and (6) clear instructions regarding when and how to get referrals.

From Picker Institute. (n.d.). *Principles of patient-centered care*. Retrieved from http://pickerinstitute.org/about/picker-principles/

---

the national level, healthcare professionals can do much to increase the level of information and skills of patients through patient education and health literacy.

Patient Education

Patient education is defined as "an individualized, systematic, structured process to assess and impart knowledge or develop a skill in order to effect a change in behavior. The goal is to increase comprehension and participation in the self-management of health care needs" (The University of Texas Medical Branch, 2014, p. 1). Patient education is mainly used by healthcare professionals to improve patients' skills caring for themselves (Fig. 3.4). Examples include a nurse teaching a newly diagnosed

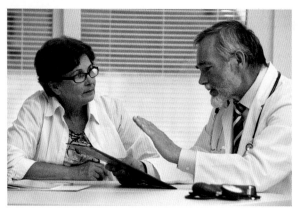

FIG. 3.4 Healthcare professionals use patient teaching to help patients improve their health literacy. (© AlexRaths/iStock/Thinkstock.)

BOX 3.4   Red Flags for Low Health Literacy

- Frequently missed appointments
- Incomplete registration forms
- Noncompliance with medication
- Unable to name medications, explain purpose, or provide dosing
- Identifies pills by looking at them, not reading label
- Unable to give coherent, sequential history
- Asks few questions
- Lack of follow-through on tests or referrals

From Davis, T., DeWalt, D., Hink, A., et al. (2015). *Health Literacy: Hidden Barriers and Practical Strategies* [Slide Presentation]. In: Brega, A. G., Barnard, J., Mabachi, et al. (2015). *AHRQ Health Literacy Universal Precautions Toolkit* (2nd Ed). AHRQ Publication No. 15-0023-EF. Rockville, MD: Agency for Healthcare Research and Quality Department of Health and Human Services (DHHS). http://www.ahrq.gov/professionals/quality-patient-safety/quality-resources/tools/literacy-toolkit/tool3a/index.html (Content last reviewed December 2017). Adapted with permission of the Agency for Healthcare Research and Quality (AHRQ); Rockville, MD.

insulin-dependent diabetic patient how, how much, and when to inject insulin or an occupational therapist teaching a patient with limited mobility how to put on her shoes using a long-handled shoe horn. Although patient education affects patients' health literacy, it is mostly associated with teaching patients how to care for their disease or injury during a clinical visit.

What Is Health Literacy?

Health literacy is "the degree to which individuals have the capacity to obtain, process, and understand basic health information and services needed to make appropriate health decisions" (Ratzan & Parker, 2000, p. vi). Because it is difficult to identify who may have low health literacy (Box 3.4), it is recommended that healthcare professionals "assume that all patients and caregivers may have difficulty comprehending health information and should communicate in ways that anyone can understand" (Brega et al., 2015, p. 1). The health literacy universal precautions that all healthcare professionals can engage in are (1) simplifying communication and confirming comprehension from all patients, (2) making the office environment and healthcare system easier to navigate, and (3) supporting patients' efforts to improve their health (Brega et al., 2015).

Low health literacy affects people's ability to: "1) navigate the healthcare system, 2) fill out complex forms and locate providers and services, 3) share personal information, such as health history, with providers, 4) engage in self-care and chronic-disease management, and 5) understand mathematical concepts such as probability and risk" (DHHS, n.d., p. 2.1). However, significant tools

have been developed to improve and compensate for low levels of health literacy. The Office of Disease Prevention and Health Promotion's *AHRQ Health Literacy Universal Precautions Toolkit* is useful in addressing health literacy issues; a link to the toolkit can be found in the Additional Resources box at the end of this chapter.

The first and last sections of the toolkit contain approaches to addressing structural barriers to health literacy. The other three sections provide approaches to addressing patients with low health literacy: spoken communication, written communication, and patient self-management and empowerment (Box 3.5). In the category of spoken communication, Tool 4: Communicate Clearly, includes strategies such as making eye contact; listening carefully; using plain, nonmedical language; using the patient's words; slowing down; and limiting and repeating content. Some strategies to address written communication include identifying poor-quality materials, considering alternatives to written materials, and providing materials in the languages your patients speak (Tool 11: Assess, Select, and Create Easy-to-Understand Materials). The final section addresses patient self-management and empowerment; strategies include asking for permission to talk about health behaviors, determining motivation, writing an action plan with the patient, assessing confidence, and identifying barriers (Tool 15: Make Action Plans).

BOX 3.5 Agency for Healthcare Research and Quality Health Literacy Universal Precautions Toolkit

Tools to Start on the Path to Improvement
Tool 1: Form a team
Tool 2: Create a Health Literacy Environment Improvement Plan
Tool 3: Raise awareness

Tools to Improve Spoken Communication
Tool 4: Communicate clearly
Tool 5: Use the teach-back method
Tool 6: Follow up with patients
Tool 7: Improve telephone access
Tool 8: Conduct brown bag medicine reviews
Tool 9: Address language differences
Tool 10: Consider culture, customs, and beliefs

Tools to Improve Written Communication
Tool 11: Assess, select, and create easy-to-understand materials

Tool 12: Use health education material effectively
Tool 13: Welcome patients

Tools to Improve Patient Self-Management and Empowerment
Tool 14: Encourage questions
Tool 15: Make action plans
Tool 16: Help patients remember how and when to take their medicine
Tool 17: Get patient feedback

Tools to Improve Supportive Systems
Tool 18: Link patients to nonmedical support
Tool 19: Direct patients to medicine resources
Tool 20: Connect patients with literacy and math resources
Tool 21: Make referrals easy

From Brega, A. G., Barnard, J., Mabachi, et al. (2015). *AHRQ Health Literacy Universal Precautions Toolkit* (2nd Ed). "Contents." AHRQ Publication No. 15-0023-EF. Rockville, MD: Agency for Healthcare Research and Quality Department of Health and Human Services (DHHS). https://www.ahrq.gov/professionals/quality-patient-safety/quality-resources/tools/literacy-toolkit/healthlittoolkit2.html (Contents last reviewed February 2015). Adapted with permission of the Agency for Healthcare Research and Quality (AHRQ); Rockville, MD.

BOX 3.6 National Action Plan to Improve Health Literacy's Seven Goals

1. Develop and disseminate health and safety information that is accurate, accessible, and actionable.
2. Promote changes in the healthcare system that improve health information, communication, informed decision-making, and access to health services.
3. Incorporate accurate, standards-based, and developmentally appropriate health and science information and curricula in child care and education through the university level.
4. Support and expand local efforts to provide adult education, English language instruction, and culturally and linguistically appropriate health information services in the community.
5. Build partnerships, develop guidance, and change policies.
6. Increase basic research and the development, implementation, and evaluation of practices and interventions to improve health literacy.
7. Increase the dissemination and use of evidence-based health literacy practices and interventions.

From Department of Health and Human Services (DHHS), Office of Disease Prevention and Health Promotion. (2010). *National action plan to improve health literacy*. Washington, DC: Author. Retrieved from https://health.gov/communication/initiatives/health-literacy-action-plan.asp.

Although healthcare professionals can address issues of health literacy with their patients and in their work institutions, a concerted national effort is necessary to improve health literacy. Some of the barriers to achieve high levels of health literacy in the population are structural in nature and require government intervention. For example, healthcare professionals can use plain language and visual aids to assist the patient's understanding of instructions, but only the government can make changes in the education system to improve people's ability to read and perform basic math computations. The current policy of the US government regarding health literacy can be found in the National Action Plan to Improve Health Literacy (Box 3.6).

CASE STUDY

Patient-Centered Care

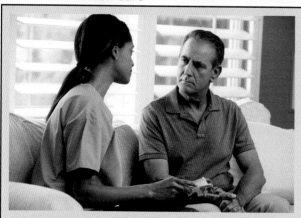

(© Monkey Business Images LtD/Monkey Business/Thinkstock.)

Mr. Ramos is a 66-year-old Honduran American man who immigrated to the United States in his 20s. He is married and has three grown children who live nearby. He has a good relationship with his wife that can be characterized as somewhat traditional. His wife works part time as a child care worker in a day care mainly serving the Latino community; he works as a butcher in a Hispanic grocery store in the neighborhood. While Mr. Ramos is financially stable and probably does not need to work, he takes pride on providing for his family and has not considered retirement yet.

Mr. Ramos is recovering from a hip fracture due to a fall at work; he was hosing down the floor of the butcher shop at the end of the evening when he slipped and fell. After the surgery, he was transferred to a nursing home to recover and initiate rehabilitation. His team included the orthopedic surgeon, a geriatrician, a dietician, a physiotherapist, a social worker and the attending nurse. Mr. Ramos's wife and children visited frequently, and usually brought him home-cooked food.

Mr. Ramos worked closely with his physical therapist, Dr. Albert Miller. The doctor developed a state-of-the-art treatment plan for Mr. Ramos and every time he would introduce a new exercise or modify an existing exercise in the treatment plan, the doctor demonstrated to Mr. Ramos and Tina, the physical therapy aide, how to perform it. Mr. Ramos was always very compliant with Dr. Miller. However, when working with the PT aide, he seemed more hesitant performing the exercises. Tina suspected Mr. Ramos was experiencing more pain than he had expressed, so she asked him. He shrugged his shoulders which she took as a "no."

Once Mr. Ramos was ready to be discharged, Dr. Miller put together a comprehensive treatment plan for his outpatient treatment. It included weekly outpatient therapy at the rehab center and a series of exercises to perform at home meant to strengthen the operated leg, increase flexibility, and regain balance. After a couple of weeks, Dr. Miller felt Mr. Ramos's progress had slowed down, so he asked Mr. Ramos if he had been doing his exercises at home. Mr. Ramos answer, "I am trying." The doctor decided to sit down with Mr. Ramos and go over the treatment plan with him. One by one, the doctor asked Mr. Ramos if he found the exercise difficult to perform and what made it difficult.

In general, the doctor learned that Mr. Ramos was not following the plan because he was still experiencing some pain performing some of the exercises; in other cases, he felt "silly" doing the exercises, especially when his wife was around. The doctor modified the treatment plan by agreeing with Mr. Ramos to a couple of the most important exercises; Dr. Miller also told him to not perform the movements to the point it hurts, and suggested Mr. Ramos could take Tylenol a half hour before exercising to control the pain. In order to address the embarrassment performing some of the exercises, using a model of the hip, the doctor explained how the exercises helped him to recover. The doctor hoped that by explaining the treatment to Mr. Ramos, it would become more meaningful to him and some of the embarrassment would dissipate. The doctor also suggested he could do the exercises in the bathroom before taking a shower, so his wife was not around.

Discussion Questions

1. What problems arose in this case study because the rehab team did not engage in patient-centered care at the beginning of the case study?
2. What were some missed opportunities in the beginning of this case study?
3. How could the team have included the family, especially his wife, on Mr. Ramos's rehabilitation? How could the involvement of the family have changed the outcome in this case study?
4. Once Dr. Miller included Mr. Ramos in the development of the new plan, what went well?
5. Besides what Dr. Miller was able to do at the end of the case study, what could have been accomplished if the team would have engaged in patient-centered care from the beginning?

ADDITIONAL RESOURCES

This chapter discussed the concepts of wellness and patient-centered care. These concepts were included in this book to provide frameworks of practice congruent with the Core Competencies of Interprofessional Collaborative Practice (IPCP). The resources in this section should help you to understand those concepts better and give you some tools you can use with your patients.

Foundational Book on Wellness

The Wellness Workbook: How to Achieve Enduring Health and Vitality (3rd ed.). Travis, J., & Ryan, R. S. (2004). Berkeley, CA: Celestial Arts.

Dr. John W. Travis is one of the founders of the wellness movement. His *Wellness Workbook* is an easy guide to personal wellness and a good resource for professionals aiming to implement wellness programs in their workplaces. The book combines assessments, activities, and theory in an accessible manner.

Organizations Working on Wellness

National Wellness Institute http://www.nationalwellness. org/

For over 40 years, National Wellness Institute has promoted wellness and the development of competent health professionals in the wellness philosophy. The Institute provides wellness resources, continuing education, professional development programs, and assessments.

Global Wellness Institute https://www.globalwellnessinstitute.org/

The mission of the Global Wellness Institute is to educate the public and private sectors about the benefits of preventive health and wellness. The Institute has projects around the world promoting and increasing expertise in Wellness.

World Health Organization (WHO) http://www.who.int/en/

The World Health Organization coordinates world-wide programs for global health and wellness including health education, health promotion and disease prevention.

U.S. Workplace Wellness Alliance http://www.prevent.org/default.aspx

This organization is a coalition of businesses, health care advocates, and nonprofit organizations dedicated to promoting health and wellness in the workforce and at the workplace. The organization focuses on the development of health and wellness policy in the workplace. Their website provides links to the coalition partners and their resources.

Organizations Working on Patient-Centered Care and Associated Documents

Picker Institute http://pickerinstitute.org/

The Picker Institute was an organization dedicated to the promotion of patient-centered care. They closed doors in 2013, but their website is still being hosted by the Institute for Patient- and Family-Centered Care. The website still contains many resources, including resources around their well-regarded Picker's Principles of Patient-Centered Care. The following are two of their most important documents:

Frampton, S. Guastello, S., Brandy, C., Hale, M., Horowitz, S., Bennett Smith, S., & Stone, S. (2008). *Patient-centered care: Improvement guide.* Derby, CT: Planetree & Camden, ME: Picker Institute. Retrieved from http://patient-centeredcare.org/

The Institute for Alternative Futures (on behalf of the Picker Institute). (2004). *Patient-centered care 2015: Scenarios, visions, goals & next steps.* Alexandria, VA: Author. Retrieved from http://www.altfutures.org/pubs/health/Picker%20Final%20Report%20May%2014%202004.pdf

The Commonwealth Fund http://www.commonwealthfund.org/

The mission of The Commonwealth Fund is to promote a high-performing healthcare system that achieves better access, improved quality, and greater efficiency, particularly for society's most vulnerable, including low-income people, the uninsured, minority Americans, young children, and elderly adults. The Fund carries out this mandate by supporting independent research on health care issues and making grants to improve health care practice and policy. The Commonwealth Fund sponsored the following report on patient-centered care:

Shaller, D., & Shaller Consulting. (2007). *Patient-centered care: What does it take?* New York, NY: The Commonwealth Fund. Retrieved from http://www.commonwealthfund.org/usr_doc/Shaller_patient-centeredcarewhatdoesittake_1067.pdf

Institute for Patient- and Family-Centered Care http://www.ipfcc.org/

Similar to the Picker Institute, the Institute for Patient- and Family-Centered Care provides educational resources for practitioners and students in the health professions around the issue of patient-centered care. Their work is worldwide.

Continued

ADDITIONAL RESOURCES—cont'd

The Josie King Foundation http://josieking.org/

The Josie King Foundation provides several resources available in their website. These resources include the book that narrates Josie's Story, a DVD of a talk her mother, Sorrel King, did at Harvard Medical School, a patient safety curriculum, and other programs. Educators and administrators trying to improve patient-centered care may find these resources particularly useful.

Resources for Health Literacy

"What Did the Doctor Say?": Improving Health Literacy to Protect Patient Safety.

https://www.jointcommission.org/assets/1/18/improving_health_literacy.pdf

This publication from The Joint Commission addresses health literacy as a systems problem rather than as a patient problem. It may be more useful for institutions rather than practitioners; however, it makes reference to tools practitioners may want to use in their practice.

AHRQ Health Literacy Universal Precautions Toolkit (2nd ed.). https://www.ahrq.gov/sites/default/files/wysiwyg/professionals/quality- patient-safety/quality-resources/tools/literacy-toolkit/impguide/healthlit-guide.pdf

This tool kit from the Agency for Healthcare Research and Quality, an office of the Department of Health and Human Services (DHHS), is very comprehensive and well regarded. It offers tools for institutions and practitioners.

Health Literacy: Hidden Barriers and Practical Strategies [PowerPoint slides]. https://www.ahrq.gov/sites/default/files/wysiwyg/professionals/quality-patient-safety/quality-resources/tools/literacy-toolkit/tool3a/literacy-tool3a.pptx

These slides from the Agency for Healthcare Research and Quality, an office of the Department of Health and Human Services (DHHS), provide a good overview about the topic of health literacy. The slides are appropriate for a lecture by educators or advanced undergraduate students studying independently.

Quick Guide to Health Literacy. https://health.gov/communication/literacy/quickguide/Quickguide.pdf

This document is a collection of fact sheets about health literacy produced by the Centers for Disease Control and Prevention (CDC). The fact sheets are designed to educate health professionals. However, some of them could be used with more functional patients.

National Action Plan to Improve Health Literacy. https://health.gov/communication/HLActionPlan/pdf/Health_Literacy_Action_Plan.pdf

This plan is pretty dense and may be more appropriate for institutions, people working on advocacy and policy, and students researching this topic in depth. Because the document is comprehensive, practitioners can find references to resources to work on health literacy with their patients.

KEY POINTS

- A comprehensive idea about wellness was first proposed in 1961 by Dunn, based on 3 decades of work at the National Office of Vital Statistics (Jordan, 2016); Dunn is widely regarded as the father of the wellness movement.
- Travis proposed the wellness paradigm, which conceptualized illness and wellness as a continuum (see Fig. 3.1) that ranges from high-level wellness to premature death (Travis & Ryan, 2004).
- Hettler developed the concept of dimensions of wellness (see Fig. 3.3). His original model had six dimensions of wellness, but his model has been expanded since then to include additional dimensions (Becker & McPeck, 2013).
- Antonovsky (1979) proposed the concept of salutogenesis (i.e., the origin of health) as a counterpart to

pathogenesis (i.e., the origin of disease); he proposed that health should be studied in the same way that disease is studied.

- Using the concept of salutogenesis, Becker added a positive health dimension to the illness–wellness continuum, producing the positive health model (see Fig. 3.2) (Becker & McPeck, 2013).
- Robbins and Hall (1970), Lalonde (1974), and Ardell (1977) proposed models to shift the healthcare system from addressing disease to preventing it.
- *Wellness* is the conscious and deliberate process of making choices to improve one's health (Johnson, 1986; Swarbrick, 2006; 2013). It is "an integrated method of functioning which is oriented toward maximizing the potential of which the individual is capable" (Dunn, 1977, p. 4).

- Illness and wellness are conceptualized as two-dimensional, with one dimension representing levels of wellness (i.e., positive health axis) and the other dimension representing levels of illness (i.e., negative health axis).
- *Salutogenesis* is the study of the origin of health. The concept of salutogenesis can best be understood in contrast to its opposite, pathogenesis, which is the study of the origin of disease.
- To maintain optimal health (first quadrant of Fig. 3.3), attention must be paid to all aspects of the human being. The Eight Dimensions of Wellness model includes occupational, physical, social, intellectual, spiritual, emotional (Hettler, 1980), environmental (Foster & Keller, 2007), and financial (Swarbrick, 2006) wellness.
- *Disease prevention* constitutes interventions aiming to reduce the impact of disease and associated risk factors (WHO, n.d.). In other words, disease prevention involves actions taken to avoid the occurrence or development of a health problem (WONCA, 2016); it includes primordial prevention, primary prevention, secondary prevention, tertiary prevention, and quaternary prevention.
- *Health promotion* is the "process of empowering people to increase control over their health and its determinants through health literacy efforts and multisectoral action to increase healthy behaviors" (WHO, n.d., par. 5).
- The World Health Organization (2016) identified three elements of health promotion: health literacy, healthy cities, and good governance for health. These three elements are associated with the three levels of intervention identified in some health promotion models: individual level, community level, and political level.
- Determinants of health "are the range of personal, social, economic, and environmental factors that determine the health status of individuals or populations. They are embedded in our social and physical environments" (Healthy People 2020, 2008, p. 21).
- Five broad categories of determinants of health are often cited: biology and genetics, individual behavior (health behaviors), social environment, physical environment, and health services (CDC, 2014).
- Biological and genetic determinants of health are extremely difficult or impossible to change—for example, age, gender, genetic disorders, or missing a limb.
- *Social determinants of health* are "the complex, integrated, and overlapping social structures and economic systems that are responsible for most health inequities. These social structures and economic systems include the social environment, physical environment, health services, and structural and societal factors" (CDC, 2014, par. 14). Social determinants of health tend to be moderate to difficult to influence.
- *Health behaviors* are "any activity undertaken by an individual, regardless of actual or perceived health status, for the purpose of promoting, protecting or maintaining health, whether or not such behavior is objectively effective towards that end" (WHO, 1998, p. 8). This determinant of health tends to be easy to moderately difficult to influence.
- *Patient-centered care* is care that is "respectful of and responsive to individual patient preferences, needs, and values, and ensuring that patient values guide all clinical decisions" (IOM, 2001, p. 6).
- The Picker Institute (n.d.) developed eight principles of patient-centered care: (1) respect for patients' values, preferences, and expressed needs; (2) coordination and integration of care, (3) information, communication, and education; (4) physical comfort; (5) emotional support and alleviation of fear and anxiety; (6) involvement of family and friends; (7) continuity and transition; and (8) access to care (see Box 3.3).
- The following barriers to patient-centered care were identified: lack of evidence about the efficacy of patient-centered care, lack of motivation to engage in patient-centered care, lack of a holistic view of the patient, lack of teamwork coordination, lack of understanding about the role of the patient in the healthcare team, lack of resources (e.g., personnel shortage, lack of time), and resistance from the leadership within the silos to engage in patient-centered care.
- *Health education* is defined as "consciously constructed opportunities for learning involving some form of communication designed to improve health literacy, including improving knowledge, and developing life skills which are conducive to individual and community health" (WHO, 1998, p. 4).
- *Patient education* is defined as "an individualized, systematic, structured process to assess and impart

knowledge or develop a skill in order to effect a change in behavior. The goal is to increase comprehension and participation in the self-management of health care needs" (The University of Texas Medical Branch, 2014, p. 1).

- *Health literacy* is "the degree to which individuals have the capacity to obtain, process, and understand basic health information and services needed to make appropriate health decisions" (Ratzan & Parker, 2000, p. vi).

REFERENCES

Antonovsky, A. (1979). *Health, stress and coping.* San Francisco, CA: Jossey-Bass Publishers.

Ardell, D. B. (1977). *High level wellness: An alternative to doctors, drugs, and disease.* Emmaus, PA: Rodale Press.

Association of Faculties of Medicine of Canada (AFMC). (n.d.). *AFMC primer on population health: An AFMC Public Health Educators' network resource.* Retrieved from https://afmc.ca/pdf/AFMC-Primer-on-Population-Health-2013-08-14.pdf.

Becker, C., & McPeck, W. (2013). *Creating positive health: It's more than risk reduction (White Paper).* Retrieved from http://www.nationalwellness.org/resource/resmgr/WhitePapers/NWIWhitePaper_BeckerMcPeck20.pdf.

Becker, C., & Rhynders, P. (2013). It's time to make the profession of health about health. *Scandinavian Journal of Public Health, 41,* 1–3.

Brega, A. G., Barnard, J., Mabachi, N. M., et al. (2015). *AHRQ health literacy universal precautions toolkit* (2nd ed.). AHRQ Publication No. 15-0023-EF. Rockville, MD: Department of Health and Human Services (DHHS), Agency for Healthcare Research and Quality. Retrieved from https://www.ahrq.gov/sites/default/files/wysiwyg/professionals/quality-patient-safety/quality-resources/tools/literacy-toolkit/impguide/healthlit-guide.pdf.

Breslow, L. (2000). The societal context of disease prevention and wellness promotion. In M. Schneider-Jamner & D. Stokols (Eds.), *Promoting human wellness* (pp. 38–43). Berkeley, CA: University of California Press.

Brunton, D. (2014). *Health and wellness in the 19th century: Health and wellness in daily life.* Santa Barbara, CA: ABC-CLIO.

Buist, M. (2016). Patient-centered care: Just ask a thoughtful question and listen. *Joint Commission Journal on Quality and Patient Safety, 42*(6), 286–287.

Canadian Interprofessional Health Collaborative (CIHC). (2010). *A national interprofessional competency framework.* Vancouver, BC, Canada: Author.

Center for the Study of Student Life, Ohio State University. (2015, January). *Assessing the nine dimensions of wellness.* Author. Retrieved from http://cssl.osu.edu/posts/documents/wellness-assessment-report-january-2015.pdf.

Centers for Disease Control and Prevention (CDC). (2014 March 10). *National Center for HIV/AIDS, viral hepatitis, STD, and TB prevention (NCHHSTP).* NCHHSTP Social Determinants of Health. Atlanta, GA: Author. Retrieved from https://www.cdc.gov/nchhstp/socialdeterminants/definitions.html.

Chambers-Clark, C. (1996). *Wellness practitioner: Concepts, research, and strategies.* New York, NY: Springer.

Crane, T., & Patterson, S. (2000). Introduction. In T. Crane & S. Patterson (Eds.), *History of the mind-body problem* (pp. 1–11). New York, NY: Routledge.

Davis, T. S., Saltzburg, S., Wellman, A., et al. (2014). *Exploring wellbeing to support success of LGBTQ and questioning students at the Ohio State University.* Columbus, OH: College of Social Work, The Ohio State University.

De Maio, F., Shah, R. C., Schipper, K., et al. (2017). Racial/ethnic minority segregation and low birth weight: A comparative study of Chicago and Toronto community-level indicators. *Critical Public Health, 27*(5), 541–553.

Department of Health and Human Services (DHHS), Office of Disease Prevention and Health Promotion. (n.d.). *Quick guide to health literacy.* Washington, DC: Author. Retreaved from https://health.gov/communication/literacy/quickguide/Quickguide.pdf.

Dunn, H. L. (1977). *High level wellness: A collection of twenty-nine short talks on different aspects of the them "High-Level Wellness for Man and Society."* Thorofare, NJ: Charles B. Slack.

Duxbury, A. (2000). Disease prevention versus health promotion. In M. Schneider-Jamner & D. Stokols (Eds.), *Promoting human wellness* (pp. 395–423). Berkeley, CA: University of California Press.

Esmaeili, M., Cheraghi, M. A., & Salsali, M. (2013). Barriers to patient-centered care: A thematic analysis study. *International Journal of Nursing Knowledge, 25*(1), 2–8.

Foster, L. T., & Keller, C. P. (2007). *The British Columbia atlas of wellness.* Retrieved from http://www.geog.uvic.ca/wellness/wellness/Atlas%20of%20Wellness%20FINAL2.pdf.

Frampton, S. B., & Guastello, S. (2014). Time to embrace a new patient-centered care rallying cry: "Why not?". *Patient, 7*, 231–233.

Gallo, K. P., Campbell Hill, L., Eaton Hoagwood, K., et al. (2016). A narrative synthesis of the components of and evidence for patient- and family-centered care. *Clinical Pediatrics, 55*(4), 333–346.

Gofrit, O. N., Shemer, J., Leibovici, D., et al. (2000, July). Quaternary prevention: A new look at an old challenge. *The Israel Medical Association Journal, 2*, 498–500.

Hafen, M. (2016). Of what use (or harm) is a positive health definition? *Journal of Public Health, 24*, 437–441.

Hales, D. (2005). *An invitation to health* (11th ed.). Belmont, CA: Thomson & Wadswoth.

Healthy People 2020 [The Secretary's Advisory Committee on National Health Promotion and Disease Prevention Objectives for 2020]. (2008). *Phase I report: Recommendations for the framework and format of Healthy People 2020.* Retrieved from https://www.healthypeople.gov/sites/default/files/PhaseI_0.pdf.

Hettler, B. (1980). Wellness promotion on a university campus. *Family and Community Health, 3*(1), 77–95.

Institute of Medicine, Committee on Quality of Health Care in America. (2001). *Crossing the quality chasm: A new health system for the 21st century.* Washington, DC: National Academy Press.

Interprofessional Education Collaborative (IPEC). (2016). *Core competencies for interprofessional collaborative practice: 2016 update.* Washington, DC: Author.

Jamoulle, M., & Roland, M. (1995, June). *Quaternary prevention.* Presentation at the 1995 meeting of the WONCA Classification Committee, Hong Kong. Retrieved from http://www.ph3c.org/PH3C/docs/27/000103/0000261.pdf.

Johnson, J. (1986). *Wellness: A context for living.* Thorofare, NJ: Slack.

Johnson, R. M. (2015). The changing face of patient care: Delivering patient-centered and culturally competent care in an evolving world. *Delaware Medical Journal, 87*(3), 85–87.

Jonas, W. B. (2005). *Mosby's dictionary of complementary & alternative medicine.* St. Louis, MO: Elsevier Mosby.

Jordan, M. (2016, Winter). Wellness: From movement to profession. *American Fitness Magazine,* 58–63.

Lalonde, M. (1974). *A new perspective on the health of Canadians: A working document.* Ottawa, Canada: Minister of Supply and Services.

Lane, E. (2016). *Optimal wellbeing: Is an absence of disease enough? Positive Health, 232.* Retrieved from http://www.positivehealth.com/article/naturopathy/optimal-wellbeing-is-an-absence-of-disease-enough.

Leddy, S. K. (2006). *Health promotion: Mobilizing strengths to enhance health, wellness, and well-being.* Philadelphia, PA: FA Davis.

Lusk, J. M., & Fater, K. (2013). A concept analysis of patient-centered care. *Nursing Forum, 48*(2), 89–98.

Marr, J. J. (2014, Winter). Fall from grace. *Pharos,* 8–13.

Massey, J. (2015). Mind-body medicine: Its history & evolution. *Naturopathic Doctor News & Review, 11*(6). Retrieved from http://ndnr.com/e-version/jun15/jun15.pdf.html.

Miles, A., & Mezzich, J. E. (2011). The care of the patient and the soul of the clinic: Person-centered medicine as an emergent model of modern clinical practice. *The International Journal of Person Centered Medicine, 1*(2), 207–222.

Mishra, B. N. (2009). Secret of eternal youth; teaching from the centenarian hot spots ("Blue Zones"). *Indian Journal of Community Medicine, 34*(4), 273–275.

National Wellness Institute (NWI). (n.d.). *The six dimensions of wellness model.* Author. Retrieved from http://c.ymcdn.com/sites/www.nationalwellness.org/resource/resmgr/docs/sixdimensionsfactsheet.pdf.

Nutbeam, D., Padmadas, S. S., Maslovskaya, O., et al. (2013). A health promotion logic model to review progress in HIV prevention in China. *Health Promotion International, 30*(2), 270–280.

Palmer, L. (2016). A retrospective on patient-centered care. *MGMA Connection, March,* 48.

Pender, N. J., Murdaugh, C., & Parsons, M. A. (2015). *Health promotion in nursing practice* (7th ed.). Upper Saddle River, NJ: Pearson Education.

Pes, G. M., Tolu, F., Poulain, M., et al. (2013). Lifestyle and nutrition related to male longevity in Sardinia: An ecological study. *Nutrition, Metabolism, and Cardiovascular Diseases, 23*, 212–219.

Picker Institute. (n.d.). *Principles of patient-centered care.* Retrieved from http://cgp.pickerinstitute.org/?page_id=1319.

Ratzan, S. C., & Parker, R. M. (2000). Introduction. In C. R. Selden, M. Zorn, S. C. Ratzan, et al. (Eds.), *National library of medicine current bibliographies in medicine: Health literacy.* NLM Pub. No. CBM 2000-1. Bethesda, MD: National Institutes of Health, U.S. Department of Health and Human Services.

Robbins, L. C., & Hall, J. H. (1970). *How to practice prospective medicine.* Indianapolis, IN: Methodist Hospital of Indiana.

Rubenstein, L. V., Stockdale, S. E., Sapir, N., et al. (2014). A patient-centered primary care practice approach using evidence-based quality improvement: Rationale, methods, and early assessment of implementation. *Journal of General Internal Medicine, 29*(Suppl. 2), S589–S597.

Seligman, M. E. P. (2008). Positive health. *Applied Psychology: An International Review, 57*, 3–18.

Sidani, S., & Fox, M. (2014). Patient-centered care: Clarification of its specific elements to facilitate interprofessional care. *Journal of Interprofessional Care, 28*(2), 134–141.

Silverman, B. D. (2012). Physician behavior and bedside manners: The influence of William Osler and The Johns Hopkins School of Medicine. *Proceedings/Baylor University Medical Center, 25*(1), 58–61.

Stokols, D. (2000). The social ecological paradigm of wellness promotion. In M. Schneider-Jamner & D. Stokols (Eds.), *Promoting human wellness* (pp. 21–37). Berkeley, CA: University of California Press.

Substance Abuse and Mental Health Services Administration (SAMHSA). (2016, July 1). *The eight dimensions of wellness. Author.* Retrieved from http://www.samhsa.gov/ wellness-initiative/eight-dimensions-wellness.

Swarbrick, M. (2006). Coping with: A wellness approach. *Psychiatric Rehabilitation Journal, 29*(4), 311–314.

Swarbrick, M. (2013). Wellness-oriented peer approaches: A key ingredient for integrated care. *Psychiatric Services, 64*(8), 723–726.

Tanenbaum, S. J. (2015). What is patient-centered care? A typology of models and missions. *Health Care Analysis, 23*, 272–287.

Travis, J., & Ryan, R. S. (2004). *The wellness workbook: How to achieve enduring health and vitality* (3rd ed.). Berkeley, CA: Celestial Arts.

University of Texas Medical Branch (UTMB). (2014). *UTMB handbook of operating procedures, policy 9.3.4: Patient/ family education.* Galveston, TX: Author. Retrieved from https://www.utmb.edu/policies_and_procedures/IHOP/ Clinical/Patient_Rights/IHOP%20-%2009.03.04%20-%20 Patient%20Family%20Education.pdf.

Wellness Center, Franklin Pierce University. (n.d.). *Seven dimensions of wellness.* Author. Retrieved from http://eraven.franklinpierce.edu/s/dept/hr/Wellness/ Wellness_Publications/Seven%20Dimensions%20of%20 Wellness.pdf.

World Health Organization. (n.d.). *Health promotion and disease prevention through population-based interventions, including action to address social determinants and health inequity.* Retrieved from http://www.emro.who.int/pdf/ about-who/public-health-functions/health-promotion-disease-prevention.pdf?ua=1.

World Health Organization. (2016, August). *What is health promotion?* Geneva, Switzerland: Author. Retrieved from http://www.who.int/features/qa/health-promotion/en/.

World Health Organization, Division of Health Promotion, Education and Communication (HEP). (1998). *Health promotion glossary.* Geneva, Switzerland: Author. Retrieved from http://www.who.int/healthpromotion/ about/HPR%20Glossary%201998.pdf.

World Organization of National Colleges, Academies, and Academic Associations of General Practitioners/ Family Physician (WONCA). (2016). *WONCA international dictionary for general/family practice.* Author. Retrieved from http://www.ph3c.org/PH3C/ docs/27/000092/0000052.pdf.

Worrall, S. (2015, April 12). *Here are the secrets to a long and healthy life. National Geographics.* Retrieved from http:// news.nationalgeographic.com/2015/04/150412-longevit y-health-blue-zones-obesity-diet-ngbooktalk/.

Foundations of Values and Ethics for Interprofessional Practice

LEARNING OUTCOMES

After studying this chapter, you will be able to:

1. Explain the differences and similarities between ethics and bioethics.
2. Differentiate between morals and values.
3. Explain the principle of "double effect."
4. Differentiate between deontology, utilitarianism, and applied ethics.
5. Discuss the use of distributive justice in health care.
6. Give an example of each of the following ethical principles: autonomy, beneficence, nonmaleficence, justice, fidelity, and veracity.
7. Use values clarification to identify your own values and those of patients and families.
8. Apply the steps of an interprofessional ethical decision-making process and rubric in making a decision.
9. Give an example of moral courage.

This chapter provides a brief overview of basic concepts associated with the Core Competency of Values/Ethics for Interprofessional Practice. Foundational concepts such as ethics, morals, and values are explained and differentiated as they pertain to health care. Six basic ethical principles are reviewed, as well as moral relativism and the principle of "double effect." Short descriptions of relevant ethical theories provide a background for the analysis of ethical issues in later chapters and in clinical practice. A discussion of Interprofessional Ethics as an emerging field with its own ethical issues and concerns concludes the chapter.

FOUNDATIONAL CONCEPTS

Ethics and Bioethics

Ethics

At its most basic, ethics is the study of right and wrong. Ethics is defined as "the rules and principles which govern right conduct" (O'Toole, 2017, p. 650). This definition can be expanded to mean a set of moral principles. A code of ethics is a set of moral principles or expected behaviors. Each profession has a specific code of ethics that each member of that profession must follow at all times.

Ethical Dilemma

Unfortunately, the answer to what is right or wrong or good or bad in a particular patient situation is often unclear. A dilemma is commonly known as a "no-win" situation. However, an ethical dilemma goes deeper than that, and "involves two (or more) morally correct courses of action that cannot both be followed" (Dougherty & Purtilo, 2016, p. 66). As a healthcare professional, you will be faced with ethical issues and dilemmas throughout your career. These issues may involve patients, families, coworkers, or the entire healthcare team. Caselet 4.1 presents a common dramatic example of an ethical dilemma (Fig. 4.1).

CASELET 4.1 The Lifeboat

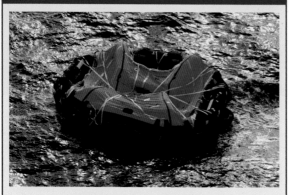

(© Panmaule/iStock/Thinkstock.)

A group of friends are taking a trip on a boat. The boat hits a submerged rock that punctures the hull. The boat is too far from land for anyone to swim back. There are eight people aboard. There is only room for five on the lifeboat. If everyone gets in the lifeboat, it will capsize and everyone will be lost. How should the group choose who will get in the lifeboat?

Discussion Questions
1. What is it that makes this a dilemma?
2. Using your current knowledge, what would you consider in making the decision?

CASELET 4.2 Life Support

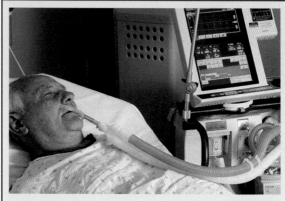

(From Adler A, Carlton R: Introduction to Radiologic Sciences and Patient Care, ed 5, St. Louis, 2012, Saunders.)

A group of people are taking a trip on a chartered boat. The weather turns stormy, and the boat collides with another boat, causing multiple serious injuries to many on board. Fortunately, the captain of the chartered boat is able to notify the Coast Guard, who airlifts the injured to the nearest hospital. Ten people require life support in the form of mechanical ventilation. Unfortunately, the small local hospital has only eight ventilators, and two are already in use for critically ill patients. The hospital is far from a large medical center. The severe weather and unstable conditions of the patients prohibit transfer to another hospital. Which patients get the ventilators?

Discussion Questions
1. What makes this an ethical dilemma?
2. How will the healthcare team decide?
3. What criteria should be used in making the decision?

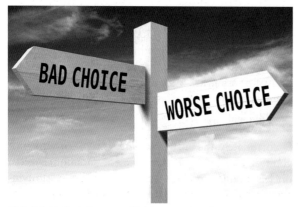

FIG. 4.1 Ethical dilemma. (© 3D generator/iStock/Thinkstock.)

Bioethics

Bioethics is the "identification, analysis, and resolution of ethical problems, issues, and dilemmas associated with the biological sciences, especially medicine, healthcare practice, and research" (Scott, 2009, p. 30). When Caselet 4.1 is put into a bioethical context, it might look like Caselet 4.2.

Values and Morals
Values

Values are personal beliefs about the worth of a given idea, attitude, custom, or object. Values vary among cultures, individuals, and even professions. Personal (and professional) values may change over time. Personal values develop through influences from family, school, religion, culture, and personal experience. Values shape the way that we view the world and determine our perspective. Values form the foundation for our judgments, decisions, and actions (Schwartz, Preece, & Hendry, 2016). It is

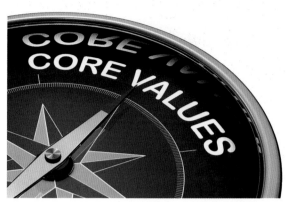

FIG. 4.2 Values. (© frankpeters/iStock/Thinkstock.)

ACTIVE LEARNING

Values Clarification

This exercise in values clarification for healthcare decision making can be used with patients, families, and within the healthcare team. Try using it to evaluate a personal decision you are faced with, even a simple one such as whether to go to a party or stay home and write a paper.

1. List alternatives. What possible courses of action are available?
2. Examine potential consequences of choices. What are the potential consequences of each choice? What are the risks and benefits to you and others?
3. Choose freely. Did you have a say in the decision? Were you given a choice? Did you feel heard? Did you feel coerced?
4. Feel good about the choice. How do you feel about the decision?
5. Affirm the choice. What will you tell others about this?
6. Act on the choice. Will it be difficult to do this or tell people what you decided? What help do you need in carrying out your decision?
7. Act with a pattern. Have you done this or something similar before? Would you do this again? Is this decision consistent with your beliefs?

important to understand that each healthcare profession may have slightly different values. Values are neither right nor wrong; they merely reflect what is important to a culture, profession, or individual.

Healthcare professionals share values acquired through their education that result in a biomedical view of health. This biomedical viewpoint is a relatively narrow one, and healthcare professionals must realize that others, especially patients and families, may have different approaches to health, prevention, and illness. It is important for healthcare professionals to identify, acknowledge, and respect value differences among themselves and their patients. The IPEC (2011, 2016) *Core Competencies for Interprofessional Collaborative Practice* may be seen as a set of values (Fig. 4.2). To become competent in interprofessional collaboration, you must value the concepts inherent in the identified Core Competencies of Values/Ethics, Teams and Teamwork, Interprofessional Communication, and Roles/Responsibilities. If you do not value interprofessional practice, you are unlikely to become skilled at interprofessional collaboration.

Values Clarification

Values clarification is an ongoing personal process that can be used to help you become aware of your own values and to recognize how they may affect your personal and professional behavior. This process requires active reflection and critical thinking. When faced with a disturbing ethical issue, use the following set of questions as a process with which to clarify your personal values related to the issue. Ask yourself: "Why does this bother me? What about it makes me uncomfortable? What would I do or

want done? Why?" A more detailed discussion regarding the process of self-reflection is found in Chapter 7. Try using the values clarification exercise in the Active Learning box as a model for values clarification in decision making in health care.

Once you learn to clarify your own values, as a healthcare professional, you can assist patients and other team members in clarifying their values. You must take care not to influence or impose your personal values on others. In interprofessional teams, it may be important to clarify the team's values to assist in decision making. All team members must be willing to consider different perspectives and values. This is necessary because "openness is a requirement of respectful interaction with others. If we permit our own value judgements to function without challenge, we risk imposing them on others" (Schwartz, Preece, & Hendry, 2016, p. 2).

Healthcare professionals are called upon to assist patients and families in decision making. It is important that the professionals provide accurate information about all available options and their potential risks and benefits to the patient. Healthcare professionals can only assist others (e.g., patients, team members) to clarify their values if they themselves have clarified their own values in relation to the issue at hand. Professionals must avoid slanting information to influence the patient's specific choice. You and the healthcare team share responsibility to assist patients in making informed decisions that are consistent with the patient's own values. You and the healthcare team must make sure the patient is informed of all available options with their pros and cons. You and the team can discuss with the patient which option you think is best and explain why, but the decision ultimately belongs to the patient. You and the other team members must be prepared to accept the patient's decision, even if it differs from what you and the team think is best. The team must support the patient's and family's decision, whatever it may be.

Morals

Morals are personal beliefs about what is right and what is wrong. Each person has his or her own individual morals. Morals are influenced by culture, religion, family teachings, and, in some cases, philosophies and world views. Like values, they differ from person to person and culture to culture. There are some morals that may be almost universal, such as the "Golden Rule": the need to treat others in the way that you would want to be treated. Because morals are personal, you should not be compelled to follow another's morality. However, everyone must follow the law (Scott, 2009). Morals can be thought of as personal ethics. It is important to consider that healthcare professionals must adhere to their profession's code of ethics regardless of their personal morals.

Moral Distress

Jameton (1984) defined moral distress as "when one knows the right thing to do, but institutional constraints make it nearly impossible to pursue the right course of action" (p. 6). It occurs when a healthcare professional is unable to act according to his or her core values and perceived obligations. A review by Ganske (2010, par. 10) noted that research findings "suggest that moral distress may be expressed through physical symptoms, such as trouble sleeping, headaches, shaking, and/or gastrointestinal changes, as well as psychological symptoms, such as feelings of anguish, frustration, anxiety, and/or guilt" (Fig. 4.3). Although first identified in nurses, moral distress was found in psychologists and academic faculty (Ganske, 2010) and most likely occurs in all

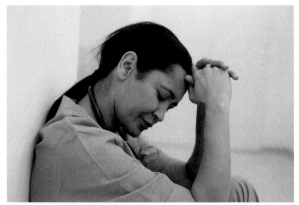

FIG. 4.3 Moral distress. (© Wavebreakmedia Ltd/Wavebreak Media/Thinkstock.)

healthcare professionals who are forced by a situation to violate their own moral beliefs. The effects of moral distress may linger; this is known as *moral residue* (Epstein & Delgado, 2010). Moral distress differs from an ethical dilemma in that there is no conflict regarding the right thing to do. The difficulty that causes moral distress is that the right thing to do is known but cannot be done. See Caselet 4.3 for an example.

OVERVIEW OF ETHICAL THEORIES

Ethical theories are useful in ethical decision making and in understanding your own ethical perspective, as well as those of others. When healthcare professionals are collaborating on an issue that has ethical implications, it is helpful to have a working knowledge of the various ethical theories, or philosophies, to better understand the perspective of individual team members (Fig. 4.4). The theories mentioned here are some of the most commonly known and applied in health care.

Deontology

Deontology is known as *duty-based ethics*. Actions are defined as right or wrong based on adherence to ethical principles. Right action is determined by examining the presence or absence of ethical principles in an individual situation, with no concern for the ultimate consequences. An act is considered moral if motives or intentions are good, regardless of outcome. In this theory of ethics, the "means justify the end." There are universal truths that determine which actions are right or wrong, no matter what; for example, *it is wrong to lie,* no matter what the

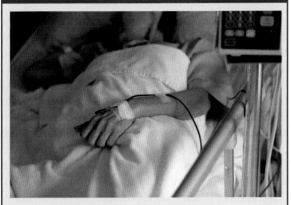

(© pat138241/iStock/Thinkstock.)

After major surgery, a patient told her nurse that she did not want her grandchildren to see her like this, with tubes and machines everywhere; "I don't want them to remember me like this, please don't let them visit." The patient took a turn for the worse and became unresponsive. The patient's daughter came to visit with her two children (the patient's grandchildren). The nurse stopped them and explained to the daughter that her mother did not want the grandchildren to visit; she also explained why. The daughter insisted on having them see their grandmother "one last time." Because there was no policy that prevented grandchildren to visit, the nurse could not stop them. The patient later died without regaining consciousness. The nurse was very upset and felt that she failed her patient in the patient's last hours of life. The nurse regretted not being able to honor this patient's last wish.

Discussion Questions

1. What is the source of moral distress in this caselet?
2. What are some residual effects of moral distress that the nurse might experience?

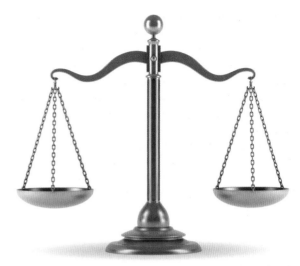

FIG. 4.4 Ethical theories can help us determine what is the right action. (© Sergey Volkov/Hemera/Thinkstock.)

went to get a special meal, a ring, and flowers, despite the consequence that it will ruin the surprise.

Utilitarianism (Consequentialism)

Utilitarianism is also known as *teleology* or *consequence-based ethics.* This type of ethics is almost the opposite of deontology. Here the emphasis is on consequences, or the "end justifies the means." Doing the greatest good for the greatest number of people is the standard used to determine right actions. The process by which the end is achieved is irrelevant. For example, if a patient has a highly contagious infectious disease, she may be placed in isolation and not allowed to leave her hospital room. Caregivers and visitors are limited and must wear personal protective equipment, including gowns, gloves, masks, and goggles. All food must be served on completely disposable tableware. This practice may violate the personal rights of the patient because the patient has no choice regarding leaving her room, whether the visitors wear protective gear, and how food will be served, but the actions are done for the good of the rest of the patients and community, to prevent the spread of disease.

Principlism

Principlism uses the key ethical principles of beneficence, non-maleficence, autonomy, and justice to resolve ethical dilemmas. Rather than strict adherence to an ethical theory or philosophy, principlism uses ethical principles to analyze ethical issues and to resolve ethical dilemmas

situation. Take the following example. A young woman is hospitalized after a motor vehicle crash. Her boyfriend has stayed with her most of the time. She falls asleep, and he leaves the room. He tells the nurse he won't be back until dinnertime because he plans to propose to his girlfriend, and is going to pick up a special meal, the ring, and some roses. He wants to surprise his girlfriend. When she wakes up, she asks the nurse if her boyfriend said where he went, and if he said what he was doing. Following deontology theory, and the idea that it is wrong to lie, the nurse must tell the patient that her boyfriend

(Black, 2011). Key ethical principles are presented later in this chapter.

Virtue Ethics

Virtue ethics relates to character traits that are considered or shown to be praiseworthy. Virtues are "tendencies to act, feel and judge that develop through appropriate training but come from natural tendencies" (Black, 2011, p. 107). Virtue ethics is largely influenced by culture because what is considered virtuous in one culture may not be considered honorable in another. The character traits of the decision maker influence the decision. A "virtuous" person will do the right thing.

Using virtue ethics, ethical reasoning (or what is considered "right wisdom") incorporates a wide range of possible actions, consequences, and societal values. When faced with making an ethical decision, the specific circumstances play a large part and are closely examined. Ethical decision making considers both the individual and society.

ETHICAL PRINCIPLES

There are six generally accepted ethical principles that guide healthcare professionals' practice, research, and education (Fig. 4.5). They are useful in ethical decision making, for understanding best practice in patient care, and in advocating for and protecting patient rights.

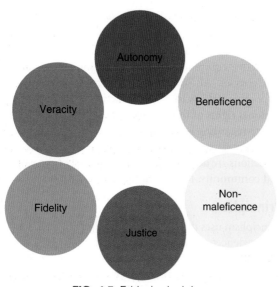

FIG. 4.5 Ethical principles.

Autonomy (Respect for Persons)

Autonomy is the right to self-determination. This means that all human beings have the right to decide what is best for them. Each person can control what is done to him or her. Individuals have the right to determine their own actions and have the freedom to make their own decisions without coercion. This principle also incorporates the need to protect those who are not capable of making a reasoned decision, such as comatose patients, children, or those who are cognitively impaired (National Commission for the Protection of Human Subjects of Biomedical and Behavioral Research, 1979). Legal guardians must be appointed for these patients, and the guardians make the decisions, not the healthcare team. It is the responsibility of the team to fully inform patients or their guardians of the risks and benefits of the treatment being offered. This is known as *full disclosure.* A patient has the right to refuse a treatment, even though the healthcare professionals believe it is best (Scott, 2009). This is often difficult for clinicians to accept because it may not be what they would choose for themselves. As long as the patient understands what is being offered, and the consequences of accepting or rejecting the treatment, the patient's decision is the only decision that counts. Consider Caselet 4.4.

Beneficence

Simply put, beneficence is the obligation to maximize the good. It means that healthcare providers must actively work to secure the well-being of the patient. This includes advocating for the patient and making sure the patient's voice and desires are heard and respected. The patient's best interests come first. Healthcare professionals must take positive action to help others.

Non-Maleficence

Non-maleficence means to do no harm. It is a corollary of the principle of beneficence. Non-maleficence addresses the obligation of healthcare professionals to avoid harm and to do everything possible to minimize the risks and adverse effects of treatment. However, many treatments may cause discomfort or even temporary injury, as in the case of surgery. The key concept here is intent. Healthcare professionals cannot *intentionally and maliciously* harm anyone in their care. This principle also applies to omissions—failure to act when one should (Scott, 2009).

CASELET 4.4 **Autonomy**

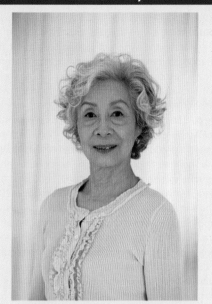

(© rakkogumi/iStock/Thinkstock.)

Daphne Washington is 70 years old and has a fractured hip. The orthopedic surgeon recommends that she have total hip replacement surgery. Ms. Washington refuses the surgery. The surgeon requests a psychiatry consult to determine whether Ms. Washington is competent to make the decision. Ms. Washington accurately explains what the surgery entails, and that she knows that without it she may never be able to walk properly. She still refuses the surgery and wants to go home to her family. She says she is not afraid of surgery, she just does not want to go through it. The psychiatrist declares her competent to make the decision. The surgeon, nurses, and social worker who comprise her healthcare team cannot understand why she would not want the surgery, but they respect her autonomy. Ms. Washington is discharged from the hospital to home that afternoon with a referral to an orthopedic specialist.

Discussion Questions
1. What are your thoughts on the patient's decision?
2. Explain how the principle of autonomy applies in the caselet.

Double Effect

Although not one of the commonly accepted ethical principles, the so-called *principle of double effect* bears mention in any discussion of ethics. The principle of double effect applies when the intent of treatment or care is to

CASELET 4.5 **Beneficence Versus Non-Maleficence and Double Effect**

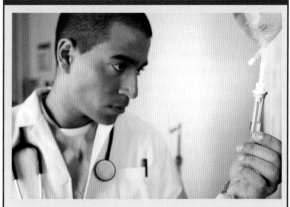

(© Hemera Technologies/AbleStock.com/Thinkstock.)

A critically ill patient is in great pain, despite a high dose of morphine. Increasing the dose would relieve his pain (do good). However, increasing the dose might cause certain side effects such as confusion, hallucination, or slowing of respirations to a point that it could compromise his ability to breathe (cause harm). The healthcare team must weigh the benefit of easing the patient's suffering by increasing the morphine, against the potentially harmful side effects. Consider also that the patient is critically ill. If the dosage is increased and the patient experiences side effects, steps could be taken to treat the side effects. If side effects do occur, it was not the *intent* of the team to cause harm.

Discussion Questions
1. What would you recommend in this situation?
2. Explain your reasoning using ethical principles and theory.

benefit the patient, but the result of treatment is unexpected harm. For example, a patient with a serious infection is given penicillin, which is known to cure the infection. The patent has no known allergies, but experiences a life-threatening allergic reaction to the penicillin and nearly dies. The intent was to help the patient, but the treatment nearly killed him. This is the principle of double effect, and it occurs often in health care. Most treatments have risks and side effects that could potentially cause harm. Caselet 4.5 illustrates the difference between beneficence and non-maleficence and the principle of double effect.

Justice

At its core, the principle of justice means fairness. Access to care is an issue that falls under the principle of justice.

Is health care a right or a privilege? In the United States, not everyone has equal access to care. The Emergency Medical Treatment and Labor Act (EMTALA) was enacted by the US Congress in 1986 to ensure public access to emergency services regardless of ability to pay. Medicare-participating hospitals that offer emergency services are required to provide a medical screening examination and provide stabilizing treatment for those with an emergency medical condition, including active labor, regardless of ability to pay (CMS, 2012). However, many such patients cannot afford follow-up care or ongoing treatment. Also included in the principle of justice are the concepts of right to privacy, confidentiality, and protection of vulnerable populations. According to the principle of justice, healthcare professionals are responsible to protect patients and population groups from exploitation. On the other hand, healthcare professionals must make sure that those from vulnerable populations are given equal opportunities for quality care and access to care. A detailed definition of *vulnerable population* is found in Box 4.1. Furthermore, the ethical principle of justice requires healthcare professionals to provide the highest quality of care possible in the situation, regardless of the background, socioeconomic status, or other characteristics of the patient.

Distributive Justice

Distributive justice is concerned with the fair allocation of resources throughout a diverse society. In health care, this raises many issues. In the case of kidney, heart, or other organ transplants, there are more people who need transplants than there are organs available for transplant. If all people are to be treated equally, how can we decide who gets the transplant? Many models exist that deal with this problem of resource allocation. Examples of such models include to each equally, to each according to merit (including past or potential contributions to society), to each according to what is available in the marketplace, to each according to need (adapted from Black, 2011). Each of these models have problems as well as merits. There is no single or easy way to ensure fair and equitable distribution of healthcare resources. Many injustices and disparities exist in all types of healthcare systems, despite efforts to adhere to the principle of justice. Caselet 4.6 provides examples of how different models of distributive justice might be applied to a healthcare decision regarding who should get an artificial liver.

BOX 4.1   Vulnerable Populations

Vulnerable populations are those who may be less able to protect their own interests and rights when these are in jeopardy and who are vulnerable and at risk for exploitation or harm (Johnstone, 2016). In terms of healthcare research, vulnerable populations "refers to but not limited to children, minors, pregnant women, fetuses, human in vitro fertilization, prisoners, employees, military persons and students in hierarchical organizations, terminally ill, comatose, physically and intellectually challenged individuals, institutionalized elderly individuals, visual or hearing impaired, ethnic minorities, refugees, international research, economically and educationally disabled and healthy volunteers" (Shivayogi, 2013, p. 53). The same populations can be considered as vulnerable and needing extra safeguards in all types of health care, not just research. People who are unable to make decisions for themselves, those who lack freedom (as in the case of prisoners or the institutionalized), and any population who is disadvantaged in any way (such as the uninsured or economically disadvantaged) may be considered vulnerable (Fig. 4.6).

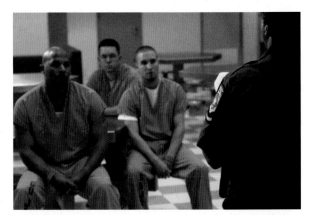

FIG. 4.6 Prisoners are considered a vulnerable population. (© Thinkstock Images/Stockbyte/Thinkstock.)

Fidelity

Fidelity means "faithfulness." It is the obligation to provide care and follow through; in essence, the nonabandonment of patients. It has to do with professional integrity. You, as a healthcare provider, cannot simply decide not to care for a patient in need. You cannot leave for vacation unless you arrange for another qualified professional to care for your patients. You cannot refuse to continue to care for a patient who is noncompliant until you provide a

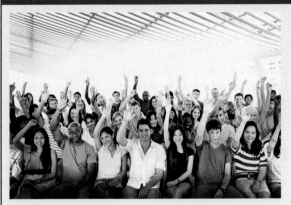

(© Rawpixel/iStock/Thinkstock.)

Artificial livers are currently in development (Mizner, Grabow, & Klammt, 2016). Suppose an artificial liver is approved by the US Food and Drug Administration (FDA). It is effective, but quite expensive. We need to distribute them to those with liver disease. Using four different models of distributive justice, this caselet illustrates how the decision would be made.

1. To each equally. Using this method, we will have a lottery. Everyone who needs an artificial liver has an equal chance of winning one. However, some will not get one, and must wait until the next lottery, when more artificial livers become available. Some of these people are critically ill and will die before the next lottery.

2. To each according to merit (including past or potential contributions to society). With this strategy, we must determine who is most deserving of an artificial liver. Is the scientist worthier to receive an artificial liver than a child? Are those who developed liver disease due to drug or alcohol use less worthy than those who live a healthy lifestyle?

3. To each according to what is available in the marketplace. Using this approach, we distribute the cheapest available artificial liver so that more can receive one, and let the best artificial livers go to those who can afford to pay more for one.

4. To each according to need. This procedure requires determining who most needs a liver. The sickest people would get the artificial liver; those who are not as seriously ill can wait for the next lot of artificial livers. The difficulty with this approach is that the sickest people may not survive as long or benefit as much from the artificial liver as those in better condition, and that there is no accurate way of predicting how long a person will live. We would have to develop a method of measuring who is "sickest."

Discussion Questions

1. Which do you think is the best method? Why or why not?
2. Which ethical theory would you apply to making this decision? Why?
3. Can you think of a better way to allocate the artificial liver? Explain.

referral to other providers or sources of care. The principle of fidelity includes being faithful to responsibilities and commitments. Fidelity also includes the need to make decisions regarding which responsibilities take precedence in certain situations. For example, a nurse feels ill halfway through her 12-hour shift. She is caring for five patients. She starts to feel worse and worse and vomits. She has a headache and feels dizzy. She takes her temperature and discovers she has a fever. She has a responsibility to care for her patients and not to abandon them. However, she also has a responsibility not to expose them to a potentially contagious disease and a responsibility to avoid making potential errors because she is ill. The nurse tells the assistant nurse manager about her illness. The assistant nurse manager tells the nurse to give him a report on her patients, go to Employee Health, and then go home. The assistant nurse manager arranges for another nurse

to come in and finish the nurse's shift. He cares for her patients until the other nurse arrives.

Fidelity forms the key foundation for the therapeutic provider–patient relationship. Fidelity is essential to effective interprofessional collaboration. It is the key to upholding most professional codes of ethics and for maintaining competence in one's profession.

Veracity

Another word for *veracity* is truth-telling. You cannot lie to or deceive patients or families. Veracity is fundamental to continued trust between people. Veracity requires full disclosure of risks and benefits of treatments, medications, and alternate therapies that are available. It requires honestly answering all patient and family questions, even if the answer may be difficult to hear. For example, in the case of certain terminal illnesses, a point may be

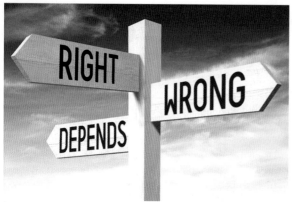

FIG. 4.7 Ethical relativism. (© 3D generator/iStock/Thinkstock.)

reached at which there is nothing left to do medically to treat the disease. This must be told to the patient and family. However, it does not mean giving up on the patient. Medications and treatments that will maintain comfort and preserve as much function as possible will be continued, and referrals may be made to hospice care and community agencies, such as family support groups.

Ethical Relativism

Ethical relativism considers that nothing is objectively right or wrong (Fig. 4.7). There are no absolute truths. Rather, what is right or wrong is relative to the norms of the society, culture, or historical period. An act or behavior may be ethical in one society, culture, or historical period and be considered unethical in another. Child labor is considered unethical in current American society. However, there was a time in American history when it was the norm. Today, child labor is still acceptable in some cultures. Decisions made using this ethical relativism will be determined by the cultural and societal norms of the time and place. This theory allows for the idea that ethics evolve and change over time and are influenced by historical events and experience. This theory applies when working with those from cultures different from your own.

APPLIED ETHICS

As the name implies, applied ethics involves the practical application of ethical and legal principles to a specific situation. It is considered by some to be more concrete and practical than some of the other ethical theories.

Using applied ethics to make ethical decisions or solve ethical dilemmas involves careful consideration of the effect on the individual and the legal aspects of the decision. Applied ethics deals with ambiguous situations; decisions are made based on facts and critical reasoning rather than theory. Decisions are made on a case-by-case basis, rather than using preexisting rules or protocols. Applied ethics are often used by healthcare teams and institutional ethics committees.

ETHICAL DECISION MAKING

Knowledge of ethical theories, principles, and one's own morals and values provides a foundation for ethical decision making. However, to make a decision when faced with an ethical issue or dilemma requires more than just foundational knowledge. It requires a process by which to analyze and examine the situation, weigh alternatives, and come up with a solution or decision that the interprofessional team finds ethically acceptable. This process must consider all stakeholders who may be affected by the decision. These stakeholders include the patient and family first and may include the institution and the population at large, as in cases of contagious disease. An ethical decision-making process for nurses was presented by Black (2011); its steps are to (1) clarify the ethical dilemma, (2) gather additional data, (3) identify options, (4) make a decision, (5) act, and (6) evaluate. There are many other ethical decision-making models and processes available in the literature, too numerous to mention. Some are discipline-specific.

The following decision-making process adapted by the author from a variety of existing models is an approach that is specific to interprofessional team-based decision making and incorporates the IPEC Values/Ethics for interprofessional collaboration competency (Fig. 4.8).

1. Identify the decision to be made. What exactly are the ethical concerns?
2. Whose decision is it to make? Is it really the interprofessional team's decision, or the patient's or family's ultimate decision? Perhaps it is the institution's ethics committee who should decide, as in the case of limited resources, or cases with legal aspects.
3. Identify the stakeholders. Who will be affected by the decision? The patient is usually always first; however, the decision may have repercussions for others, such as the family, the institution, healthcare professionals, caregivers, and even the community

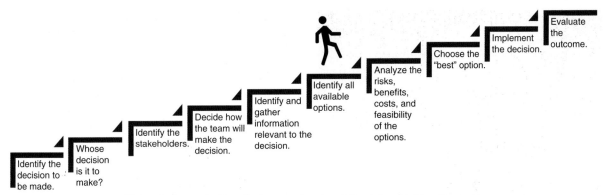

FIG. 4.8 Steps in Reed's Interprofessional Decision-Making Process.

at large. Some ethical decisions may not involve specific patients at all, as in the case of impaired professionals or unethical professional behavior.

4. Decide how the team will make the decision. Will it be based on ethical principles? What process will be used? Will a vote be taken? What is the deadline for determining the solution? How will the stakeholders participate and/or be heard?

5. Identify and gather information relevant to the decision. Identify what is known and what additional information is needed. The patient's and family's wishes may need to be determined and clarified. Are there legal, cultural, or spiritual factors to be considered? This will require brainstorming, discussion, and fact-finding on the part of the team. It is important to protect the confidentiality of those involved when gathering information.

6. Identify all available options. Based on the information from the first four steps, what options are available?

7. Analyze the risks, benefits, costs, and feasibility of the options. Triple Aim operates here; the quality and cost of care and the patient experience must be factored into the decision. The effects on the stakeholders and community must also be considered.

8. Choose the "best" option. Information from the first six steps must be considered, and each team member must have the opportunity to weigh in. The unique cultures, values, roles and responsibilities, and expertise of other healthcare professionals must be respected. All team members must be able to "live with" the decision. Often there is no clear right answer, and all options seem lacking in one way or another; however, a decision must be agreed upon. Discussion

of ethical principles and values clarification may need to take place.

9. Implement the decision. The team must decide which team members are to carry out specific aspects of the decision, including who will communicate with the stakeholders and other necessary persons. If community arrangements must be put in place, who will manage that? This step requires working in cooperation with those who receive care, those who provide care, and others who contribute to or support the delivery of prevention and healthcare services.

10. Evaluate the outcome. After the decision is made, the team should gather information regarding the outcome of the decision and evaluate the effectiveness of the decision. The team's decision-making process should also be evaluated. The evaluation should be done in the spirit of "What can we do better?" instead of "Where did we go wrong?"

MORAL COURAGE

Resolution of ethical issues is a complex process. To remain true to your own professional code of ethics, personal morals, and function as an effective member of an interprofessional team, and as an advocate for patients and families, you may be called upon to demonstrate moral courage. Rushworth Kidder (2005) wrote a landmark book defining and outlining the process of moral courage. Moral courage comes from "an ethical commitment, a kind of inner moral compass calibrated by a set of core values" (p. viii). According to Kidder, ethical issues arise for two reasons. The first is being tempted to violate core values, such as engaging in cheating to get a better grade or lying to protect a co-worker. The second is facing

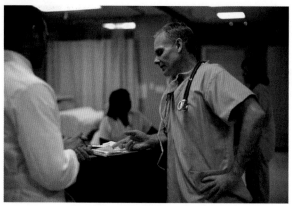

FIG. 4.9 Speaking out against injustice requires moral courage. (© Thomas Northcut/DigitalVision/Thinkstock.)

a dilemma in which "two deeply held values are in opposition. Fairness, perhaps versus compassion" (p. viii). These two reasons may be characterized as "right versus wrong" and "right versus right."

Moral courage is having the will to speak out and do the right thing (Fig. 4.9). It requires turning principles into action, actually having the courage to *do* something. It often involves choosing the "hard right" over the "easy wrong" (Kidder, 2005). Moral courage is standing up for principle. Moral courage can (and should) be demonstrated in daily encounters; it does not necessarily involve a major crisis. For example, in the breakroom of the Emergency Department, staff members are discussing a patient. "Did you get a load of that guy in room 3? Looks like he's been living in a tent for years." Another staff member responds, "Yeah, smells like it too!" The other one says, "I wonder if he came in to get free food or drugs, probably both, or a sheet for a new tent!" Both laugh. A third team member states, "You don't know this person. You have no idea what his situation is. He may be seriously ill. He has the same right to health care as anyone else. We all need to treat him with the same respect as we would a wealthy person or anyone else. I won't tolerate making fun of any patient. Please stop this right now." To stand up for the principle of justice in this situation may risk alienating colleagues (the hard right) and requires moral courage. The easy wrong is to say nothing. Moral courage requires more than *having* morals and values; it requires *living* them.

There is always some sort of risk involved in situations requiring moral courage. Healthcare professionals (and

everyone) must carefully assess the situation, the principles, and the actions involved; assess the risks versus the benefits of taking action; plan the action; and be prepared to endure the hardships involved. The processes of values clarification and ethical decision making also apply in situations involving moral courage.

✳ ACTIVE LEARNING
Moral Courage

Think of an experience in your daily life in which you demonstrated (or could have demonstrated) moral courage.
1. What were the risks to you of taking action?
2. What values or principles were involved?
3. Was it a right versus wrong or right versus right issue? Explain.
4. What were some inhibitors or barriers to taking action?
5. Applying the information you learned in this chapter, would you have acted differently? Why or why not?

INTERPROFESSIONAL ETHICS AS AN EMERGING FIELD

Interprofessional ethics is an emerging field. A new paradigm is needed to prepare professionals to resolve ethical issues within an interprofessional context. Each profession brings its own perspective to patient-centered interprofessional care, and all professionals desire to practice to the full extent of their legal scope of practice. Because there may be considerable overlap in skills, conflict may arise (Engel & Prentice, 2013). Adding to the potential tension is that "roles, tasks, and accountabilities are guided by values and beliefs that are particular to disciplines" (Engel & Prentice, 2013, p. 427); beliefs about right and wrong, good and bad, and what constitutes beneficence may differ between disciplines.

Interprofessional ethics can serve to prevent or avoid interprofessional conflict and enhance collaboration. Keep in mind that "ethics education shares a single groundwork: helping students sharpen the processes by which they reason through complex issues and prioritize certain concerns over others in taking action" (Caldicott & Braun, 2011, p. 145). This transcends the narrower focus of a single discipline. With the increasing focus on interprofessional care and teamwork in the current healthcare environment, diverse professionals must be able to work together in an atmosphere of mutual respect and understanding toward a common goal of ethically sensitive, quality health care. To do so requires preparation for interprofessional teams to work through and resolve the difficult ethical situations that are inevitable in health care. This entails more than knowledge of ethics and your professional code of ethics. Interprofessional ethics is an emerging field that requires applying the Core Competencies of Interprofessional Collaboration to the resolution of ethical issues in health care.

✴ ACTIVE LEARNING
Interprofessional Oath

Carefully read the interprofessional oath in the Research Highlight box.
1. What are your thoughts about it?
2. Is it consistent with your personal morals and professional ethics? Give an example.
3. Would you change it in any way, add or subtract any statement? Explain your reasons.
4. Would you be willing to take such an oath? Why or why not?

◢ RESEARCH HIGHLIGHT
Proposed Interprofessional Oath

Brown, Garber, Lash, & Schnurman-Cook (2014) used qualitative research to identify shared values based on the IPEC (2011) Core Competencies of Values/Ethics and Teamwork. Eighteen oaths were developed by interprofessional teams. The researchers identified themes and used them to develop an interprofessional oath based on common values shared by participants.

Proposed Interprofessional Oath

We make this oath in due faith and we recognize the unique role of being a healthcare professional and the associated responsibilities which include honesty, faithfulness, compassion and collaboration.

We pledge to promote health in individuals and the community rather than just treating the sick. We will protect privacy and confidentiality.

The patient is the ultimate priority and focus of our care. Our role is to empower, teach and promote health in the patient, treating all persons equally and appropriately. The patient is more than a body and we will benefit the patient rather than harm.

Our care will be of the highest quality, safe, and based on evidence. We will seek to provide care within our scope of practice with ever-growing knowledge and skills.

We will work with others to provide care, recognizing the unique skills of each and we will seek to collaborate effectively on the healthcare team.

Brown, S., Garber, J., Lash, J., et al. (2014). A proposed interprofessional oath. *Journal of Interprofessional Care*, 28(5), 471-472.

📄 ADDITIONAL RESOURCES

Chapters 4 and 5 provide the foundations of values and ethics and highlighted specific perspectives and behaviors needed for interprofessional collaboration. These chapters focus on working with patients, families, and other team members in an atmosphere of trust and mutual respect. The following resources are provided to assist you when exploring the concepts of interprofessional values and ethics.

Professional Codes of Ethics. To locate the Code of Ethics for a health profession, go to that profession's professional organization's website. A list of links for these websites is located in Appendix A.

CITI Training for Research with Human Subjects. CITI Training is required by many institutions to conduct research with human subjects. The training modules are online and in a self-learning format. This site provides comprehensive information for use by all professions and students regarding the ethical conduct of healthcare research. A certificate indicating successful completion of the training is available, and professional continuing education contact hours are available for select professions for a fee. It contains information about ethical principles. https://about.citiprogram.org/en/homepage/

Continued

📄 **ADDITIONAL RESOURCES—cont'd**

The Hastings Center. "Founded in 1969, The Hastings Center is the world's first bioethics research institute. It is a nonpartisan, nonprofit organization of research scholars from multiple disciplines, including philosophy, law, political science, and education. Our team includes other staff members with expertise in communications, publishing, and finance and a worldwide network of elected Fellows, an active board, and an advisory council. The Hastings Center and its scholars produce books, articles, and other publications on ethical questions in medicine, science, and technology that help inform policy, practice, and public understanding" (Hastings Center, 2017, par. 1). This is an interprofessional resource site for bioethics research. http://www.thehastingscenter.org/who-we-are/

The Joint Centre for Bioethics. This organization is a collaboration of the University of Toronto and several affiliated health organizations, including the World Health Organization. The Joint Centre for Bioethics is one of six member bioethics centers in the Global Network of WHO Collaborating Centres for bioethics. The Centre is dedicated to the advancement of education, research, and the practice of bioethics. Their website provides some free resources, especially in the Community Tools section. http://jcb.utoronto.ca/index.shtml

Cultural Competence for Health Professional. This is an online, self-paced course designed for health professions students (including dental students) to provide a foundation in cultural competence and strategies to appropriately address cross-cultural issues in clinical settings. The University of Minnesota provides the course with a free registration. https://learning.umn.edu/search/publicCourseSearchDetails.do?method=load&courseId=1408677

KEY POINTS

- It is important for healthcare professionals to understand key theories of ethics and bioethics because everyone will experience ethical issues and ethical dilemmas during their careers. Members of the healthcare team may come from differing ethical perspectives. It is helpful to understand what these are to work together effectively and resolve differences.

- It is necessary for you as a healthcare professional to use values clarification to identify your own values and those of patients and families. Healthcare professionals should assist patients and families in making informed decisions

- The ethical principles of autonomy, beneficence, non-maleficence, justice, fidelity, and veracity are key foundational concepts necessary for understanding and achieving the IPEC (2011; 2016) Core Competency and Sub-competencies of Values/Ethics in Chapter 5.

- You and the healthcare team share responsibility to assist patients in making informed decisions that are consistent with the patient's own values. You and the healthcare team must make sure the patient is informed of all available options with their pros and cons. You and the team can discuss with the patient which option you think is best and explain why, but the decision ultimately belongs to the patient and must be accepted and supported.

- To make a decision when faced with an ethical issue or dilemma requires a process by which to analyze and examine the situation, weigh alternatives, and come up with a solution or decision that the interprofessional team finds ethically acceptable. This process must consider all stakeholders who may be affected by the decision. The healthcare team should use a formal model or method of ethical decision making to resolve ethical issues and dilemmas.

- To remain true to one's own professional code of ethics and personal morals, function as an effective member of an interprofessional team, and advocate for patients and families, you may need to demonstrate moral courage. Moral courage is having the will to speak out and do the right thing. It requires turning principles into action, actually having the courage to *do* something.

- Although each healthcare profession has its own code of ethics to which all members of that profession must adhere, there is a need to develop interprofessional ethics to maintain a climate of mutual respect and shared values. This is explored further in Chapter 5.

REFERENCES

Black, P. (2011). Ethics: Basic concepts for nursing practice. In K. Chitty & B. Black (Eds.), *Professional nursing: Concepts and challenges* (pp. 99–125). Maryland Heights, MO: Saunders Elsevier.

Brown, S., Garber, J., Lash, J., et al. (2014). A proposed interprofessional oath. *Journal of Interprofessional Care, 28*(5), 471–472.

Caldicott, C., & Braun, E. (2011). Should professional ethics education incorporate single-professional or interprofessional learning? *Advances in Health Science Education, 16*, 143–146.

Centers for Medicare & Medicaid Services (CMS). (2012). *Emergency Medical Treatment & Labor Act (EMTALA)*. Retrieved from https://www.cms.gov/Regulations-and-Guidance/Legislation/EMTALA.

Dougherty, R., & Purtilo, R. (2016). *Ethical dimensions in the health professions*. St. Louis, MO: Elsevier.

Engel, J., & Prentice, D. (2013). The ethics of interprofessional collaboration. *Nursing Ethics, 20*(4), 426–435.

Epstein, E. G., & Delgado, S. (2010). Understanding and addressing moral distress. *OJIN: The Online Journal of Issues in Nursing, 15*(3), Manuscript 1.

Ganske, K. M. (2010). Moral distress in academia. *OJIN: The Online Journal of Issues in Nursing, 15*(3), Manuscript 6.

Interprofessional Education Collaborative Expert Panel (IPEC). (2011). *Core competencies for interprofessional collaborative practice: Report of an expert panel.* Washington, DC: Interprofessional Education Collaborative.

Interprofessional Education Collaborative. (2016). *Core competencies for interprofessional collaborative practice: 2016 update.* Washington, DC: Interprofessional Education Collaborative.

Jameton, A. (1984). *Nursing practice: The ethical issues.* Englewood Cliffs, NJ: Prentice Hall.

Johnstone, M. (2016). *Bioethics: A nursing perspective* (6th ed.). Chatsworth, Australia: Elsevier Australia.

Kidder, R. (2005). *Moral courage.* New York: Harper Collins.

Mizner, S., Grabow, N., & Klammt, S. (2016). Artificial liver treatment, when and which one? In C. Doria (Ed.), *Contemporary liver transplantation* (pp. 1–18). Cham (ZG), Switzerland: Springer International Publishing AG.

National Commission for the Protection of Human Subjects of Biomedical and Behavioral Research. (1979). *The Belmont Report: Ethical principles and guidelines for the protection of human subjects of research.* Washington, DC: United States Government Printing Office.

O'Toole, M. (Ed.). (2017). *Mosby's medical dictionary* (10th ed.). St. Louis, MO: Elsevier.

Schwartz, L., Preece, P., & Hendry, R. (2016). *Medical ethics.* Philadelphia: Saunders Elsevier.

Scott, R. (2009). *Promoting legal and ethical awareness: A primer for health professionals and patients.* St. Louis, MO: Mosby Elsevier.

Shivayogi, P. (2013). Vulnerable population and methods for their safeguard. *Perspectives in Clinical Research, 4*(1), 53–57.

5

The Competency of Values/Ethics

LEARNING OUTCOMES

After studying this chapter, you will be able to:

1. Place the interests of patients and populations at the center of interprofessional health care delivery and population health programs, with the goal of promoting health and health equity across the lifespan.
2. Respect the dignity and privacy of patients while maintaining confidentiality in the delivery of team-based care.
3. Embrace the cultural diversity and individual differences that characterize patients, populations, and the health team.
4. Respect the unique cultures, values, roles and responsibilities, and expertise of other health professions and the impact these factors can have on health outcomes.
5. Work in cooperation with those who receive care, those who provide care, and others who contribute to or support the delivery of prevention and health services and programs.
6. Develop a trusting relationship with patients, families, and other team members.
7. Develop high standards of ethical conduct and quality of care in contributions to team-based care.
8. Manage ethical dilemmas specific to interprofessional patient/ population centered care situations.
9. Act with honesty and integrity in relationships with patients, families, communities, and other team members.
10. Maintain competence in your own profession appropriate to your scope and level of practice.

This chapter explains and operationalizes the Core Competency of Values/Ethics for Interprofessional Practice and its related Sub-competencies, as defined by the Interprofessional Education Collaborative Expert Panel (IPEC, 2011; 2016). Current issues in values/ethics are presented in terms of application to practice. Foundational concepts presented in Chapter 4 are integrated and applied to situations that may be encountered in practice.

Each specific Sub-competency of the Values/Ethics for Interprofessional Practice competency is explained. A case study model is used for the illustration and operationalization of selected Sub-competencies; self-evaluation exercises are included for each Sub-competency. You are encouraged to apply each Sub-competency to examples from your own experience or professional practice to increase your understanding of how interprofessional collaboration in the domain of values and ethics can improve patient-centered and population-focused care.

After the presentation of the Values/Ethics (VE) Core Competency Statement and specific Sub-competencies, case studies and caselets are used as appropriate to set the stage and illustrate each specific behavior. Please note that not every possible profession or team member is involved in the provided patient care scenarios. Additional case studies are provided in Chapter 6. You are encouraged to apply each specific Sub-competency to examples in your own clinical practice and experience to determine any missed opportunities for Interprofessional Collaborative Practice. An exemplar case study is provided at the conclusion of the chapter to illustrate successful application of the Values/Ethics Core Competency.

THE VALUES/ETHICS CORE COMPETENCY STATEMENT

Work with individuals of other professions to maintain a climate of mutual respect and shared values (IPEC, 2016, p. 11).

THE SUB-COMPETENCIES OF VALUES/ETHICS FOR INTERPROFESSIONAL PRACTICE

All healthcare professionals, regardless of discipline, face ethical issues and dilemmas throughout their careers. Addressing ethical dilemmas that arise while collaborating with team members is key to successful resolution. To collaborate effectively, you must be able to reflect on your own personal and professional values. As a healthcare professional, you must be able to identify how your values and those of other team members impact team functioning and ethical decision-making ability (University of Toronto, 2008).

Interprofessional values and ethics are "patient centered with a community/population orientation, grounded in a sense of shared purpose to support the common good in healthcare, and reflect a shared commitment to creating safer, more efficient, and more effective systems of care" (IPEC, 2011, p. 17). The focus on population health is even stronger in the IPEC (2016) update, along with emphasis on the triple aim of (1) improving the experience of care, (2) improving the health of populations, and (3) reducing the per capita cost of health care. The "new" healthcare professional develops professional values that are based on ensuring public trust. In addition to adhering to and incorporating the code of ethics specific to the individual's discipline, the modern professional must apply values and ethics in an interdisciplinary practice environment. Without attention to values and ethics, the patient experience in the Triple Aim (Berwick, Nolan, & Whittington, 2008) cannot be fully realized. Promoting population health while respecting the needs of the individual may give rise to ethical issues or dilemmas; how do we ethically give the best treatment? Another potential ethical concern is how to provide optimal care while achieving cost reductions.

The approach recommended by the 2011 IPEC panel and reinforced in the 2016 update focuses on the values that form the foundation of interprofessional relationships, relationships with patients and families, interprofessional communication, and ethical issues related to health policy and programs. Essential among these values is that of mutual respect among professionals, patients, families, and communities (IPEC, 2011; 2016). According to the Interprofessional Education Collaborative Panel (2011), "Mutual respect and trust are foundational to effective interprofessional working relationships for collaborative care across the health professions. At the same time, collaborative care honors the diversity that is reflected in the individual expertise each profession brings to care delivery" (p. 18). Interprofessional collaboration must be based on mutual respect and trust to be effective. The expertise that each professional brings to the team, as well as the perspective of the recipients of care, is seen as essential to promote optimal outcomes. This diversity and respect creates a team in which the whole is greater than the sum of its parts. The trust among interprofessional team members makes collaborative decision making around value-laden or complex ethical decisions possible and effective. Interprofessional communication skills are necessary to identify values and articulate ethical aspects of care. Box 5.1 contains the Sub-competencies of Values/Ethics for Interprofessional Practice (IPEC, 2016).

VE1: Place the Interests of Patients and Populations at the Center of Interprofessional Health Care Delivery and Population Health Programs, With the Goal of Promoting Health and Health Equity Across the Lifespan

The first Sub-competency in the IPEC (2011; 2016) Competency of Values/Ethics places the interests of patients and populations at the center of interprofessional health care delivery. The patient or population is the focus of care; the patient may be an individual, a family, a community, or a population. Patient-centered care is emphasized in the Institute of Medicine's (IOM, 2001a) report, *Crossing the Quality Chasm: A New Health System for the 21st Century*. This report defines patient-centered care as "providing care that is respectful of and responsive to individual patient preferences, needs, and values, and ensuring that patient values guide all clinical decisions" (IOM, 2001a, p. 40). Patient-centered care is one of six specific aims that should form the core of a restructured healthcare system, according to this report. Healthcare planning and decision making should be based on meeting

BOX 5.1   The Sub-Competencies of Values/Ethics for Interprofessional Practice

VE1. Place the interests of patients and populations at the center of interprofessional health care delivery and population health programs, with the goal of promoting health and health equity across the lifespan.

VE2. Respect the dignity and privacy of patients while maintaining confidentiality in the delivery of team-based care.

VE3. Embrace the cultural diversity and individual differences that characterize patients, populations, and the health team.

VE4. Respect the unique cultures, values, roles/responsibilities, and expertise of other health professions and the impact these factors can have on health outcomes.

VE5. Work in cooperation with those who receive care, those who provide care, and others who contribute to or support the delivery of prevention and health services and programs.

VE6. Develop a trusting relationship with patients, families, and other team members CIHC, 2010).

VE7. Demonstrate high standards of ethical conduct and quality of care in contributions to team-based care.

VE8. Manage ethical dilemmas specific to interprofessional patient/ population centered care situations.

VE9. Act with honesty and integrity in relationships with patients, families, communities and other team members.

VE10. Maintain competence in one's own profession appropriate to scope of practice.

From Interprofessional Education Collaborative Expert Panel (IPEC). (2016). *Core competencies for interprofessional collaborative practice: 2016 update.* Washington, DC: Interprofessional Education Collaborative.

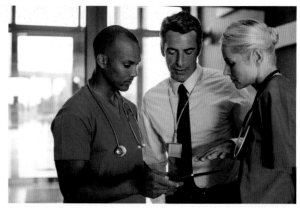

FIG. 5.1 The best interests of the patient are the primary concern of the healthcare team. (© Ridofranz/iStock/Thinkstock.)

🌐 GLOBAL PERSPECTIVE

The Canadian Interprofessional Health Collaborative (CIHC) stated the following about patient-centered care:
- It requires a balance between the professional knowledge of care providers and the personal knowledge of the patient and their family.
- It ensures the patient is listened to, valued, and engaged in conversation and decision-making about his or her own healthcare needs.
- It focuses on the patient's goals and the professional expertise of the team.
- It adds the knowledge of all team members to the patient's self-knowledge and self-awareness.

(CIHC, 2010a, p. 1)

patient needs in the safest, most effective way that takes into account patient values, culture, spiritual needs, and preferences. In planning care, the interprofessional team must consider patient values, culture, spiritual needs, and preferences (Fig. 5.1). Consider Case Study: Maria Sanchez, Part 1.

The other aspect of this Sub-competency emphasizes the community or population as the center of care. Populations are made up of individuals, and by placing the individual's interest at the center of care, we also affect population health. However, ethical issues sometimes arise when weighing what is best for a population versus what is best for, or preferred by, an individual. An example is the issue of mandatory immunizations for employees in a given healthcare setting. Mandatory immunizations are responsible for dramatic reductions in serious communicable disease, such as measles and polio. Although they protect the population at large, immunization regulations may infringe upon individual autonomy. Most healthcare facilities require healthcare professionals involved in direct patient care to have certain immunizations, such as hepatitis B and annual influenza immunizations. The policy of mandatory immunizations illustrates placing the interests of the population at the center of care (Fig. 5.2).

Self-Evaluation of VE1

Place the interests of patients and populations at the center of interprofessional health care delivery and

CASE STUDY

Maria Sanchez, Part 1

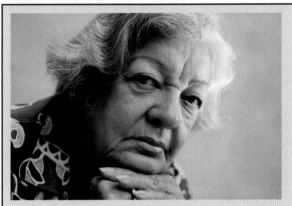

(© diego_cervo/iStock/Thinkstock.)

Maria Sanchez is a 66-year-old widow who lives alone. She has a daughter who lives in a different city, 16 hours away by car. The rest of Mrs. Sanchez's relatives are in Puerto Rico. She experiences progressive difficulty breathing, shortness of breath, and fatigue. Her ankles are swollen, and she has difficulty walking. She asks a neighbor to drive her to the Emergency Department of her local hospital. She is diagnosed with congestive heart failure (CHF), a chronic illness that will require lifestyle changes and follow-up visits to her physician. Mrs. Sanchez has Medicare as her insurance. Medicare pays the hospital for a certain number of days for the diagnosis of CHF. If her hospital stay exceeds that number, the hospital will lose money. On the other hand, if she stays less than that number of days the hospital will make money. It is in the financial best interest of the hospital to discharge her as soon as possible.

Mrs. Sanchez informs her daughter that she is in the hospital, and they decide to wait until they know when she will be discharged and what will be required before making arrangements for the daughter to visit. Mrs. Sanchez is prescribed several medications and given medication education information written in Spanish. She is seen by a nutritionist and told she must modify her diet and limit fluids. The sample diet and recommendations include few foods she actually eats and is not tailored to her cultural diet. She is told she must exercise and lose weight. She must also control her cholesterol and blood pressure. Mrs. Sanchez is overwhelmed and scared and has difficulty taking in all of this information. Although she does feel somewhat better, she is still quite fatigued. She asks her daughter to come. It will take her daughter several days to make arrangements to get there.

Mrs. Sanchez is told she can go home. She is given several prescriptions to fill and told to follow up with her doctor. The social worker gives her a voucher to pay for a taxi, and she is sent home. She arrives home alone, with no one to assist her. She has no follow-up appointments and does not clearly understand what she is supposed to do. In tears, she calls her daughter saying she does not know what to do.

Discussion Questions

1. Were Mrs. Sanchez and her specific needs the center of care delivery? Consider that her medical condition was treated according to guidelines.
2. What could be done differently to ensure a more positive outcome?
3. How could interprofessional teamwork ensure that the patient is the center of care delivery?

---

population health programs, with the goal of promoting health and health equity across the lifespan.

1. Reflect on the policy of mandatory immunizations for healthcare professionals and employees.
2. Discuss with a peer how your own beliefs about immunizations might conflict with such a mandate.
3. Identify how such policies put individual patient needs at the center of care while promoting population health.

When you can consistently place the interests of patients and populations at the center of interprofessional health care delivery, with the goal of promoting health

and health equity across the lifespan, you have demonstrated Sub-competency VE1.

VE2: Respect the Dignity and Privacy of Patients While Maintaining Confidentiality in the Delivery of Team-Based Care

Human beings have a basic right to privacy. Sub-competency VE2 addresses the many tasks that healthcare professionals must perform during the delivery of care that have the potential to violate privacy and dignity if care is not taken to respect patient rights. In healthcare

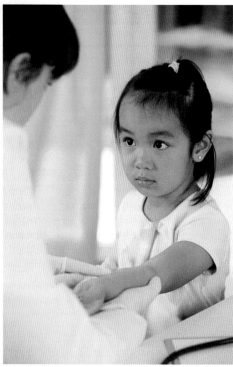

FIG. 5.2 Immunizations place the best interests of the population at the center of health care. (© KatarzynaBialasiewicz/iStock/Thinkstock.)

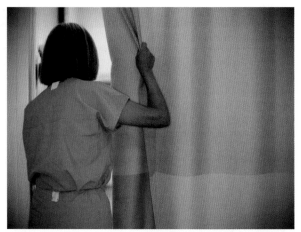

FIG. 5.3 Respecting patient privacy and dignity. (© ERproductions Ltd/Blend Images/Thinkstock.)

✳ ACTIVE LEARNING

Patient-Centered Care

Mrs. Infield brings her children to the neighborhood children's clinic for routine health care. She tells you that after reading the possible side effects of the measles vaccinations and what she has seen on the Internet about the negative effects of immunizations, she is not sure whether she should have her children get the measles vaccine.

Discussion Question
1. How would you make Mrs. Infield (your patient) the center of care, while also considering the population as center of care?

---

facilities, it is often difficult to maintain patient privacy; however, it can be done if all healthcare workers make a conscious effort to do so. Think about the experience of being a patient in an acute care hospital. The person may be required to share a room and bathroom with a stranger. There is often only a fabric curtain separating the roommates (Fig. 5.3). The patient is confined to bed most of the time and must wear a hospital gown or sleepwear. Healthcare professionals often must examine private body parts and touch patients in sensitive areas. You might say the entire experience of being a hospital patient can be undignified. Healthcare professionals must realize this and take steps to actively protect patient privacy and dignity. Knocking on the door and requesting permission to enter displays respect for patient privacy. For example, sitting down to speak with the patient instead of standing over him or her puts you both at the same level and implies that you will take time to listen. Making sure the door is closed and the curtain is drawn before examining the patient is essential, even if you will only need a few minutes. The same is true in outpatient settings, such as a busy public health dental clinic with several dental chairs in one large room. Keeping your voice low when discussing care or waiting until the patient's roommate is out of the area or asleep may help protect privacy and confidentiality. Always tell the patient what you are going to do before touching him or her, and expose as little skin as possible.

It is important to know that you may not release patient information to anyone without the patient's written permission. This includes the patient's family members, other healthcare facilities, and, in certain cases, other members of the healthcare team. For example, a surgeon may not release the operative report to the patient's primary care physician without the patient's written permission, even though they are both members of the patient's team and the primary care provider will be responsible for ongoing care after the patient is discharged from the hospital.

Most healthcare professionals are required to use electronic medical records (EMRs) in the delivery of care. The issue of the privacy and confidentiality of electronic medical information is complex. It is unethical for healthcare professionals to access the EMR of any person unless they are directly involved in the person's care or have an administrative reason to access the information. It may be tempting to look at the EMR of someone you know, but it is both unethical and illegal and is usually grounds for immediate dismissal and possible legal action, as illustrated in Caselet 5.1.

CASELET 5.1   Electronic Medical Records and the Mayor

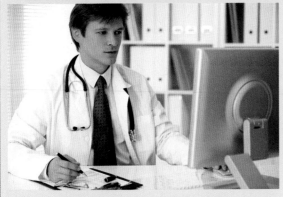

(© Andrei_r/iStock/Thinkstock.)

The mayor of a major city was involved in a motor vehicle crash and was transported to a local hospital. The news media covered the incident, so the hospital to which the mayor was admitted was public knowledge. A healthcare professional working at the hospital, but not involved in the mayor's care, was curious about the mayor's condition and accessed the mayor's electronic medical record (EMR). EMR access requires a password and is electronically recorded. The hospital's privacy officer checked to see who accessed the mayor's record, and the healthcare professional was immediately fired.

Discussion Questions

1. Was the hospital justified in firing the employee? Explain why or why not.
2. Was the mayor's dignity, privacy, and confidentiality violated? Explain.

E-mail and texting present other issues regarding patient privacy and confidentiality. Healthcare team members often use e-mail and texting to communicate with one another. E-mail may be seen by others or accessed by information technology (IT) personnel. It is best to keep identifying information out of e-mail or use other means of communication. For example, you might mention "the patient we discussed earlier" or "the patient in room 123." Texting provides an easy form of communication between team members. It may be tempting to text a social worker with a question about discharge plans or a physician to obtain orders. This may violate privacy and confidentiality. Texting is best used to alert members of the team to an immediate need to contact you or to access the patient's EMR for pertinent information, without providing specific patient information in the text. Many institutions issue telephones at the beginning of each shift for ease and efficiency of communication. Care must be taken not to discuss identifiable patient information within earshot of others. Each facility has a specific policy regarding the use of these phones. It is inappropriate and a violation of patient privacy and confidentiality to post photographs or other patient information on any form of social media. Although it may be tempting to take a "selfie" with a patient and post it, this is a privacy violation.

Before communicating any patient-related information, stop a moment and think about whether you may be violating confidentiality. Before interacting with a patient or performing a treatment, be sure the environment is such that you will not risk compromising patient privacy.

Some may question whether there is a risk that patient confidentiality may be compromised during team-based care. Remember that the patient is also an important member of the healthcare team. The patient must be kept informed and participate in his or her care. The United Kingdom based Medical Defence Union offers this advice regarding confidentiality and the healthcare team: "Tell patients why, when, and with whom information will be shared" (Medical Defence Union, 2017, par. 2). It is important that patients are oriented to the concept of team-based care (Schottenfeld, 2016). This can be done formally through brochures and admission materials, and informally through discussions with the patient and family. Most healthcare facilities and providers have patients sign a form that indicates specific family members or friends allowed to receive information from providers about the patient's care or condition. All members of the team should be aware of and respect this.

Self-Evaluation of VE2

Respect the dignity and privacy of patients while maintaining confidentiality in the delivery of team-based care.

1. Think of a situation in your clinical practice or in your personal experience in which you may have violated someone's confidentiality or did not provide enough privacy, or when you did take steps to protect patient privacy and dignity. What was the outcome for the other person?
   a. How did you feel?
   b. How did it affect your relationship with the other person?
   c. What will you do in the future to ensure dignity, privacy, and confidentiality in patient care?

If you respected the dignity and privacy of a patient while maintaining confidentiality in the delivery of team-based care, you have demonstrated Sub-competency VE2 in this situation.

VE3: Embrace the Cultural Diversity and Individual Differences That Characterize Patients, Populations, and the Health Team

Note that the first word in the VE3 Sub-competency is "embrace." This is critical to understanding this Sub-competency. To embrace is to welcome, incorporate, or support. It does *not* mean merely to tolerate, accept, put up with, or endure cultural differences. To meet this Sub-competency, you must truly celebrate such differences and welcome the opportunity to learn from and with those who may be different from you; this includes members of the healthcare team. Culture may be defined as "that complex whole which includes knowledge, beliefs, arts, morals, laws, customs, and any other capabilities and habits acquired by [a human] as a member of society. The term sub-culture is used to refer to minority cultures within a larger dominant culture" (UNESCO, 2016, par. 1). Consider Caselet 5.2.

Healthcare professionals' cultural backgrounds influence how they see their patients, in the same way that the culture of patients influences the way they see healthcare professionals. Also notice that VE3 calls for "embracing the cultural diversity" of the healthcare team. This includes the culture of the organization, the healthcare professionals, the community, and the patient.

CASELET 5.2   Embracing Cultural Differences

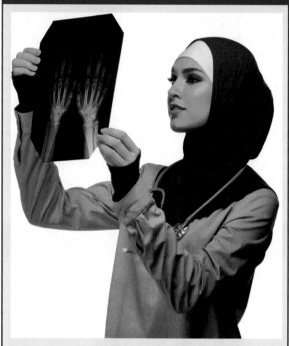

(© rbv/iStock/Thinkstock.)

Two healthcare professionals share a small office. One of them tells the other he is going to the cafeteria to bring back lunch and asks her if she wants anything. She says no, and explains that she is observing Ramadan and is fasting from dawn to sunset during the month-long holiday. Her officemate is unfamiliar with the holiday and its observance and asks her to explain it to him, which she does. As a result, he learned about another culture, and was able to support and respect his colleague by not eating or drinking in the office in front of her during her fast.

Discussion Question

Think of an opportunity you had to educate another person about your culture or learn about his or hers.
1. How did this enhance your relationship and your understanding of other cultures?

Each individual is culturally unique, and beliefs and practices vary within every culture. It may be useful to have a member of the healthcare team perform a cultural assessment with the patient to determine the specific needs of that individual. Ask the individual about his or her cultural beliefs and practices regarding health

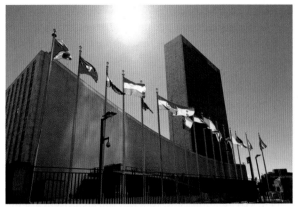

FIG. 5.4 The United Nations Educational, Scientific, and Cultural Organization (UNESCO) issued a declaration on cultural diversity in 2001. (© mizoula/iStock/Thinkstock.)

and illness, treatment, diet, and communication. Assess for biological variations and susceptibilities. Be aware of culturally compatible resources available within the organization and community, such as cultural centers, charitable organizations, spiritual and religious resources, and support services targeted toward specific groups, such as older adults or African Americans.

To embrace cultural diversity is to appreciate differences among individuals and cultural groups. Cultural groups can be related to ethnicity, religion, race, geography, socioeconomics, class, occupation, ability or disability, sexual orientation, belief systems, or other characteristics. Healthcare professionals must be prepared to accept and work with individuals from varied backgrounds, whether they are patients, other professionals, or entire populations (e.g., the Lesbian Gay Bisexual Transgender [LGBT] community, or people with disabilities) to provide care in a culturally sensitive, caring, nonjudgmental way. The ethical principle of justice requires fair and equitable treatment of all patients.

In 2001, the United Nations Educational, Scientific, and Cultural Organization (UNESCO) issued a Universal Declaration on Cultural Diversity (Fig. 5.4). Box 5.2 contains excerpts that will help you understand the true meaning of cultural diversity within the global community.

To embrace cultural diversity, it is necessary to avoid stereotyping. Stereotyping is the assumption that all people in a similar group are alike and share values, beliefs, behaviors, and attributes. Each person is culturally unique, and beliefs and practices vary within every culture. The best way to avoid stereotyping is to treat each person as

---

BOX 5.2 United Nations Educational, Scientific, and Cultural Organization (UNESCO) Universal Declaration on Cultural Diversity Excerpts

Firstly, the Declaration promotes the principle that "culture takes diverse forms across time and space. This diversity is embodied in the uniqueness and plurality of the identities of the groups and societies making up humankind. As a source of exchange, innovation and creativity, cultural diversity is as necessary for humankind as biodiversity is for nature. In this sense, it is the common heritage of humanity and should be recognized and affirmed for the benefit of present and future generations." (Article 1)

Secondly, the Declaration emphasises [sic] the understanding of moving from cultural diversity to cultural pluralism. "In our increasingly diverse societies, it is essential to ensure harmonious interaction among people and groups with plural, varied and cultural identities as well as their willingness to live together. Policies for the inclusion and participation of all citizens are guarantees of social cohesion, the vitality of civil society and peace. Thus defined, cultural pluralism gives policy expression to the reality of cultural diversity. Indissociable [sic] from a democratic framework, cultural pluralism is conducive to cultural exchange and to the flourishing of creative capacities that sustain public life." (Article 2)

Thirdly, the Declaration delineates cultural diversity as a factor in development. "Cultural diversity widens the range of options open to everyone; it is one of the roots of development, understood not simply in terms of economic growth, but also as a means to achieve a more satisfactory intellectual, emotional, moral and spiritual existence." (Article 3)

Finally, cultural diversity presupposes the respect for human rights. "The defence [sic] of cultural diversity is an ethical imperative, inseparable from respect for human dignity. It implies a commitment to human rights and fundamental freedoms, in particular the rights of persons belonging to minorities and those of indigenous peoples. No one may invoke cultural diversity to infringe upon human rights guaranteed by international law, nor to limit their scope." (Article 4)

From UNESCO. (2016). Cultural diversity. Retrieved from http://www.unesco.org/new/en/social-and-human-sciences/themes/international-migration/glossary/cultural-diversity/

a unique individual and directly ask each person whether he or she has any cultural or spiritual needs or preferences. Madeleine Leininger developed the classic theory of transcultural nursing. She recommended that, when faced with unfamiliar ethnic or cultural health practices, healthcare professionals should preserve practices that promote health, accommodate practices that are not harmful, and restructure potentially harmful practices by negotiating better practices (Leininger, 2002).

Be aware of culturally compatible resources available within the organization and community. The only way to truly embrace differences is to be willing to learn and to directly ask patients and families how the healthcare team can best meet their cultural (and spiritual) needs. In this way care becomes individualized and patient centered. Also, be aware that you and the members of your interprofessional team have your own cultural biases, and that some of these are related to your professional culture. Let's return to Case Study: Maria Sanchez, Part 2.

CASE STUDY

Maria Sanchez, Part 2

Mrs. Sanchez was given standard dietary and nutritional education that did not account for her cultural diet. Most foods that she ate daily were not included in the information, so it was essentially useless to her. Because she was Hispanic and spoke with an accent, it was assumed she required information written in Spanish. However, she learned to read in an American elementary school. Although she speaks Spanish fluently, she cannot read Spanish. Materials written in English would be much more useful to her. In this example, Mrs. Sanchez was not the center of care, and her cultural needs were not addressed. This failure may lead to negative health outcomes.

Discussion Questions

1. How could the team demonstrate that they appreciate her cultural differences?
2. What evidence of stereotyping can you find in this scenario?
3. What could be done in this situation to avoid stereotyping and meet individual needs?

Self-Evaluation of VE3

Embrace the cultural diversity and individual differences that characterize patients, populations, and the health team.

1. Think about colleagues or fellow students who have a different cultural background from yours. If you have clinical experience, think about a patient or client who had a different cultural background.
   a. What do you know about their cultural beliefs and practices?
   b. How do you know this? Are you assuming based on stereotypes, or have you taken the time to learn about them as individuals?
   c. Reflect on your own cultural biases and beliefs.

When you are consistently able to embrace the cultural diversity and individual differences that characterize patients, populations, and yourself, you are demonstrating Sub-competency VE3.

🌐 GLOBAL PERSPECTIVES

The Need for a Global Ethic

"All ethics so far evolved rest upon a single premise: that the individual is a member a community of interdependent parts" (Leopold, 1940 in Goldberg & Patz, 2015, p. 1973). Think back to some of the ethical theories presented in Chapter 4. Each one considers not just one individual, but others as well. Goldberg and Patz (2015) stated that "Applied to global health, the health of each of us is linked to the health of all the rest." This is the basis for a need for a global ethic, one that transcends individuals, communities, and countries, and considers ethical issues in terms of the world as a whole (Goldberg & Patz, 2015). A true global ethic must transcend economics, allocation of resources, and politics. It must become a way of thinking and evaluating all health care. Goldberg and Patz (2015) contend that "each and every one of us, individually and through our relationships, will experience an intense consciousness of health—whether we live in a city in Africa or the woods of Wisconsin. Perhaps this shared reality might yet inspire the development of a global health ethic that all of society eventually embraces" (p. 1973).

VE4: Respect the Unique Cultures, Values, Roles/Responsibilities, and Expertise of Other Health Professions and the Impact These Factors Can Have on Health Outcomes

Each individual healthcare profession has its own culture, values, roles/responsibilities, and expertise. You must respect these factors to collaborate effectively and achieve positive patient outcomes. People brought up in the same

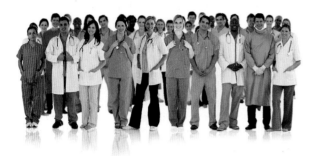

FIG. 5.5 Respect the unique cultures, values, roles and responsibilities, and expertise of other healthcare professions. (© Wavebreakmedia Ltd/Wavebreak Media/Thinkstock.)

culture tend to share a common set of core values and sense of morality (Beauchamp & Childress, 2013). This is true for professions as well. Each profession has its own culture, norms, and set of values. Each profession also has its own set of skills and standards, although some specific skills may be shared with other professions (Fig. 5.5). For example, almost all healthcare professionals are trained in pain assessment and are able to measure vital signs such as blood pressure and heart rate. However, the focus and total education of each profession add up to a unique area of expertise. Members of healthcare professions must respect the culture, values, and expertise of other healthcare professions. Although medicine may be seen as having a culture based on curing and nursing as having a focus on caring, this does not mean that physicians are not caring or that nurses are not interested in curing. Although speech language pathologists and physical therapists are focused on rehabilitation, this does not mean that their skills cannot be helpful in end-of-life care to assist with swallowing difficulties and to prevent painful contractures. Although dental care is often seen as an outpatient service, a dental consult may be indicated for a patient who has difficulty chewing or poor oral hygiene.

Each profession has its own code of ethics that all members of that profession must follow unconditionally. Although some elements of each profession's code of ethics may be similar to those of your own profession, others may differ slightly. The importance lies in recognizing that each professional has an obligation to practice according to the specific ethical guidelines of his or her profession, and in respecting this obligation. Beware of professional ethnocentrism. Ethnocentrism is the belief that one's own cultural beliefs and practice are superior to those of others (O'Toole, 2017).

✴ ACTIVE LEARNING

Professional Codes of Ethics

Look up the professional code of ethics for your chosen profession and that of another healthcare profession on the Internet.
1. Compare and contrast the codes of ethics.
2. What are the commonalities?
3. How do they differ?

Differences in professional cultures may affect healthcare outcomes. This effect may be positive, if professionals respect the unique cultures, values, roles/responsibilities, and expertise of other health professions, or negative if they do not. Consider Caselet 5.3.

Self-Evaluation of VE4

Respect the unique cultures, values, roles/responsibilities, and expertise of other health professions and the impact these factors can have on health outcomes.
1. Think of a situation in which the culture of one profession conflicted with that of another profession. If you cannot think of an actual situation in the healthcare setting, think of a potential or hypothetical situation in your personal life.
    a. How was the situation approached?
    b. How was the healthcare outcome affected?
    c. Did you think that one profession's expertise or values were superior to the others, or were you able to see both perspectives as equally important?

When you consistently show respect for the unique cultures, values, roles/responsibilities, and expertise of other health professions and the impact that these factors can have on health outcomes, then you have demonstrated the VE4 Sub-competency.

VE5: Work in Cooperation With Those Who Receive Care, Those Who Provide Care, and Others Who Contribute to or Support the Delivery of Prevention and Health Services and Programs

Although the part of health care delivery that relies on the unique expertise of each healthcare profession lends

CASELET 5.3 Ms. Williams

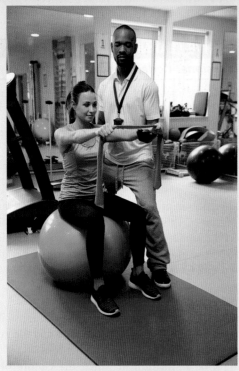

(© monkeybusinessimages/iStock/Thinkstock.)

Ms. Williams is a patient in an inpatient rehabilitation center after spinal fusion surgery. She experiences nausea and vomiting and is having pain. Her nurse contacts the physician and gets an order for medication to relieve the nausea. They are waiting for it to come from the pharmacy, so that she can then take her pain medication. The physical

therapist encourages Ms. Williams to attend therapy, and Ms. Williams says she does not feel up to therapy, but wants to comply. The nurse is focused on the immediate symptoms. The nurse and physical therapist discuss the situation with Ms. Williams. They respect each other's perspectives, and agree Ms. Williams should forego physical therapy that morning. Ms. Williams receives her medication and begins to feel better. The nurse encourages her to attend her afternoon physical therapy session, which she does. The nurse was focused on the nursing and medical care of the patient, whereas the physical therapist was focused on the rehabilitation goals. Both were correct, but by understanding the need for the patient to get her immediate symptoms under control, and also the need for therapy, the nurse and the physical therapist were able to work together, using their unique areas of expertise to improve the patient outcome. Ms. Williams felt better, got her nausea and pain under control, and only missed one therapy session.

Discussion Questions
1. How might the outcome in this caselet differ if the patient, nurse, and physical therapist had not collaborated?
2. Why was it important to involve Ms. Williams in the discussion?

---

itself to operate in isolation, effective, comprehensive health care can only happen when those providing and receiving care work in cooperation. Those who receive care may be individuals, families, communities, or entire populations. Those who provide care may include family members; community agencies; home health agencies; primary, secondary, and higher education facilities; and public health agencies. Outreach workers, transportation companies, and sanitation workers also perform services needed to protect the health of the population. Pharmacies provide immunizations and health education. Clinics may be located within schools, supermarkets, or workplaces.

As a healthcare professional, you must learn to work cooperatively with those who receive care, provide care,

prevent illness, and promote health to achieve the best possible healthcare outcomes. This may mean a primary care provider having office hours in the evening or on weekends to accommodate patients who work. It may also mean providing healthcare education for groups of patients with a specific health condition or who are at risk for a certain illness. Healthcare professionals can support the delivery of prevention and health services and programs by referring patients and posting or otherwise providing information to those who may benefit from such resources. For example, primary care providers can refer patients to smoking cessation programs. Information about flu immunization sites can be posted in rehabilitation facilities, and therapists can ask patients whether they received a flu shot for that year. It also means working with and considering the needs of those who provide care. Care providers may be family members, community agencies, or other healthcare professionals. They may benefit from participating in community support groups or professional conferences, respectively. Volunteering your services to community agencies, health fairs, and screenings and offering educational activities are just a few ways you can support health services and programs and disease prevention. Working cooperatively with other healthcare professionals is a theme that runs throughout this entire book, with many different aspects addressed in depth in different chapters.

A good example is Caselet 5.3 of Ms. Williams, which demonstrates not only respect for different professional cultures but also how to work cooperatively and collaborate interprofessionally to maximize patient outcomes.

Self-Evaluation of VE5

Work in cooperation with those who receive care, those who provide care, and others who contribute to or support the delivery of prevention and health services and programs.

1. Think of a time when you worked in cooperation with those who receive (e.g., as a provider) or who provide care (e.g., as a patient or family of a patient) to support the delivery of prevention and health services and programs. As a provider of care, this may have included delivering health education to the public or other professionals; referring patients, families, or other professionals to health services; or making them aware of specific programs (Fig. 5.6). As a recipient of care this could have meant remaining in contact with your healthcare providers, asking questions during visits, and seeking assistance from your social network. It may also have included getting involved in the care of a family member or friend, pointing out gaps in care, or advocating for better health policies. Reflect on the following:
    a. How did you or could you have cooperated to support the delivery of prevention services?
    b. How did you or could you have cooperated to support the delivery of health services?
    c. How did you or could you have cooperated to support the delivery of programs?

When you can demonstrate the ability to work in cooperation with those who receive care, those who provide care, and others who contribute to or support

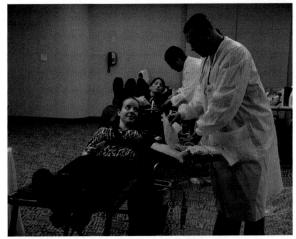

FIG. 5.6 Volunteering for community health fairs is a way that professionals can contribute to or support the delivery of prevention and health services and programs. (Cowperthwaite, L., & Lones, E. (2008). "Share Your Passion, Illuminate Our Profession" Congress Highlights. AORN Journal, 87(6), 1079-1087.)

the delivery of prevention and health services and programs, you have met the VE5 Sub-competency.

VE6: Develop a Trusting Relationship With Patients, Families, and Other Team Members

This Sub-competency addresses the need to develop a trusting relationship with patients, families, and other team members. It was adopted from the Canadian Interprofessional Health Collaborative's 2010 (CIHC, 2010b) National Interprofessional Competency Framework, in which it exists as a Sub-competency of Interprofessional Communication. This Sub-competency highlights the need for open and honest communication among healthcare professionals, patients, families, and other team members to build trust. It requires truth-telling (veracity) and keeping to your word (fidelity). To develop a trusting relationship, you must listen to what others are saying and take time to clarify meaning to foster understanding. Likewise, it requires you to believe (trust) that others are telling the truth. Building a trusting relationship requires focusing on patients as people first, including paying attention to their problems and concerns, without minimizing their importance.

Sub-competency VE6 requires full disclosure of information regarding risks and benefits of procedures and obtaining informed consent for procedures. You cannot withhold information from patients or team members. You must be honest about risks, benefits, and alternative treatments.

You must be honest with patients who may ask you to keep a secret that may affect care. You must tell them that you are required to share this information with the interprofessional team involved in their care, but will not disclose the information to others. Building a trusting relationship takes time and effort. If you are truthful and honest in your communication, and do what you say you will in terms of actions, it will enhance trust. Building a trusting relationship includes avoiding making promises you can't keep and avoiding statements like "it will all be okay" if the outcomes are not assured. You should not join in if a patient criticizes another member of the team; rather, you should encourage the patient to address the problem directly with that team member.

Developing trusting relationships with other healthcare workers requires trusting they will do a good job and complete their tasks. In return, when the other healthcare professionals follow through with their tasks, it will help you increase your trust in them, therefore making the relationship closer. Similarly, when you complete your tasks in a timely and efficient manner, you will be increasing the trust that other healthcare professionals put in you. Sharing decision making requires trust that each member of the team has something valuable to contribute; it also increases the trust among the people making the decision. If team members are trusted, then they will feel valued, which leads them to trust the team even more. The more people trust and are trusted, the more they feel involved. With this sense of involvement comes increased trust and openness. Fig. 5.7 illustrates the cycle of trust, which involves openness to trust, willingness to delegate, shared decisions, feeling valued, and a sense of involvement.

Interprofessional communication is essential to building a trusting relationship. It is important to understand that there are times that you may not be able to form a trusting relationship with some people due to their personal issues, past experiences, or general mistrust of the healthcare system and healthcare professional. Still, it is your obligation to continue to try and not give up.

Self-Evaluation of VE6

Develop a trusting relationship with patients, families, and other team members (CIHC, 2010b).

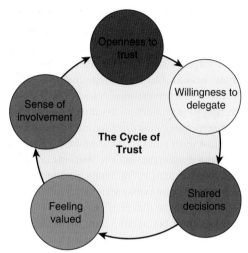

FIG. 5.7 The cycle of trust.

Consider the following questions:
1. Do your patients or team members call you when they have needs, questions, or concerns?
2. Do you take more time listening than talking in interactions?
3. Are others forthcoming with information?
4. Are you able to speak freely with patients, families, and other members of the team?
5. Are you comfortable asking each other questions and admitting that you don't know something?
6. Are you able to focus on patient and family and team needs rather than your own?

These questions may help you evaluate whether you have developed a trusting relationship.

When you are consistently able to develop trusting relationships with patients, families, and other team members, you are demonstrating the VE6 Sub-competency (Fig. 5.8).

VE7: Demonstrate High Standards of Ethical Conduct and Quality of Care in Contributions to Team-Based Care

When working with an interprofessional team, it is essential to demonstrate high standards of ethical conduct and quality of care. This requires adhering to the ethical principles of respect for persons, beneficence, nonmaleficence, fidelity, veracity, and justice (discussed in Chapter 4) when contributing to team-based care. You cannot relax and expect that someone else will point out an ethical issue or handle a difficult patient situation. You

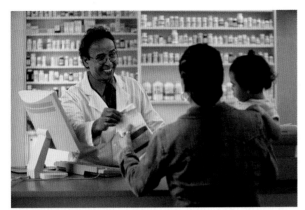

FIG. 5.8 Develop a trusting relationship with patients, families, and team members. (© Jose Luis Pelaex Inc./ Blend Images/Thinkstock.)

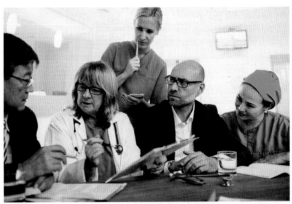

FIG. 5.9 Demonstrating high standards of ethical conduct and quality of care in contributions to team-based care requires commitment, respect for others, trust, and a nonjudgmental attitude. (© Rawpixel/iStock/Thinkstock.)

RESEARCH HIGHLIGHT

Pharmacy Community Relationships

A study involving 74 mental health consumers (patients) and caregivers used focus groups and interviews to explore the perceptions of and relationships with pharmacy staff. It highlighted the importance of patient-centered care and trusting relationships. Researchers found that trusting relationships among consumers, caregivers, and community pharmacy staff were seen as important in mental health care and contributed to views of the pharmacy as a safe healthcare space by both patients and caregivers. Formation of relationships were strongly influenced by participants' experiences in the pharmacy. "Positive experiences were identified as the main facilitator to (a) forming initial rapport, and (b) nurturing a relationship over time through open engagement and the development of trust" (Mey et al., 2013, p. 284). Positive experiences were also related to knowledgeable pharmacy staff and feeling welcome in the pharmacy. "Community pharmacy services that included core elements of patient-centred [sic] care appeared to facilitate relationship formation and associated benefits" (Mey et al., 2013, p. 281).

must be ready to provide your professional expertise and sometimes may need to question suggestions for care that are not based in evidence. You must follow your professional code of ethics at all times, while respecting that other professionals must follow theirs. Be prepared to offer an evidence-based rationale for your plan of care to ensure quality of care, and do not be afraid to ask for evidence when others suggest interventions. Acting

according to high ethical standards means keeping your commitment to the team and the patient, telling the truth, treating others fairly, and respecting others (Fig. 5.9).

An effective team "does not offer judgments but engages in reflection, open dialogue, and presents an openness to others" (Jason, Royeen, & Purtilo, 2010, p. 249). This represents a high standard of ethical conduct. Open reflection and dialogue with other team members help ensure quality of care. Dougherty and Purtilo (2016) developed a list of reasonable expectations for interprofessional team relationships. These expectations are based on the ethical principle of fidelity. They are listed in Box 5.3.

Treating other members of the interprofessional team (including the patient and family) respectfully and ethically is a theme that runs through this text and the IPEC Competencies of Interprofessional Collaboration. Chapter 13 is devoted to the foundations of teams and teamwork, and Chapter 14 operationalizes the competency of teams and teamwork. Rather than acting individually, respecting other members of the team and allowing them to use their expertise, voice their opinions, and enter into discussions about care, results in better patient outcomes. This professional collaboration ensures quality of care.

Self-Evaluation of VE7

Demonstrate high standards of ethical conduct and quality of care in contributions to team-based care.
1. Think of times when you had to work in a team.
   a. Were you able to meet the expectations listed in Box 5.3 consistently?

BOX 5.3   **Expectations of Team Relationships Based on the Ethical Principle of Fidelity**

1. Collegial trust, mutual respect, and the shared goal of a caring response
2. Substantive assistance from teammates regarding questions about good patient care or other matters of professional judgment
3. A willingness by all teammates to be flexible and carry a fair share of the workload
4. Sympathetic understanding regarding work-related stresses
5. An environment conducive to a high level of functioning and one that fosters work satisfaction for everyone involved, not just some members of the team
6. A commitment by everyone to respect differences in values and contributions of other team members and to embrace each person's unique gifts
7. Encouragement to develop both professionally and personally within the work environment
8. A commitment to establishing ways of communicating and working together that includes negotiating and developing roles with each other to support the team's work

From Dougherty, R. & Purtilo, R. (2016). *Ethical dimensions in the health professions.* St. Louis, MO: Elsevier.

b. Did you consciously adhere to the ethical principles of respect for persons, beneficence, non-maleficence, fidelity, veracity, and justice?
c. Was your team able to reflect and discuss potential decisions?
d. Was quality of care the ultimate goal?

When you consistently practice using high standards of ethical conduct and quality of care in contributions to team-based care you have demonstrated the VE7 Sub-competency.

VE8: Manage Ethical Dilemmas Specific to Interprofessional Patient/ Population Centered Care Situations

An ethical dilemma specific to interprofessional patient- or population-centered care situations is any ethical dilemma that arises during the team-based care of an individual or population. Managing ethical dilemmas in healthcare situations is a difficult skill to develop. It requires understanding that you as a healthcare professional are not working in isolation; you have a team to draw upon. It requires an understanding of basic ethical principles and theories discussed in Chapter 4. To effectively manage ethical dilemmas, you and the healthcare team must actively use an agreed-upon formal ethical decision-making model. One is presented in Chapter 4; there are many others available. You may not have the luxury of a great deal of time in which to ponder ethical dilemmas, so it is a good idea to have an ethical decision-making process ready for use, should the need arise. One of the first issues is to determine exactly what the dilemma is, and whose decision it is to make. The decision may not be yours, and the problem may be that you do not agree with or have difficulty accepting the decision that was made.

Use available resources to assist in managing the ethical dilemma. You might discuss the situation with a supervisor or another member of the healthcare team, being careful not to violate confidentiality. Most hospitals and healthcare facilities have an ethics committee that could be called upon to assist with the patient-care dilemma. Some facilities have anonymous "ethics lines," which employees can use to anonymously report suspected or observed ethical violations without fear of reprisal. The situation is then investigated and addressed by appointed representatives in the facility. It is your responsibility to be aware of the resources available in your team and workplace and be able to access them. It is best to be informed about such resources *before* you need them instead of waiting until you are faced with an ethical dilemma in an actual care situation.

If you face a situation in which your personal values are in conflict with your professional responsibilities in care delivery, you are obligated to follow the code of ethics of your profession, state and federal laws, and facility policies. All of these should be known to you in advance of any ethical issue. Treat such a conflict as an ethical dilemma and utilize the strategies previously presented. Have a frank discussion within your healthcare team. It is always best to be proactive if you know that such conflicts are likely to arise. For example, if participating in an abortion procedure is against your religious beliefs, then you should not seek employment in a facility or unit in which abortions are commonly performed. Make such issues known to your supervisor and the healthcare team before a situation arises so that you are not assigned to a case that violates your beliefs.

✳ **ACTIVE LEARNING**

Managing Ethical Dilemmas

Pick a case study from Chapter 6 or one from your own experience. Use the ethical decision-making process outlined in Chapter 4 or a different one of your choice to work through the case and make a decision that resolves the ethical dilemma.

Self-Evaluation of VE8

Manage ethical dilemmas specific to interprofessional patient/population-centered care situations.

Use the Active Learning activity to evaluate your performance in this Sub-competency:

1. What were the resources available to you in managing this ethical dilemma?
2. What was the decision-making process you used to manage the ethical dilemma?
3. Describe your participation in the decision-making process? Did you fully participate in the discussion, or were there things you did not get to say?
4. Were you satisfied with the outcome of the process? Why or why not?
5. How could the ethical dilemma have been managed more effectively?

When you can manage ethical dilemmas specific to interprofessional patient/population-centered care situations, you have demonstrated the VE8 Sub-competency.

VE9: Act With Honesty and Integrity in Relationships With Patients, Families, Communities, and Other Team Members

Acting with honesty and integrity in relationships requires adherence to the ethical principles discussed in Chapter 4. It requires adherence to state and federal laws and institutional policies. It requires ethical professional behavior and cultural sensitivity. It also involves the application of Sub-competencies VE1 through VE8. Sub-competency VE9 means to nurture relationships through being trustful and reliable with patients, families, and team members and following through with responsibilities.

Honesty is related to the ethical principle of veracity. It not only means to tell the truth to colleagues, patients, families, and communities, but also includes the absence of deception. It also requires that information be freely given and not withheld. It requires transparency in all

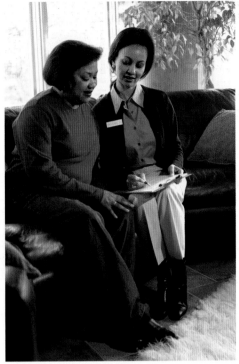

FIG. 5.10 Acting with honesty and integrity requires giving full information. (© Thinkstock/Stockbyte/Thinkstock.)

that you do as a healthcare professional (Fig. 5.10). Acting with integrity means to act with high moral and ethical standards and to consistently "do the right thing." It means to live and act according to your own values and ethics and those of your profession.

Sub-competency VE9 is quite similar to Sub-competency VE6 but focuses on honesty and integrity in *relationships,* not only with patients and team members, but also with the community. Acting with honesty and integrity is the foundation of forming a trusting relationship with stakeholders. After establishing a trusting relationship (VE6), acting with honesty and integrity is essential to maintaining and strengthening that relationship. Dishonest or unethical actions on the part of professionals have the opposite effect. For example, there are certain healthcare providers in some communities who are known to prescribe narcotics or other drugs with an abuse potential to anyone who will pay. Although these practitioners are few, their actions erode trust toward healthcare providers in the community. Likewise, if homeless or poor people or people of certain cultures are not treated respectfully in emergency departments,

CASELET 5.4   An Ethical Dilemma: Acting With Integrity

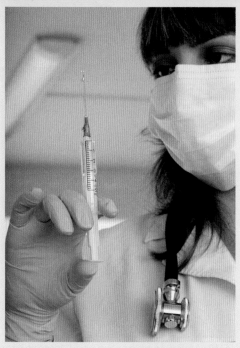

(© targovcom/iStock/Thinkstock.)

Rajesh Patel is a registered nurse who works in a busy medical unit of an acute care hospital. He is concerned about another nurse who works on the unit, Marta Wosniak. Mr. Patel notes that often the narcotics count does not add up correctly when she is on duty. She often volunteers to do the count, to go to the pharmacy to pick up patient medications, and to give medication to other nurses' patients, saying, "I'll help because you seem so busy, let me just give this pain medication for you." She seems moody, sometimes short-tempered and snappy, and other times in a daze. She recently made several minor errors, and her performance seems to have gone downhill. Other members of the healthcare team have noticed these behaviors and suspect that she may be using drugs. Mr. Patel becomes quite upset when a patient tells him that he thinks that Ms. Wosniak is not giving him his full dose of pain medication because it doesn't seem to give the same relief as when other nurses administered it. Mr. Patel has not actually seen Ms. Wosniak use drugs, and does not want to get her in trouble. On the other hand, he is concerned for patient safety.

Discussion Questions

1. How would you go about resolving this dilemma if you were Mr. Patel?
2. Use the ethical decision-making process from Chapter 4 (or another of your choice) and work through each of the steps to resolve the dilemma in this Caselet.
3. What is your decision?

---

hospitals, or clinics, they may be less likely to access care when needed. Actions of individual professionals may contribute to a wider perception within the community regarding the trustworthiness of healthcare professionals and institutions in general. Caselet 5.4 demonstrates an ethical dilemma faced by a healthcare professional.

Using the ethical decision-making process from Chapter 4, let's work through Caselet 5.4.

1. Identify the decision to be made. The decision here is whether to report Ms. Wosniak's suspected drug use to the nurse manager, and how to ensure that the patient's complaint is investigated and addressed.
2. Whose decision is it to make? In this case, it is ultimately Mr. Patel's responsibility to report the patient's complaint. It is the team's (including the nurse manager) responsibility to decide how to address the patient complaint.

3. Identify the stakeholders. The patient who made the complaint is the first stakeholder. Another person affected by the decision is Ms. Wosniak. Ms. Wosniak's patients both now and in the future may also be affected. The healthcare team on the unit is also affected because patient outcomes are involved. The decision also affects Mr. Patel and his relationship with Ms. Wosniak. It has implications for patient safety because patients could ultimately be affected by impaired practice and improper dosages. The hospital could also be affected by reduced quality of care related to impaired practice.
4. Decide how the team will make the decision. The team decides to base its decision on the facts available and to work through the decision-making process. They decide the overriding issue is patient safety.

5. Identify and gather information relevant to the decision. Mr. Patel reviews the professional nursing literature for signs of chemical impairment in nurses and writes down his specific observations of Ms. Wosniak's behavior. He also reviews his hospital's policy for reporting suspected impaired practice. He reviews the American Nurses' Association Code of Ethics (ANA, 2015). Mr. Patel reports this information back to the team.

6. Identify all available options. The team has three possible options: (1) Have the nurse manager formally report and investigate the team's observations, following hospital policy. (2) Wait until they have concrete evidence and not report Ms. Wosniak now. (3) Confront Ms. Wosniak directly with their observations.

7. Analyze the risks, benefits, costs, and feasibility of the options. (1) Reporting Ms. Wosniak could cost her her job and possibly her nursing license, but only if she is found to be using drugs; if Ms. Wosniak is found to be using drugs she can receive treatments and rehabilitation to prevent further consequences to her and her patients. (2) Delay or failure to report could negatively affect patient safety and quality of care. If Ms. Wosniak is using drugs and makes a serious error, it could cost lives and result in financial loss to the institution. (3) Confronting Ms. Wosniak directly could ruin their relationship with her and affect the team's dynamics.

8. Choose the "best" option. The team decides that the nurse manager should report and investigate Ms. Wosniak. Review of the hospital policy assured them that the report is anonymous. The team also found that their state participates in an Alternative to Discipline Program, which means that nurses who are found to be or admit to using drugs may agree to participate in a rehabilitation program. The goal of this program is to help impaired nurses stop using drugs (including alcohol), retain their licenses, and return to work with support and monitoring. The team considers that reporting Ms. Wosniak is the ethical thing to do because it upholds the principle of doing no harm to patients (non-maleficence). It also upholds the principles of veracity (truthfulness) and fidelity, because by reporting potentially impaired practice they are honoring their commitment to patient safety.

9. Implement the decision. The nurse manager reported the patient complaint and the team's observations according to institutional policy.

10. Evaluate the outcome. The eventual outcome was that Ms. Wosniak left her hospital job and entered the alternative program. Her nursing license was temporarily suspended. After 2 years of treatment and monitoring, her license was reinstated and she returned to work at the hospital as a case manager, where she has no access to narcotics. She continues to attend support groups and participate in voluntary urine testing. She often tells others that she wishes she knew who reported her because that person saved her life and her career. Patients in the unit received prescribed doses of pain medication, and patient safety was protected. The team developed experience acting with honesty and integrity in relationships with patients, families, communities, and other team members and in managing ethical dilemmas.

Self-Evaluation of VE9

Act with honesty and integrity in relationships with patients, families, communities, and other team members.

1. Reflect on your interactions with patients, families, communities, and other team members. If you do not have clinical experience yet, reflect on your interactions with members of a team you have been part of. Do you consistently act with honesty and integrity?

2. Think of an interaction or situation in which your actions could have contributed to a wider perception of healthcare professionals in the community. Did you demonstrate honesty and integrity?

When you can demonstrate honesty and integrity in relationships with patients, families, communities, and other team members, you have demonstrated the VE9 Sub-competency.

VE10: Maintain Competence in One's Own Profession Appropriate to Scope of Practice

Maintaining competence in your own profession within your scope of practice is an ethical obligation. The science of health care is changing rapidly, with new developments in medication, technology, and treatment strategies occurring with increasing frequency (Fig. 5.11). Each healthcare profession fulfills a specific need of society; patients, families, and other team members depend on healthcare professionals executing their duties competently. Each healthcare professional is accountable to consumers for the provision of high-quality care with predictable outcomes. Most healthcare professions require a certain number of continuing education credits or hours

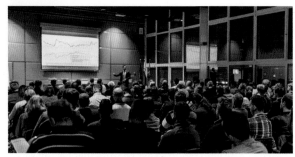

FIG. 5.11 Attending professional conferences is a way to maintain competence in your profession. (© kasto80/ iStock/Thinkstock.)

✳ ACTIVE LEARNING

Maintaining Professional Competence

Go online to your state licensing agency for your profession and another healthcare profession and look up the license renewal requirements.
1. Are there any continuing education requirements?
2. How do they differ between the two professions?
3. How are they the same?

---

to renew their licensure or certification. This underscores the importance of keeping up to date in your profession. The practice of each healthcare profession is different today than it was 20, or even 10, years ago. You have a moral obligation to your patients, team members, and the community to maintain competence and develop new skills throughout your career. The public trusts that

healthcare professionals are knowledgeable and current in their respective professions.

Self-Evaluation of VE10

Maintain competence in one's own profession appropriate to scope of practice.

Do a self-check related to your maintenance of professional competence:
1. How do you maintain competence in your profession?
2. Do you regularly read journals, participate in in-service or continuing education activities, and attend workshops or professional conferences?
3. What are the continuing education requirements of your profession for state licensure and specialty certification (as applicable)?
4. How do you, or will you, keep accurate ongoing records of these activities and continuing education credits?

When you can maintain competence in your profession, appropriate to your scope of practice, you have demonstrated the VE10 Sub-competency.

DEMONSTRATING THE SUB-COMPETENCIES OF VALUES/ETHICS FOR INTERPROFESSIONAL PRACTICE

The Exemplar Case Study: Maria Sanchez demonstrates how incorporating the Sub-competencies of Values/Ethics in practice can lead to positive patient outcomes. Compare and contrast the outcomes in Exemplar Case Study: Maria Sanchez with those previously encountered in Case Study: Maria Sanchez Parts 1 and 2.

◎ EXEMPLAR CASE STUDY

Maria Sanchez

Maria Sanchez is a 66-year-old widow who lives alone. She has a daughter who lives in a different city, 16 hours away by car. The rest of her relatives are in Puerto Rico. She experiences progressive difficulty breathing, shortness of breath, and fatigue. Her ankles are swollen and she has difficulty walking. She asks a neighbor to drive her to the Emergency Department of her local hospital. She is diagnosed with congestive heart failure (CHF), a chronic illness that will require lifestyle changes and follow up visits to her physician. Mrs. Sanchez has Medicare for health insurance. Medicare pays the hospital for a certain number of days for the diagnosis of CHF. If her hospital stay exceeds that number, the hospital will lose money. On the other

hand, if she stays less than that number of days the hospital will make money. It is in the financial best interest of the hospital to discharge her as soon as possible.

As part of the admission assessment, the admitting nurse conducts a psychosocial, cultural, spiritual needs assessment, as well as medication history, allergies, and nursing physical assessment. The medical resident conducts a medical history and physical [VE1, 3, 5]. As a result of these assessments, arrangements are made for a Catholic priest to visit Mrs. Sanchez, since she expressed a desire to see one [VE1, 3, 4]. Since she lives alone and has no family in the area, the team discusses the need to involve a social worker/case manager, and to take special

◎ **EXEMPLAR CASE STUDY**

Maria Sanchez—cont'd

care that Mrs. Sanchez understands how to care for herself after discharge [VE1, 4, 5]. They also decide to add a nutritionist to Mrs. Sanchez's interprofessional healthcare team, after discussing the need for dietary changes with her [VE1, 4, 5].

Mrs. Sanchez informs her daughter that she is in the hospital and they decide to wait until they know when she will be discharged and what will be required before making arrangements for the daughter to visit. Mrs. Sanchez is seen by a nutritionist and told she must modify her diet to reduce dietary fat and calories and to limit fluids [VE5]. The nutritionist asks her what foods she likes and dislikes and performs a dietary assessment that includes what she eats on a normal day [VE1, 3, 5, 6]. Together, Mrs. Sanchez and the nutritionist plan a diet that Mrs. Sanchez feels able to follow [VE1, 3, 5, 6]. Specific instructions for limiting fluids, and what counts as a fluid, such as gelatin and ice cream, are discussed. The nutritionist returns later and uses the "teach-back" method, in which Mrs. Sanchez is asked to describe to the nutritionist how to incorporate recommended restrictions [VE1, 5, 7]. The nutritionist asks her whether she can read and whether she prefers written materials in Spanish or English [VE1 3, 5]. Mrs. Sanchez is given several handouts written in English (her stated preference) to take home. The nutritionist gives her his card and encourages her to call if she has questions when she returns home [VE1, 3, 5, 6, 9].

The healthcare team recommends that Mrs. Sanchez start a regular exercise program. She must control her cholesterol and blood pressure. She is started on medications to help with this and told that diet and exercise will also help [VE4, 5, 7]. The registered nurse explains her new medications, including their dosage, timing, purpose, and side effects. The nurses frequently assess the effects of these medications. Each nurse identifies each medication whenever it is given [VE1, 5, 7, 10]. During her stay, Mrs. Sanchez is encouraged to identify each medication and its purpose when it is given [VE1, 5, 6]. A social worker–case manager is assigned to Mrs. Sanchez's team to assist with discharge planning and to ensure her needs will be adequately met once she leaves the hospital [VE1, 4, 7]. Together they discuss how and where she can get regular exercise [VE1, 5]. The case manager finds that the senior center in her neighborhood has daily exercise classes that are appropriate for Mrs. Sanchez's age and condition [VE 5, 10]. The classes are free of charge, and Mrs. Sanchez say she thinks she would enjoy going to the center and can get a ride there from her neighbor, who regularly goes to the senior center [VE1, 5, 6, 9].

The interprofessional team meets, and the physician says that medically, Mrs. Sanchez is ready to go home. The nurse states that Mrs. Sanchez appears to understand her medications. The nutritionist reports that Mrs. Sanchez should be able to adapt to her dietary restrictions. The case manager asks what follow-up care will be needed. She requests time to make these follow-up appointments and arrange for transportation, at times that are acceptable to Mrs. Sanchez. When this is done, she will contact the nurse, who will notify the physician or resident that the discharge orders can be written. The nurse states she will go over the medications again with Mrs. Sanchez and suggest she use a pill container that she can fill with a week's worth of pills [VE1, 4, 5, 6, 7, 9].

The case manager meets with Mrs. Sanchez and tells her the team feels she is ready to go home. Together they call and make follow-up appointments with Mrs. Sanchez's primary care physician and new cardiologist [VE1, 5, 7, 9]. The case manager arranges for transportation to these appointments through a free county senior transport program, in which she registers Mrs. Sanchez. The program is described to her, and printed information is given to her in her preferred language, English [VE1, 3, 5, 9]. The nurse meets with Mrs. Sanchez and verifies her understanding of her medications [VE1, 4, 5, 7]. The nurse then notifies the resident to write the discharge orders. He visits Mrs. Sanchez and asks how she feels about going home [VE1, 5, 6, 9]. She says she is still a little tired but feels ready to go home. After he leaves, Mrs. Sanchez calls her daughter, and they make arrangements for the daughter to visit for the weekend.

At the time of discharge Mrs. Sanchez is given several prescriptions to fill. She is given printed information about her medications and written information about the date, time, location, and doctors' names of her follow-up appointments. She also has contact information for the nutritionist and case manager. The case manager gives her a voucher to pay for a taxi. On the way to the taxi, the nurse's aide stops at the hospital outpatient pharmacy with Mrs. Sanchez to fill her prescriptions, so she will have medication to take home with her. She waits with her for the taxi [VE1, 2, 5, 7, 9].

Upon arrival home, Mrs. Sanchez calls her neighbor to say she is home. She then calls her daughter. Mrs. Sanchez explains all the follow-up and healthcare plans to her daughter, and together they plan for the daughter's weekend visit. Mrs. Sanchez is excited to be home and feels that she can maintain and maybe even improve her health.

KEY POINTS

- The patient is the center of all care, and the patient's needs come before those of the institution, providers, or other stakeholders. The recipient of care may be an individual, family, community, or population.
- Interprofessional values and ethics are part of a professional identity that is both professional and interprofessional in nature. Almost all healthcare professionals will face ethical issues and dilemmas during their careers.
- Healthcare professionals have a responsibility to promote population health as well as individual patient health.
- Patient dignity, privacy, and confidentiality must be protected at all times. Patient information may not be released to anyone without the patient's written permission. This includes the patient's family members, other healthcare facilities, and, in certain cases, other members of the healthcare team.
- Cultural groups can be related to ethnicity, religion, race, geography, socioeconomics, class, occupation, ability or disability, sexual orientation, belief systems, or other characteristics. Healthcare professionals must be prepared to embrace and work with individuals from varied backgrounds, whether they are patients, other professionals, or entire populations.
- Developing a trusting relationship with patients, families, and other team members is essential to achieve effective, quality health care and positive patient outcomes.
- Interprofessional collaboration must be based on mutual respect and trust to be effective. The expertise that each professional brings to the team and the perspective of the recipients of care are seen as essential to promote optimal outcomes.
- Diversity, trust, and respect create a team in which the whole is greater than the sum of its parts.
- Managing ethical dilemmas specific to interprofessional patient/population-centered care situations requires knowledge of basic ethical principles, use of a formal ethical decision-making model agreed upon by the team, and familiarity with and use of available resources.
- Acting with honesty and integrity in relationships requires adherence to basic ethical principles, state and federal laws, institutional policies, and your professional code of ethics. It requires ethical professional behavior and cultural sensitivity.
- Maintaining competence in your own profession within your scope of practice is an ethical obligation. Each healthcare professional is accountable for the provision of high-quality care with predictable outcomes to consumers.

REFERENCES

American Nurses Association (ANA). (2015). *Code of ethics for nurses with interpretive statements*. Retrieved from http://nursingworld.org/DocumentVault/Ethics-1/Code-of-Ethics-for-Nurses.html.

Beauchamp, T., & Childress, J. (2013). *Principles of biomedical ethics* (7th ed.). New York: Oxford University Press.

Berwick, D., Thomas, W., Nolan, T., et al. (2008). The Triple Aim: Care, health, and cost. *Health Affairs, 27*(3), 759–769.

Canadian Interprofessional Health Collaborative (CIHC). (2010a). *CIHC fact sheets: What is patient centered care*. Retrieved from http://www.cihc.ca/resources/toolkit.

Canadian Interprofessional Health Collaborative (CIHC). (2010b). *A National interprofessional competency framework*. Vancouver, Canada: Author.

Dougherty, R., & Purtilo, R. (2016). *Ethical dimensions in the health professions*. St. Louis, MO: Elsevier.

Goldberg, T., & Patz, J. (2015). The need for a global ethic.[comment]. *The Lancet Commission*, 1973. Retrieved from http://dx.doi.org/10.1016/S0140-6736(15)60757-7.

Institute of Medicine (IOM). (2001a). *Crossing the quality chasm: A new health system for the 21st century*. Washington, DC: National Academies Press.

Interprofessional Education Collaborative Expert Panel (IPEC). (2011). *Core competencies for interprofessional collaborative practice: Report of an expert panel*. Washington, DC: Interprofessional Education Collaborative.

Interprofessional Education Collaborative Expert Panel (IPEC). (2016). *Core competencies for interprofessional collaborative practice: 2016 update*. Washington, DC: Interprofessional Education Collaborative.

Jason, G., Royeen, C., & Purtilo, R. (2010). Interprofessional ethics in rehabilitation: The Dreamcatcher journey. *Journal of Allied Health, 39*(Suppl. 1), 246–250.

Leininger, M. (2002). Culture care theory: A major contribution to advance transcultural nursing and practices. *Journal of Transcultural Nursing, 13*(3), 189–192.

Medical Defence Union (MDU). (2017). *Confidentiality and the healthcare team*. Retrieved from https://www.themdu. com/guidance-and-advice/guides/the-healthcare-team.

Mey, A., Knox, K., Kelly, F., et al. (2013). Trust and safe spaces: Mental health consumers' and carers' relationships with community pharmacy staff. *Patient, 6*, 281–289.

O'Toole, M. (Ed.). (2017). *Mosby's medical dictionary* (10th ed.). St. Louis, MO: Elsevier.

Schottenfeld, L. (2016). *Creating patient-centered team-based primary care*. Agency for Healthcare Research and Quality, U.S. Department of Health and Human Services: Rockville, MD. Retrieved from https://pcmh.ahrq.gov/ page/creating-patient-centered-team-based-primary-care.

United Nations Educational, Scientific, and Cultural Organization (UNESCO). (2016). *Cultural diversity*. Retrieved from http:// www.unesco.org/new/en/social-and-human-sciences/ themes/international-migration/glossary/ cultural-diversity/.

University of Toronto. (2008). Competency framework. *Advancing the Interprofessional Education Curriculum 2009: Curriculum overview*. Toronto: University of Toronto Office of Interprofessional Education.

6

Values/Ethics Case Studies

LEARNING OUTCOMES

After successfully working through the case studies in this chapter, you will be able to:

1. Demonstrate the ability to apply the Interprofessional Values/Ethics Sub-competencies to problem-based case studies.
2. Operationalize the behaviors of Interprofessional Values/Ethics Sub-competencies through case study application.

3. Demonstrate Interprofessional Values/Ethics Core Competency in simulated interprofessional collaboration through case study discussions or role-play.

This chapter presents several patient- /population-based case studies involving challenges to values/ethics for interprofessional practice (IPEC, 2011; 2016). They can be used in group discussions or debates, as role-playing exercises, or as individual learning experiences. The authors acknowledge that all four competencies may apply to each case; however, the focus of the case studies in this chapter is on Values/Ethics (Box 6.1). There are discussion questions at the end of each case study; however, you are encouraged to ask your own questions and further investigate the issues involved. As in ethical dilemmas and most ethical issues in health care, there is no single correct answer. It is strongly recommended that you use a specific ethical decision-making process to work through the cases. The interprofessional ethical decision-making process, discussed in Chapters 4 and 5, is included in Box 6.2.

CASE STUDY: MEDICAL MARIJUANA

Specific Sub-competencies to consider and apply: VE1, VE4, VE6, VE7.

Jennifer Green is 15 years old and was recently diagnosed with leukemia. She is currently being treated with chemotherapy. Based on research, there is a very good chance that the leukemia can be cured, but she will have to undergo some form of treatment for 3 years with frequent monitoring in the form of blood tests and other procedures. The oncologist (physician who specializes in cancer treatment) on her healthcare team receives a phone call from Mrs. Green, Jennifer's mother. Mrs. Green inquires about the possibility of getting a prescription for medical marijuana for Jennifer. She says that since the last chemotherapy, Jennifer experienced severe nausea with occasional vomiting and is not eating much at all. The anti-nausea medication she has does not seem to work very well. Jennifer also has difficulty sleeping and feels anxious for 2 days after treatment due to the steroids that are administered prior to chemotherapy. The family is distraught seeing Jennifer suffer so much. Jennifer's aunt Alice Reston brought over brownies she baked that contained marijuana. Ms. Reston said that her friend's daughter, who also has cancer, got great relief from medical marijuana. Because Jennifer was suffering, they allowed her to have a brownie. It really helped decrease her nausea, increased her appetite, and calmed her. The oncologist explained that medical marijuana is not legal in their state, nor is recreational marijuana. He cautioned against giving Jennifer any more marijuana and said that he will consult the pharmacist

BOX 6.1 Values/Ethics Core Competency and Sub-Competencies (IPEC, 2016, p.11)

Core Competency: Values/Ethics. Work with individuals of other professions to maintain a climate of mutual respect and shared values.

VE1. Place the interests of patients and populations at the center of interprofessional health care delivery and population health programs, with the goal of promoting health and health equity across the lifespan.

VE2. Respect the dignity and privacy of patients while maintaining confidentiality in the delivery of team-based care.

VE3. Embrace the cultural diversity and individual differences that characterize patients, populations, and the health team.

VE4. Respect the unique cultures, values, roles/responsibilities, and expertise of other health professions and the impact these factors can have on health outcomes.

VE5. Work in cooperation with those who receive care, those who provide care, and others who contribute to or support the delivery of prevention and health services and programs.

VE6. Develop a trusting relationship with patients, families, and other team members (CIHC, 2010).

VE7. Demonstrate high standards of ethical conduct and quality of care in contributions to team-based care.

VE8. Manage ethical dilemmas specific to interprofessional patient/population centered care situations.

VE9. Act with honesty and integrity in relationships with patients, families, communities and other team members.

VE10. Maintain competence in one's own profession appropriate to scope of practice.

From Interprofessional Education Collaborative Expert Panel (IPEC). (2016). *Core competencies for interprofessional collaborative practice: 2016 update.* Washington, DC: Interprofessional Education Collaborative.

BOX 6.2 Interprofessional Ethical Decision-Making Process

1. Identify the decision to be made.
2. Whose decision is it to make?
3. Identify the stakeholders.
4. Decide how the team will make the decision.
5. Identify and gather information relevant to the decision.
6. Identify all available options.
7. Analyze the risks, benefits, costs, and feasibility of the options.
8. Choose the "best" option.
9. Implement the decision.
10. Evaluate the outcome.

dronabinol (Marinol), a legal medication derived from marijuana, that is approved for pediatric use to treat chemotherapy-related nausea and vomiting and is also effective as an appetite stimulant. The oncologist recommends that they try the new medication suggested by the pharmacist.

To the oncologist's surprise, Sara White, the Greens' social worker, becomes quite upset. She states that the Greens should be reported to the state child protection service for child endangerment because they gave Jennifer illegal drugs. Reporting the Greens could result in them being declared unfit parents and Jennifer being placed in foster care. Sara also states that the Greens and Alice Reston should be reported to the police for possession of illegal drugs. The rest of the team disagrees, noting that this was a one-time occurrence, and that the Greens have been responsible, caring parents throughout Jennifer's illness. The nurse points out that Mrs. Green was honest about giving Jennifer a marijuana-laced brownie, and that she agreed not to give her any more, but the nurse disagrees about prescribing the dronabinol because it is derived from marijuana. The nurse fears it may lead to Jennifer using marijuana later on. The physical therapist states that it would be cruel to make the family undergo a child endangerment investigation after all they are going through with Jennifer's illness. Such an investigation may be emotionally devastating to Jennifer and the Greens, and foster care would not be in her best interest. Sara White insists that it is her legally mandated obligation to report the Greens, and that she will do so anonymously, whether or not the team agrees.

to see what legal medications could be prescribed to help Jennifer's nausea, appetite, and anxiety. Mrs. Green agrees and says she really hopes the team can help Jennifer.

When the healthcare team meets to discuss Jennifer's case, the oncologist tells them about the phone conversation described previously. The oncologist states that he consulted the pharmacist who recommended

Discussion Questions

1. What is the ethical issue/dilemma facing the team?
2. What actions would serve the best interests of the patient, Jennifer Green?
3. How should the team respond to Sara White's decision to report the Greens to the child protection agency?
4. What evidence is there that the Greens have a trusting relationship with members of the team, and how would reporting them affect this relationship?
5. What evidence is there that the team members have trusting relationships with each other?

CASE STUDY: RISK TO PUBLIC HEALTH[1]

Specific Sub-competencies to consider and apply: VE1, VE2, VE5, VE8, VE9.

Ann Singer was first diagnosed with tuberculosis (TB) in February and immediately began treatment. In June of that year she was diagnosed with multidrug-resistant tuberculosis (MDR-TB), a strain of TB that is resistant to treatment using "first-line" drugs that are usually effective against TB. She was advised by county public health officials not to fly via commercial airlines because she would be putting others at risk. She was scheduled to be married in June, and then take an extended honeymoon throughout Europe. Despite the public health risk, she decided to go through with her plans. When she was in Paris, France, she was contacted by a representative from the United States Centers for Disease Control and Prevention (CDC), who advised her that it was discovered that she had extremely drug-resistant tuberculosis (XDR-TB). XDR-TB is very contagious and is extremely difficult to treat. Mrs. Singer was told that she was put on a no-fly list, and the only way she could fly back to the United States would be to charter a private plane. Mrs. Singer then booked a commercial flight that left earlier than the one she originally booked, flew to Denmark, and then to Canada, where she and her husband rented a car and drove to the United States. Despite an alert attached to her passport, she was not detained at the Canadian border. Mrs. Singer then voluntarily checked into a Denver hospital for treatment.

All passengers on all flights with Mrs. Singer were identified, contacted, and required to undergo TB testing.

French public health officials asserted that the United States did not contact them in a timely fashion. The case made national and international news. Mrs. Singer considered suing the CDC for revealing her name and breaching her privacy.

Discussion Questions

1. How were the interests of Mrs. Singer and population health involved in this case?
2. There was no evidence of team-based care in this case. How do you think team-based care could have affected this case?
3. How could cooperation among healthcare professionals involved in this case (nationally and internationally) have been improved?
4. Do you think Mrs. Singer had a trusting relationship with the public health representatives? Explain why or why not and how this may have affected the outcome.
5. Is there an ethical dilemma present in this case? How would you manage the dilemma?
6. Did the various people involved in this case act with honesty and integrity in their relationships? Explain.

CASE STUDY: CONFIDENTIALITY AND TEEN PREGNANCY

Specific Sub-competencies to consider and apply: VE2, VE5, VE6, VE9.

Yasmine Kamal is a 14-year-old high school student. She is being treated for major depressive disorder at an outpatient mental health facility. She currently sees a psychologist for weekly therapy sessions, but has made little progress. The psychologist refers her to the psychiatric nurse practitioner (NP) to determine whether antidepressant medication might be beneficial. The patient and her mother discuss the issue with the NP, and they all decide that a trial of a low-dose antidepressant is warranted. Prior to prescribing medication, the NP orders routine laboratory work according to the facility's protocol, which includes a pregnancy test for any female of childbearing age. The laboratory results are all within normal limits, and the pregnancy test is positive. The law of the state in which the case occurred requires written permission from any patient age 14 years and older to discuss information with a parent. Yasmine has not signed the permission form. On the follow-up visit, the NP sees Yasmine alone and explains the results of her pregnancy

---

[1]This case is based on a real-life situation. Names and details have been changed to protect the privacy of individuals.

test. Yasmine bursts into tears and begs the NP not to tell Mrs. Kamal, Yasmine's mother. The Kamal family is of Egyptian descent and very active in their church. They believe it is important that a girl remain a virgin until marriage. Yasmine feels that she cannot face her parents, and that it was a one-time consensual sexual encounter with her boyfriend. She is ashamed and does not know what she wants to do. The NP calls in the psychologist and they discuss with Yasmine the pros and cons of Yasmine telling her mother about her pregnancy, but Yasmine still insists that she does not want her mother to know yet. The NP explains that she will not prescribe an antidepressant at this time, and that it is extremely important that Yasmine continue to see the psychologist to discuss her options, and to continue psychotherapy to treat her depression. Yasmine promises that she will keep seeing the psychologist. After determining that Yasmine is not in danger of harming herself, the NP and psychologist agree that she can leave after making an appointment to see her the following week. The NP and psychologist discuss the case and decide that they should meet with the facility's medical director for further advice. The next day, there is a phone message for the NP from Mrs. Kamal inquiring why Yasmine did not get an antidepressant prescription.

Discussion Questions

1. How did the NP and psychologist respect the patient's confidentiality?
2. Is discussion of the case with the medical director a breach of confidentiality? Why or why not?
3. How can the NP and psychologist maintain a trusting relationship with both Yasmine Kamal and her mother without violating confidentiality?
4. How should the NP respond, with honesty, to Mrs. Kamal's question regarding why no antidepressant was prescribed?

CASE STUDY: PUBLIC HEALTH VERSUS INDIVIDUAL FOCUS OF CARE

Specific Sub-competencies to consider and apply: VE1, VE2, VE5, VE7.

Kevin O'Brien is studying for his Master of Science Degree in Public Health (MSPH). As part of his clinical practicum he works with patients in the tuberculosis (TB) clinic. Patients with active TB are instructed not to work handling food (among other restrictions), to prevent

contagion, until they have completed a full course of treatment and are medically cleared. One evening, Kevin and his roommate order a pizza to be delivered. Much to his surprise, the pizza is delivered by one of the patients who Kevin knows from the TB clinic. The patient recognizes him as well. Kevin says, "You know, you're not supposed to work with food." The patient says, "I know, but I don't handle the food directly. I just deliver it. Hey man, don't say anything to the clinic, okay? I really need this job, I have a family to feed." Kevin says nothing in response, pays for the pizza, and tips the "patient/delivery man." Kevin wonders whether he should even eat the pizza, and whether he should communicate his concern to his roommate. He is also conflicted about whether to report the incident to his instructor or preceptor at the clinic, or both. Kevin also was unsure whether "handling food" includes delivery, or what is involved in the patient's job.

Discussion Questions

1. Which should be the main consideration in this case, the potential for the public's exposure to a contagious disease or the patient's need for a job? Explain your decision.
2. Should Kevin O'Brien share his concern about the possible contamination of the pizza with his roommate? Why or why not?
3. Should Kevin report the incident to his instructor and/or the clinic staff? Why or why not?
4. Should Kevin enter into a more direct discussion with the patient/delivery man?

CASE STUDY: SUSPECTED DRUG ABUSE

Specific Sub-competencies to consider and apply: VE2, VE6, VE7, VE9.

Gertrude Schmidt is a dental hygienist in a family outpatient dentistry practice. One of her adult patients has been coming in regularly to have her teeth cleaned since she was a teenager. Ms. Schmidt has noticed a marked deterioration in her patient's oral hygiene. She is shocked at the number of new dental caries and the worsening of others. The patient also displays symptoms of gum disease, which was not noted on previous visits. Ms. Schmidt also notes that the patient appears to have lost a great deal of weight since her last visit a year ago. The patient is fidgety, speaks rapidly, and has dilated pupils despite the overhead light. Ms. Smith suspects that the patient may be using amphetamines because she displays many symptoms, including the beginnings of "meth mouth," which is distinguished by severe tooth decay and gum disease (American Dental Association, 2017). Ms. Schmidt completes her assessment of the patient's dental health and begins to clean the patient's teeth. As she works, she wonders whether she should ask the patient directly about her suspected amphetamine use. Ms. Schmidt plans to tell the patient to make an appointment with the dentist as soon as possible, to treat the decay and potential gum disease. She decides to take a break from the cleaning to contact Dr. Melville, the dentist, to discuss her suspicions about the patient's drug use, her concern about the patient's severely deteriorated dental health, and to create a plan of care to present to the patient before the patient leaves. Together, they decide to meet with the patient after her cleaning is complete, discuss their concern about her dental health, make an appointment with the dentist, and possibly provide education about amphetamine use and its consequences on dental health.

Discussion Questions

1. Did Gertrude Schmidt, the dental hygienist, respect the patient's dignity, privacy, and confidentiality in this case? Explain, giving examples.
2. How did the dentist and dental hygienist work to maintain a trusting relationship with the patient?
3. How did team-based care contribute to acting with high ethical standards in this case?
4. Did the professionals in this case act with integrity and high ethical standards? Explain your answer.
5. What is your opinion of the dental team's decision to provide education and dental treatment rather than confront the patient with their suspicions that she was using amphetamines?

CASE STUDY: TRAUMA AND TRANSPLANT

Specific Sub-competencies to consider and apply: VE1, VE7, VE8.

Cherry and Merry Richards were 12-year-old identical twin sisters. Tragically, on the way home from school, the car in which they were riding (driven by their mother) was hit by a car driven by a drunk driver. Cherry sustained severe trauma as a result of the motor vehicle crash, while Merry sustained only minor injuries. Cherry was hospitalized in the pediatric trauma unit for several weeks. She sustained kidney damage, and her kidneys shut down. She required dialysis treatments three times a week. She slowly began to recover, and it became clear that she would need to have dialysis for the rest of her life unless she received a kidney transplant. Cherry had a rare blood type, and Mr. and Mrs. Richards were told by the trauma team that it would probably be quite some time before a kidney became available. In the meantime, Cherry would continue dialysis three times a week, along with physical and occupational therapy. A dietician was part of Cherry's interprofessional team to counsel the patient and family on dietary restrictions related to her renal (kidney) condition and dialysis. The plan was to eventually transfer Cherry to a pediatric rehabilitation hospital, where tutoring would begin so that she could keep up with her schoolwork.

Cherry and Merry were very close. Merry visited Cherry almost daily. She repeatedly expressed her wish to help Cherry in any way possible and couldn't understand why this happened to her sister while she was spared. When she told this to Cherry's nurse, the nurse consulted the team, and it was suggested that the girls receive psychiatric assessments. The Richards agreed, and after the assessment, the psychiatrist recommended individual counseling for each of the girls in combination with family counseling. A counseling social worker was brought into the team. Cherry told her they were waiting for a match before she could get a kidney. Together, the girls looked up information on the Internet and formed the idea that Merry would probably be a good match for a kidney. Merry said she would gladly give Cherry a kidney. The girls approached the parents with their idea, and the Richards' agreed to discuss the idea with Cherry's healthcare team. They approached the nephrologist (kidney specialist) with Merry's offer to donate a kidney to her sister.

At this point in her care, Cherry's team consisted of her family, trauma physician, nephrologist, primary nurse, dietician, social worker, psychologist, occupational therapist, physical therapist, and transplant nurse. The team met to discuss Cherry's plan of care and progress, and the nephrologist presented the idea of having Merry donate a kidney. Several issues were discussed. First, Merry is a minor and cannot give legal consent, although her parents could give their consent. Some members of the team feel that this is acceptable, but others do not think that the parents are able to make an unbiased decision in this case. Merry will be left with only one kidney for the rest of her life, which she may later regret. Second, the surgical procedure presents a risk to Merry, with the only benefit being her contribution to her sister. Third, there is the chance that the kidney will be rejected anyway, which may cause psychological harm to both sisters and the parents. The team is faced with the difficult decision regarding whether to allow Merry to donate a kidney to Cherry, with the parents' consent, after all members of the family are educated on the risks, benefits, and implications of the transplant and surgery.

Discussion Questions

1. Who is the center of care in this case? Whose best interests take precedence? Why?
2. Use a formal ethical decision-making process to work through this case. Determine at least two alternative solutions.
3. Role play with others as various members of the healthcare team, including the patient and family.
4. What solution by the team demonstrates acting with high ethical standards? Explain your answer and why this is the best ethical alternative.

CASE STUDY: END-OF-LIFE CARE

Part I

Specific Sub-competencies to consider and apply: VE3, VE5, VE7, VE10.

Steven Johnson is a 76-year-old retiree receiving Social Security and Medicare who suffered a severe cardiovascular accident (CVA) (commonly known as a stroke) while playing golf. His fellow golfers called 911, and Mr. Johnson was transported to the city medical center, where he was admitted. He is now on a ventilator, unable to communicate or breathe on his own. He does not have a living will, and his 71-year-old wife, Nancy, states that she wants everything possible done. Mrs. Johnson calls their pastor and asks him to pray for Mr. Johnson's recovery. The Johnsons are planning to celebrate their 50th wedding anniversary in 3 months and Mrs. Johnson insists that her husband will get well in time for that. The Johnsons have two adult children who live within an hour's drive of the Johnsons.

Mr. Johnson's healthcare team consists of a respiratory therapist, hospitalist physician, neurologist, nurse, and pharmacist. They decide to include a social worker/case manager on the team.

It becomes clear that Mr. Johnson will not recover enough to have any quality of life. He has severe, irreversible brain damage, with no possibility of meaningful recovery. He will never be able to communicate, nor will he be able to breathe on his own. The team agrees that it would be in Mr. Johnson's and his family's best interest to remove him from life support and let him die peacefully. The team decides that the social worker should arrange for a meeting with the interprofessional team, including the family, to explain the options and the team's recommendations.

The meeting takes place in the hospital family meeting room. Mrs. Johnson and both of her children are present. The neurologist explains Mr. Johnson's condition and the likelihood that he will never improve, and that the team recommends removal from the ventilator, which will most likely result in death within hours, although it may take longer. He reassures the family that Mr. Johnson will be kept comfortable and free from pain. Mrs. Johnson becomes angry and vehemently refuses to consent to have him removed from the ventilator, insisting he *will* get better and attend their 50th anniversary party. Mr. Johnson's children inquire about the cost to keep him on the ventilator and are told that most Medicare plans will pay 80% of the cost, with the family being responsible for 20%, if the ventilator is deemed medically necessary, but that he will find out the details regarding what Mr. Johnson's plan will and will not cover. The social worker tells the family that there are no facilities in the area for ventilator-dependent patients, including hospice care. Mr. Johnson could go home on the ventilator but would need 24-hour care, and the family would need to rent a ventilator, which would require a physician prescription stating it was medically necessary, and only certain conditions are covered for ventilator use. Overall, the cost of Mr. Johnson's continued care would deplete the Johnsons' resources with little to no chance of Mr. Johnson improving. Mrs. Johnson's children try to convince her that the best thing for everyone is to remove him from the ventilator, but she refuses, and the meeting ends with the team stating their availability to discuss matters further at a later date if the family desires.

After the meeting, the Johnson children contact the social worker/case manager and ask him how they can force their mother to "do the right" thing. The social worker states that it is their mother's decision as she is next of kin and in her "right mind." There is nothing the team can do other than present her with the options and their recommendation. He suggests that Mrs. Johnson and her children take some time to let the information sink in and to discuss it further with Mrs. Johnson's pastor.

Discussion Questions

1. Did the nurse and the healthcare team place Mr. Johnson and his family at the center of care? Explain your answer.
2. Were Mr. Johnson's dignity, privacy, and confidentiality respected in this scenario? Explain your answer.
3. How did the nurse demonstrate high standards of ethical conduct in this situation?
4. How did the team respect and embrace the individual differences of Mr. Johnson's family members?
5. How did the team members behave with honesty and integrity according to high ethical standards in this situation?
6. Work through the case using an ethical decision-making process. Consider role-playing with others taking the roles of the healthcare professionals and family members.

Part II

Specific Sub-competencies to consider and apply: VE1, VE2, VE7.

While Mrs. Johnson is visiting her husband, the monitor alarm goes off and the nurse rushes in. Mrs. Johnson asks, "What's wrong?" The nurse says, "He's having a cardiac arrest." Mrs. Johnson yells, "Save him, please save him!" The nurse calls a code, initiates cardiopulmonary resuscitation (CPR), and asks Mrs. Johnson to step outside while the team works on her husband. Mrs. Johnson calls her children and tells them to come to the hospital as soon as they can. The code team restores Mr. Johnson's cardiac rhythm. While waiting outside the room when the nurse and the certified nurse assistant (CNA) care for Mr. Johnson and straighten up the room, Mrs. Johnson overhears the nurse tell the CNA how terrible she feels putting Mr. Johnson through cardiac resuscitation when there is no hope for him to ever regain consciousness and have any quality of life. The CNA asks why they have to call a code, and the nurse explains that they must adhere to the wife's wishes.

Discussion Questions

1. Did the nurse and the healthcare team place Mr. Johnson and his family at the center of care? Explain your answer.

2. Were Mr. Johnson's dignity, privacy, and confidentiality respected in this scenario? Explain your answer.
3. How did the nurse demonstrate high standards of ethical conduct in this situation?

Part III

Specific Sub-competencies to consider and apply: VE4, VE5, VE10.

When Mr. and Mrs. Johnson's children arrive at the hospital, Mrs. Johnson says she was thinking that it may not be the best thing for Mr. Johnson to continue on life support because it seems that it may only be prolonging his suffering. It took the cardiac arrest situation for her to finally realize that her husband will never recover. The family asks to speak to the healthcare team about removing Mr. Johnson from life support. The social worker, hospitalist, nurse, and respiratory therapist (RT) are available to meet with the family. They explain what to expect once Mr. Johnson is removed from life support, and that the family can arrange for it to be done whenever they want. Mrs. Johnson says she would like their pastor present. Arrangements are made to remove Mr. Johnson from the ventilator later that afternoon. Mrs. Johnson asks the nurse if she will be the one who will remove the life support. The nurse has never done this before and is uncomfortable. She says, "I will be present if you want me to be there with you." The nurse then privately discusses the situation with the respiratory therapist. She has never removed someone from life support and is uncomfortable doing so for the first time in this situation. The RT says removing life support is part of RT training, and he has done so in a number of cases. He suggests that he remove Mr. Johnson from the ventilator while explaining what he is doing to the family, and the nurse can observe and offer support. Afterward, he and the nurse can meet and discuss the process so the nurse can learn. The hospitalist will be present when Mr. Johnson's life support is terminated, and he can also be available to talk with the nurse and RT afterward.

Discussion Questions

1. How did the team members respect each other's roles, responsibilities, and expertise in Mr. Johnson's case?
2. Using this case, give examples of how team members worked together with each other and the Johnson family.
3. The nurse in this case study demonstrated how interprofessional collaboration can help professionals

maintain competence within their scope of practice. Can you think of other ways in which the various professionals could collaborate to learn from one another?

CASE STUDY: DEMENTIA

Specific Sub-competencies to consider and apply: VE2, VE6, VE8.

John Beauford is a 77-year-old divorced male. He moved to Florida after his divorce and has no contact with his former wife. He has no children, and his only sister lives in a distant state. They talk weekly on the phone but have not seen each other in several years. He attends church and volunteers at a community organization. He has several acquaintances but no close friends. Recently he has become increasingly forgetful but passes it off as a sign of aging. He is staying home alone more and more frequently, and often cannot remember whether he ate. He missed several meetings at the community agency because he forgot. When someone from the agency called him about his absence, he became angry and defensive, stating nobody told him there was a meeting. While driving home from church one day on a route he had taken numerous times, he became disoriented and lost. Trying to find his way home, he drove for more than 2 hours, failed to notice a traffic light, and was involved in a motor vehicle collision. He is transported to the emergency department of the closest hospital. He is unable to answer questions about his health history and becomes belligerent when different staff members ask him the same questions. However, he does not have life-threatening injuries, only some minor contusions. The emergency department staff find his driver's license and Medicare card in his wallet, but no health information is available. There are business cards from the community agency. There is no information about Mr. Beauford in the computer system of the medical center. The healthcare team needs more information about his health history, current medications, allergies, and emergency contact(s). A computerized tomography (CT) scan of the head shows no head injury that would explain his behavior. A psychiatrist and social worker are consulted.

Discussion Questions

1. How can the healthcare team obtain necessary information without breaching confidentiality?
2. What are some ways the healthcare team can use to attempt to establish a trusting relationship with Mr. Beauford?
3. Use a formal ethical decision-making process to determine what should be done regarding Mr. Beauford's case and eventual discharge.

REFERENCES

American Dental Association. (2017). *Meth mouth: How methamphetamine use affects dental health.* Retrieved from http://www.mouthhealthy.org/en/az-topics/m/meth-mouth.

Canadian Interprofessional Health Collaborative (CIHC). (2010). *A national competency framework.* Vancouver, BC: CIHC.

Interprofessional Education Collaborative Expert Panel (IPEC). (2011). *Core competencies for interprofessional collaborative practice: Report of an expert panel.* Washington, DC: Interprofessional Education Collaborative.

Interprofessional Education Collaborative Expert Panel (IPEC). (2016). *Core competencies for interprofessional collaborative practice: 2016 update.* Washington, DC: Interprofessional Education Collaborative.

7

Foundations of Professional Roles and Responsibilities

LEARNING OUTCOMES

After studying this chapter, you will be able to:

1. Identify the basic concepts associated with the Core Competency of Roles/Responsibilities.
2. Differentiate between professional roles and responsibilities and scope of practice.
3. Identify the most common healthcare providers and their roles.
4. Describe the process of professional identity development.
5. Explain the use of self-reflection in the identification of professional strengths and limitations.
6. Demonstrate self-reflection as a tool for self-awareness.
7. Discuss roles and responsibilities in the context of interprofessional teamwork.

This chapter introduces the basic concepts associated with the Core Competency of Roles/Responsibilities (IPEC, 2011; 2016). Descriptions of the most common healthcare professions and occupations are provided. Readers are provided with information related to obtaining valid and reliable information about the roles and responsibilities as well as the legal scope of practice of the most common healthcare professions and are introduced to the skills necessary to understand their own and others' roles and responsibilities. Collaboration between interprofessional team members is introduced as it relates to individualized role performance in specific patient care situations.

BASICS OF PROFESSIONAL ROLES

Healthcare professionals, as members of interprofessional healthcare teams, have specific roles in each patient care situation. The word *role* is generally used to refer to a set of behaviors that fit together into a unified whole; it is those behaviors that characterize a person's expected actions in a given context. The word *role* also can be used to refer to the duty that one has or is expected to have. In health care, for example, we refer to the role of the physician or the role of the nurse. Based on our observations of those professionals, we assume we know what their roles are; however, these roles can overlap with each other and with those of other professionals. Although we think we know the roles and responsibilities of professions other than our own, we may not have a true and clear understanding.

Healthcare professionals become socialized to their professional roles in educational programs designed specifically to prepare them for the behaviors and skills expected of members of that profession. Traditionally this basic preparation has been delivered in what have been referred to as *silos,* educational arenas where students learn with other students preparing for the same profession and who are taught, for the most part, by members of the profession they are being prepared to enter.

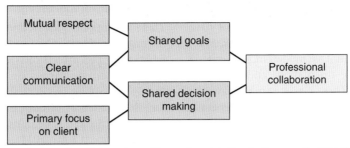

FIG. 7.1 Characteristics of collaboration. (From Arnold, E., & Boggs, K. [2016]. *Interpersonal relationships,* ed 7. St. Louis: Saunders.)

Although students acquire what is needed to be professional within these silos, it is no longer enough for healthcare providers to simply be professional. In the current global climate, healthcare workers also need to be interprofessional and function fully as part of interprofessional teams (WHO, 2010).

Public health "promotes and protects the health of people and the communities where they live, learn, work and play" (APHA, 2017, par. 1). Public health is concerned with improving access to health care; health promotion; preventing and controlling infectious disease; and reducing environmental hazards, violence, substance abuse, and injury. There are specialized degrees in the field of public health. A variety of qualified healthcare professionals specialize in the field of public health, which is focused on population health rather than the care of individuals. Examples of healthcare professionals who work in the public health field include, but are not limited to, epidemiologists, nurses, social workers, biostatisticians, infectious disease specialists, physicians, health educators, and field workers.

Fig. 7.1 illustrates the characteristics of collaboration. Interprofessional collaboration begins with mutual respect, clear communication, and a focus on the patient as the center of care. These characteristics are necessary to the development of shared goals and shared decision making. The end result is collaboration among professionals that results in optimal patient and population care.

Efficiently functioning interprofessional teams are needed to meet the complex patient and population care demands in today's healthcare system. Interprofessional teams are made up of healthcare professionals from two or more healthcare disciplines or professions whose purpose is collaboration to provide optimal health outcomes. Interprofessional team members work together closely and communicate frequently to optimize patient

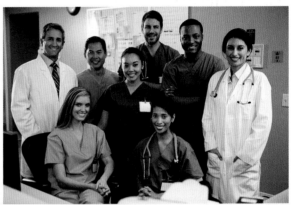

FIG. 7.2 An interprofessional healthcare team consists of people from a variety of disciplines whose roles often overlap. (© monkeybusinessimages/iStock/Thinkstock.)

care that is collaborative, creative, caring, and safe. Each patient care situation is unique, and the roles of healthcare professions often overlap. Each professional brings the knowledge, skills, expertise, and perspective of his or her profession to the patient care situation. True Interprofessional Collaborative Practice and teamwork requires a clear understanding of your own professional role and responsibilities as well as those of other professionals participating in the care. It requires knowledge of how the roles of all healthcare professionals on the team complement each other in the provision of optimal patient-centered care (IPEC, 2011). This knowledge is essential in clarifying patient care responsibilities and serves to increase collegiality, trust, and respect among healthcare team members (Fig. 7.2).

What Is a Profession?

A *profession* is defined as "a calling requiring specialized knowledge and often long and intensive academic preparation" (Merriam-Webster, 2015). There are several classic models of a profession with criteria that have evolved over time (Bixler & Bixler, 1945; Flexner, 1915; Pavalko, 1971). Some, but not all, models include criteria such as altruism, service orientation, and a distinct professional subculture. These classic models have the following criteria in common that comprise the generally accepted criteria for a profession:

Education

Education is extended, is standardized, and takes place in institutions of higher learning. Professions are intellectual and learned but involve skills that are practical rather than merely theoretical (Flexner, 1915). There are varying educational requirements for healthcare professions and occupations. See Table 7.1 for some examples.

TABLE 7.1   Minimum Educational Requirements for Entry Into Practice

Minimum Educational Requirements	Examples
Vocational education	Certified nursing assistant, emergency medical technician, paramedic, medical coder and biller, licensed practical nurse
Associate's degree (2–3 years at a community college)	Registered nurse (RN), radiologic technician, respiratory therapist, dental hygienist, surgical technologist, OT or PT assistant
Bachelor's degree (4 years at a college or university)	RN with a Bachelor of Science in Nursing
Master's degree (2 or more years postbaccalaureate at a college or university)	Occupational therapist, speech language pathologist, nurse practitioner, physician assistant
Practice doctorate degree (2–6 or more years postbaccalaureate education at a college or university)	Physician, dentist, physical therapist, audiologist, pharmacist

Unique Body of Knowledge

There is a unique body of knowledge that is specific to the professional discipline and serves as the basis for the practice of the profession (Birden et al., 2014). This knowledge can be learned and is refined and expanded through discipline-specific research (Flexner, 1915). This knowledge consists of both theoretical knowledge and technical skills and is demonstrated through evidence-based practice (Chitty, 2011).

Service

A specific need of society is served by the profession. Professions are characterized by their service. There is "a sense of calling to the discipline, a sense of mission, and a responsibility to the public" (Chitty, 2011, p. 62).

Autonomy

Autonomy is defined as the quality or state of being self-governing (Merriam-Webster, 2015). Self-governing, or self-regulation, means that it is only members of the profession themselves who decide what is required educationally and legally to become and remain a practitioner of that profession. For example, in the United States, Boards of Nursing are responsible for licensing and disciplining nurses, not Boards of Medicine. Healthcare professions accomplish self-regulation through professional licensing bodies, accrediting bodies, and other professional organizations. Professions regulate their own practice by creating and adhering to standards of practice, standards of care, licensure requirements, and various types of certification. In the United States, state licensure and state practice acts define the legal requirements to practice a specific healthcare profession and what a professional may not do in that state. Licensure and practice acts vary. It is the responsibility of all professionals to be knowledgeable about and adhere to the practice act of the state in which they are licensed to practice. Some states have compact agreements that allow professionals who are licensed in one state of the compact to practice in the other states in the compact. Professionals may not legally practice in a country, state, province, or other location in which they do not have a license.

Code of Ethics

Members of a profession identify a code of ethics for practice that outlines the standards of behavior and values held by that profession (Birden et al., 2014). A code of ethics is a written document "encompassing the set of rules based on values and the standards of conduct to which practitioners of a profession are expected to conform" (Mosby, 2012, p. 395). A code of ethics acts as a framework for decision making and is an example of a standard for practice. It is nonnegotiable. This means that one's professional code of ethics takes precedence over institutional policies and personal values (ANA, 2015).

Scope of Practice

Scope of practice denotes those activities that members of a specific profession are legally allowed to do as a result of their education, although it is often incorrectly used to denote professional roles and responsibilities. Legal scope of practice results from legislation enacted to define practice boundaries in individual states in the United States.

Representatives from six healthcare regulatory organizations collaborated to develop guidelines for changing their existing scopes of practice (NCSBN, 2009). They articulated several basic assumptions regarding scope of practice. Three are of special interest in understanding Interprofessional Collaborative Practice and the relationship of scope of practice to overlapping roles and responsibilities. They are summarized here:

- "Collaboration between healthcare providers should be the professional norm" (NCSBN, 2009, p. 10). This articulates the expectation that competent healthcare professionals will refer to other professionals in situations outside of their own expertise (Fig. 7.3). "Overlap among professions is necessary" (NCSBN, 2009, p. 10).

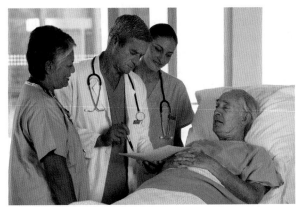

FIG. 7.3 Collaboration between healthcare providers. (© claudiobaba/iStock/Thinkstock.)

- No single profession owns a specific skill or activity. It is the entire scope and focus of activities within a profession that differentiates one profession from another.
- "No professional has enough skills or knowledge to perform all aspects of the profession's scope of practice. For instance, physicians' scope of practice is 'medicine,' but no physician has the skill and knowledge to perform every aspect of medical care" (NCSBN, 2009, p. 11). For example, an oncologist (cancer specialist) may not have adequate knowledge and skills to manage a difficult birth. All professional scopes of practice include advanced skills that new practitioners have not acquired. "As professions evolve, new techniques are developed; not all practitioners are competent to perform these new techniques" (NCSBN, 2009, pp. 10–11).

There are many skills and procedures that fall within the roles and responsibilities of multiple professions. Each profession is guided by its own legal scope of practice. Professional roles and responsibilities, as well as the legal scope of practice of each healthcare professional on the interprofessional team, need to be considered in identifying responsibilities for care.

HEALTHCARE PROFESSIONS AND OCCUPATIONS

The healthcare workforce is large and complex. Healthcare careers include those careers that focus on the promotion and maintenance of the health and condition of the human body (both mentally and physically). See Box 7.1 for a list of 43 healthcare occupations from the US Bureau of Labor Statistics (BLS) (2015). Although not listed by the BLS (2015), social workers, psychologists, and public health personnel are also considered healthcare professionals. Many healthcare professionals choose to work in the field of behavioral health, where interprofessional collaboration is as important as it is in other healthcare specialties. Other members of the healthcare team may include those who work in healthcare finance, education, sales, equipment, bioengineering, housekeeping, or research.

Healthcare professions have different minimum educational requirements for entry into practice depending on which profession is chosen. For example, a clinical doctorate is required to become a physical therapist (DPT) or an audiologist (AuD), whereas a master's degree is

BOX 7.1   Healthcare Occupations Listed by the United States Bureau of Labor Statistics (2015)

Athletic trainer and exercise physiologist
Audiologist
Chiropractor
Dentist
Dental assistants
Dental hygienist
Diagnostic medical sonographer, cardiovascular technician, vascular technologist
Dietician or nutritionist
Emergency medical technician or paramedic
Genetic counselor
Health and safety technician
Home health aide
Licensed practical or vocational nurse
Massage therapist
Medical assistant
Medical or clinical laboratory technologist or technician

Medical records and health information technician
Medical transcriptionist
Nuclear medicine technologist
Nurse anesthetist, nurse midwife, nurse practitioner
Nursing assistant; orderly
Occupational health and safety specialist
Occupational therapist
Occupational therapy assistant or aide
Optician dispensing
Optometrist
Orthotist or prosthetist
Personal care aide
Pharmacist
Pharmacy technician

Phlebotomist
Physical therapist
Physical therapy assistant or aide
Physician assistant
Physician or surgeon
Podiatrist
Psychiatric mental health technician or aide
Radiation therapist
Radiologic and magnetic resonance imaging technologist
Recreational therapist
Registered nurse
Respiratory therapist
Speech language pathologist
Surgical technician

⊕ GLOBAL PERSPECTIVES ON HEALTHCARE PROFESSIONALS

We are witnessing the migration of healthcare professionals in what is now a global market for their talents. An international shortage of healthcare professionals, combined with the maldistribution of professional talent, has resulted in a global call for change in healthcare systems, in the roles of healthcare professionals, and in the design of healthcare professional education programs (Crisp & Chen, 2014). Healthcare professionals should meet universal standards of education that support the cross-national transfer of technology, expertise, and services (Crisp & Chen, 2014).

required to become a physician assistant (MSPA) or occupational therapist (MSOT), although a clinical doctorate in occupational therapy (OTD) is available. Many professions require a single minimum degree for entry into practice and may offer specific higher degrees for those who satisfactorily complete approved further higher education programs. Nursing, unlike most professions, offers several paths to entry-level registered nurse (RN) practice.

Educational requirements vary by profession and among individual schools, colleges, universities, or educational programs. Most professional education programs require students to undergo a criminal background check and drug testing to practice in clinical areas as students or clinicians and for state licensure. All healthcare professionals are required to pass a national examination and may need to meet additional requirements for state licensure to practice. Some related careers do not meet criteria to be considered true professions; they do not require advanced education or licensure. It is the responsibility of each professional to understand licensure and/or certification processes, scope of practice, and legislation related to their profession in the geographic location in which they practice.

Appendix A contains information about the roles, responsibilities, and educational requirements of some of the most common healthcare professions and related careers. The information is specific to the United States and is meant to serve as a general guide.

PROFESSIONAL IDENTITY DEVELOPMENT

Part of the professionalization process is the development of your own professional identity. Professional identity can be defined as one's professional self-concept based on attributes, beliefs, values, motives, and experiences (Ibarra, 1999; Schein, 1978). The development of a professional identity is important in the formation of new healthcare professionals (Gibson et al., 2010; Johnson et al., 2012; Trede et al., 2012); in addition, a positive and flexible professional identity has been associated with the ability of professionals to function at a high level, benefiting not only the healthcare professional but also patients and other healthcare workers (Johnson et al., 2012).

Professional identity development is a lifelong process. For example, professional identity development can begin even before you enter professional education. Lordly and MacLellan (2012) found that the professional identity of dietetic students began with their early experiences with food. It was these early experiences that then evolved into a professional identity with the structure of professional education, including observation, exposure, practice, and expectation (Lordly and MacLellan, 2012).

Once individuals start a formal professional education, they experience an ongoing process of identity "construction and deconstruction" (Johnson et al., 2012). This means that you will be adopting and discarding values, jargon, and ways of doing things throughout your professional education and early career; this is similar to how teens develop their identity, by trying new things. This process happens through contact with peers, teachers, mentors, and professionals in your field, as well as by learning the culture and skills of your profession (Johnson et al., 2012). Your professional identity will be fairly formed by the time you start practicing; however, you will continue to adjust your professional identity throughout your professional life.

There are three recognized phases of professional identity development (Gibson et al., 2010). In the first phase, the identity of the students is held externally by authority figures and experts. In the second phase, students start to internalize the professional identity through feedback from supervisors and other professionals. Finally, in the third phase, "the new professional is able to self-evaluate, integrating experience with theory to merge personal and professional identities" (Gibson et al., 2010, p. 22). Self-reflection is a desired outcome of a successfully integrated professional identity; throughout their careers, healthcare professionals must demonstrate the ability to critically reflect on and incorporate new information (Trede et al., 2012).

⁂ ACTIVE LEARNING

Think about your own professional identity in terms of the three phases identified by Gibson et al. (2010).
1. Describe your experience of professional identity development.
2. Which phase are you in now?

PROFESSIONAL IDENTITY AND INTERPROFESSIONAL COLLABORATIVE PRACTICE

When healthcare professionals work with one another, they must make adjustments in their professional identity to accommodate other healthcare professionals. This happens because each healthcare profession has its own jargon, culture, and way of doing things, so when two or more healthcare professionals work together, each of them has to accommodate the other. For example, Meyer et al. (2015) found that "medical residents and nurse practitioner trainees were invested in negotiating their individual professional identities to create a meaningful group dedicated to the common goal of improving patient care" (p. 806).

The best time to make adjustments to your professional identity and to become truly interprofessional is when you are a student with sufficient professional identity to "represent [your] discipline but [be] flexible enough that [you] will not resist collaborative practice" (D'Amour et al., 2005, p. 125). Healthcare professionals who did not have the opportunity to experience Interprofessional Education (IPE) as students may need to experience a resocialization of the way in which they practice after graduation. This means that they will need to work in an environment that fosters collaborative practice so they can integrate this way of practice into their identity (D'Amour et al., 2005).

SELF-REFLECTION AS A LEARNING TOOL

Self-reflection can be defined as the ability to engage in introspection with the willingness to learn something

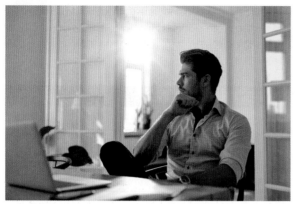

FIG. 7.4 Self-reflection is a tool for learning. (© Jacob Ammentorp Lund/iStock/Thinkstock.)

about oneself in the process and the desire to grow and change (Fig. 7.4). Philosophers have argued for centuries that self-reflection is part of the human condition, and as such, we sometimes engage in self-reflection spontaneously. "A typical example is that situation when you are standing in the shower, driving home from work or trying to get to sleep when you suddenly start thinking about the patient you saw earlier today" (Bostock-Cox, 2015, par. 4). However, as healthcare professionals, we need to develop self-reflection as a systematic and intentional process.

The first component of self-reflection, introspection, is the examination of our own feelings and thoughts. It is a process of self-scrutiny through personal observation or dialogue with the self (Watts, 2012). Introspection is a cognitive task that requires a certain level of intentionality because it can be susceptible to several barriers. One barrier is that self-scrutiny can be threatening to the self; therefore some people want to avoid it (Watts, 2012). For example, examining your role in a medical error can be emotionally difficult and threatening to your self-concept (Durgahee, 1997). Another barrier is that when things are going well, you may not see a need for self-examination (Watts, 2012). Overcoming barriers to introspection is important because, as you will see, there is a role for introspection throughout the professional life of the healthcare professional.

The second component of self-reflection is the willingness to learn something from engaging in introspection. The examination of the self alone may or may not lead to learning; however, when introspection is done with the intention of learning something about yourself, then you are engaging in self-reflection. Again, this suggests the process requires a level of intentionality on your part.

All healthcare professions try to incorporate self-reflection into their educational programs. For example, it is common for psychology, counseling, and social work students to record some of their sessions to review with their supervisors. Some healthcare professions, such as nursing, have formally integrated self-reflection in their training and practice; in fact, the concept of reflective practice is ubiquitous in nursing, to the point that is part of nursing's standards of practice (Gouylet, Laure, & Anderson, 2015). "Reflective practice is the ability to examine one's actions and experiences with the outcome of developing their practice and enhancing clinical knowledge" (Caldwell & Grobbel, 2013, p. 319). In other words, reflective practice is the ability to learn from experience. Reflective practice is believed to help with the integration of theory and practice and improve practice (Enuku & Evawoma-Enuku, 2015).

Skills Needed for Self-Reflection

Several skills were identified as necessary to engage in self-reflection; these include awareness, description, critical analysis, synthesis, and evaluation (Bulman & Schutz, 2013); action or intervention has also been suggested by some as another needed skill (Sherwood & Horton-Deutsch, 2012).

Awareness means being conscious of oneself, including beliefs, values, qualities, strengths, and limitations (Enuku & Evawoma-Enuku, 2015). For example, the skill of awareness applied to clinical practice may involve recognizing that your experience in sports make you especially well suited to working with athletes, or that because it is difficult for you to see children suffer, you could not work in a pediatric trauma center.

Description refers to the ability to state the characteristics of something (e.g., idea, object, person, situation) in a nonjudgmental manner (Enuku & Evawoma-Enuku, 2015). This skill is essential for self-reflection because it is difficult to critically examine something that you are not able to describe. For example, if you try to reflect on your role in a medical error, the self-reflection requires a complete and accurate description of the event(s) that led to and constituted the error.

Critical analysis is the ability to examine the components, internal structure, and interactions of a whole to understand it (Enuku & Evawoma-Enuku, 2015). In terms of healthcare practice, this may mean the ability to examine all the elements involved in a medical error. Many medical errors are the sum of a series of events, for example, breakdowns in communication, lack of ignoring redundancy in procedures, and lack of resources (e.g., expertise, time), among others.

Synthesis is the ability to form a single coherent idea out of several different elements (e.g., ideas, opinions, experiences) (Enuku & Evawoma-Enuku, 2015). Once an issue has been analyzed critically, synthesis is then used to formulate a solution or new perspective on the issue. For example, critical analysis of an outpatient rehabilitation patient falling at home may suggest that an occupational therapist was needed on the care team.

Evaluation is the ability to pass judgment over something using a set criteria or standard (Enuku & Evawoma-Enuku, 2015). Once a solution or new perspective is developed, it is necessary to evaluate how appropriate it is to the situation. It is possible to lack the appropriate resources to implement the best solution, or the time to implement the solution may have passed.

Action or intervention is the ability to decide whether and how to take action, once a new perspective has been developed through self-reflection (Sherwood & Horton-Deutsch, 2012). Action or intervention would be the logical culmination of the self-reflection process. Once the solution or new perspective is defined, it is important to know when and how it is appropriate to implement it in the future.

Tools to Develop Self-Reflection

A significant number of strategies have been proposed for the development of self-reflection skills in student healthcare professionals; many of them are also recommended for practicing healthcare professionals. In general, these strategies require the instructor, student, or clinician to be intentional about developing these skills. It also requires a support structure; for beginners it may be a supervisor; for practitioners, it may mean having time to reflect on their own practice. Table 7.2 provides a list of common strategies for the development of self-reflection skills.

The development of your self-reflection skills can be facilitated in the classroom, during supervision, or during other less-formal learning opportunities. Guiding questions can focus on skills—for example: "What were you good at, even as a child?" or "What skill(s), with just a little bit of practice or more training, could rapidly improve?" or "What did you learn about yourself that

helped you to improve?" (Watts, 2012). The questions can also focus on feelings, such as: "How did you feel about the call?" or "What do you think made you feel that way?" (Turner, 2015). The guiding questions can also focus directly on your practice, such as: "What happened?"; "What are the factors that affected this patient's care?"; and "How will you use this information next time?" (Willis, 2010).

Self-Awareness of Strengths and Limitations

Self-awareness is the ability to be an observer and critic of your own inner life (e.g., thinking, feelings); it is related to, but separate from, self-reflection. It can be developed in several ways. First, engaging in self-reflection will improve your self-awareness because it forces you to practice being an observer of your own thoughts and feelings (Watts, 2012). Another way to improve self-awareness is by receiving feedback from a trusted source such as teachers, colleagues, or supervisors (Watts, 2012). Receiving feedback about our actions as healthcare professionals helps us to understand ourselves better by providing information about ourselves. For example, feedback can point out to us the behaviors, thoughts, and feelings to which we may be blind.

Self-awareness is a necessary skill for healthcare professionals to assess their own strengths and limitations; this is especially true if they take time to self-reflect on those aspects of their practice. Self-awareness helps healthcare professionals to decide for which cases they have the necessary skills and experience to work by themselves, for which cases they might need consultation, and for which cases they need a more experienced colleague or supervisor to assist. Healthcare professionals have to evaluate their qualifications in terms of a wide range of aspects: having the necessary knowledge to treat a specific disorder, having the appropriate personality to work with a type of patient (e.g., the elderly), or having reservations about engaging in a treatment that is morally unacceptable to them (e.g., providing in vitro fertilization to a lesbian couple). In these situations, self-awareness can prevent errors and delay of treatment.

ROLES AND RESPONSIBILITIES IN THE CONTEXT OF TEAMWORK

What Is a Healthcare Team?

A group can be defined as "two or more individuals who are connected to one another by social relationships"

TABLE 7.2 Strategies to Develop Self-Reflection Skills

Supervised clinical experiences	The most common strategy you will experience to develop your self-reflection skills, as a student or a trainee, is some kind of supervised clinical experience. In this context, you can reflect on your clinical practice with guidance and feedback from your clinical supervisor, usually an experienced clinician. In some healthcare professions this experience is more formal and structured than in others.
Collaborative reflective training	In this strategy, a team of experienced healthcare professionals (i.e., supervisors) would observe you engaging in some kind of intervention, often a simulation. After the intervention is over, the team of supervisors will debrief the experience in front of you. This provides you with the opportunity to observe how experienced healthcare professionals reflect on a clinical situation and allows you to see your clinical performance from their point of view. This approach minimizes the power differential between you and your supervisors and gives you the opportunity to reflect on the feedback without being required to respond (Kim et al., 2016).
Reflection groups	These tend to be small groups facilitated by an experienced supervisor, in which trainees can share their emotional reaction to their clinical practice (Pololi et al., 2001). The structure of these groups is similar to the clinical group supervision that mental health workers in training (e.g., psychology, social work, and counseling) would have; however, the groups tend to focus more on the emotional aspect than on the actual practice.
Structured reflective models	These models tend to provide a series of questions that will guide your reflection. For example, Turner (2015) described a structured reflective model for paramedics. This model has eight questions in a specific sequence that would lead you to identify the best solution for a specific clinical problem.
Reflective journaling	This technique works by providing you with the opportunity to reflect on your practice. The journaling can be structured in many ways; for example, the reflective journaling described by Brathovde et al. (2013) uses Watson's science of caring theory. In another example, Pololi et al. (2001) asked students to focus their journaling by reflecting on a problem that they had in clinical practice and their personal reaction to that problem.
Creative reflective writing	The purpose of creative reflective writing is to provide you with the opportunity to reflect on the experience of clinical practice. Creative reflective writing can be open or structured; however, it tends to focus on significant experiences with patients, colleagues, and teachers. The writing styles used include poetry, short stories, skits, and critical incident essays, among others (Shapiro et al., 2006).
Reflective assignments	Assignments are another vehicle for learning self-reflection that you may encounter. They tend to have a narrow focus, but the focus of these assignments can vary widely. For example, Josephsen (2013) discussed two types of assignments. In one assignment, students were asked to reflect on "the changing role of nurses"; in another assignment, students were asked to identify and reflect on the assumptions that affected their clinical practice.
Courses focusing on self-reflection and reflective practice	Several educational institutions have developed whole courses for the development of self-reflective skills (Hannah & Carpenter-Song, 2013; Pololi et al., 2001).

(Forsyth, 2006, p. 3); however, a group in itself does not necessarily constitute a team (Deepa, 2016). Traditionally, groups of healthcare personnel involved in the provision of care to a patient have been called *teams,* whether or not they actually collaborate in providing that care. Grumbach and Bodenheimer (2004) offered the following definition of a team: "A team is a group with a specific task or tasks, the accomplishment of which requires the interdependent and collaborative efforts of its members" (p. 1247). An important difference between a group of providers and a collaborative team is that the team works together and shares responsibility for making decisions to develop and deliver a plan of care; a "group of providers" does not (Dufour & Lucy, 2010).

An *interprofessional collaborative healthcare team* is defined as a team that engages in cooperation, coordination, and collaboration that is characterized by the relationships between the professionals involved in the delivery of patient-centered care (IPEC, 2011). This means that interprofessional teamwork involves collaboration among team members to reach a common goal. A foundation of mutual trust and respect is essential for this collaborative partnership.

Clarifying Roles in Healthcare Teams

Simply bringing healthcare providers from different disciplines to work together within a team does not mean they will complement one another when providing care. When healthcare professionals do not provide interprofessional collaborative patient-centered care, they run the risk of duplicating care; for example, two providers may order the same diagnostic study. Similarly, the healthcare professionals can provide conflicting care, as would be the case when two healthcare professionals unknowingly prescribe medications that interact negatively with each other. In the first case, the professionals would be wasting resources; in the second case, the conflict could harm the patient.

All team members must be able to explain team roles and responsibilities, for themselves and for other team members, as a precursor to clarifying how the team will work together in a specific patient care situation. This clarification of specific roles and responsibilities for the patient's care is essential in light of the overlapping knowledge, skills, and abilities of professionals providing care to the same patient. This may include deciding who will share responsibilities and perform overlapping skills and responsibilities in a plan of care.

It is important to be clear about roles and responsibilities within the context of the interprofessional team. The composition of the team and the needs of the patient will influence the distribution of tasks and responsibilities. Some roles are *differentiated* roles; that is, they exist when team members have separate and distinct responsibilities by virtue of their knowledge, skills, and abilities (MacNaughton et al., 2013). This means the differentiated roles and responsibilities of the healthcare professional are clear for the case at hand. Sometimes, though, roles and responsibilities are not as clearly designated to a specific team member because the role or task is not unique to one profession. These roles are referred to as *interchangeable* or *overlapping* roles (MacNaughton et al., 2013). Caselet 7.1 provides an example of areas where professional roles may overlap.

In the case of Mr. Jackson, the management of the diabetes mediation falls within the scope of practice of the primary care physician, the endocrinologist, and the nurse practitioner (i.e., overlap); all three of them should not attempt to undertake the same role and responsibility for Mr. Jackson's medication management. It is worth remembering that roles and responsibilities in a specific case is different from scope of practice. All three healthcare professionals here are legally able to manage the diabetes medication of Mr. Jackson (i.e., scope of practice); however, only one of them should manage the diabetes medication (i.e., role and responsibility). Clarification of roles and responsibilities for medication management is vital to avoid errors that may result from the duplication of services and conflict of treatment.

Consider that, in this case, the assignment of responsibility for medication management was influenced by contextual factors, not legal scope of practice boundaries. This means that in a different context, a different healthcare professional may have been assigned the responsibility for managing the diabetes medication; however, the scope of practice of the three healthcare professionals is not affected by the context because it is set by the law.

An interprofessional team that is working collaboratively would quickly and seamlessly clarify which professional would be assigned the responsibility for any overlapping roles (Fig. 7.5). This is true because all of the professionals on the team would demonstrate high levels of cooperation, coordination, and collaboration, allowing them to recognize who is best situated to take responsibility for an overlapping role. Identifying the overlapping responsibilities of various team members

CASELET 7.1   Mr. Jackson

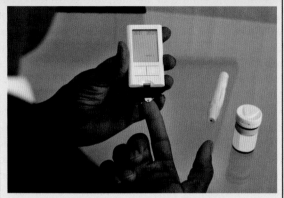

(Photo © AndreyPopov/iStock/Thinkstock.)

Mr. Jackson in a 48-year-old African American man with uncontrolled type 2 diabetes. The team involved in the management of his diabetes includes a primary care physician and his office nurse (an RN), an endocrinologist and the nurse practitioner in that practice, a nutritionist in a community diabetes care center, an ophthalmologist, and a podiatrist. He also interacts with a phlebotomist for frequent blood work and with his mail order pharmacy service. Mr. Jackson has bloodwork performed every 3 months to monitor his diabetes, which is followed by adjustment to his diabetes medication as indicated as a result of the laboratory work.

Discussion Questions
1. Can you predict any areas where professional roles will overlap in Mr. Jackson's care?
2. Describe at least two consequences of not addressing these overlapping roles in Mr. Jackson's care.
3. What can be done by the healthcare team to address overlapping roles?

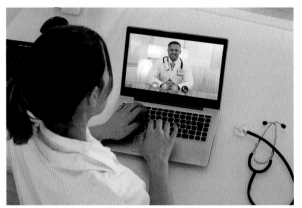

FIG. 7.5 It is important to clarify roles within the health-care team. (© AndreyPopov/iStock/Thinkstock.)

provides an avenue to streamline and enhance the continuity of team-based care. MacNaughton et al. (2013) viewed overlapping responsibilities as opportunities for "alleviating the burden of their workload" (p. 8). Frequent team interactions and the transparent sharing of information enhances trust and respect between members and promotes collaboration (MacNaughton et al., 2013).

Barriers to the Clarification of Roles in Healthcare Teams

A significant barrier to interprofessional collaboration is the perception of power imbalances between team members. Professionals may be reluctant to share power with others in developing a plan of care, particularly if their professional education occurred within discipline-specific "silos." Dufour and Lucy (2010) emphasized the importance of role clarification, role valuing, and power sharing within the interprofessional team. Historically, many interprofessional relationships involved such power imbalances, with physicians having most of the power. It is essential that each team member be valued for his or her unique and essential contributions to patient care.

Rigid adherence to total professional autonomy is a barrier to collaboration. Successfully clarifying roles necessitates finding the balance between autonomy and collaboration, instead of hierarchical interactions. Collaboration includes elements of assertiveness and cooperativeness so that parties arrive at mutually compatible solutions recognizing the concerns of all professionals involved. In one example, there is evidence that collaboration among advanced practice nurses and physicians improves quality and cost of care (Maylone et al., 2011).

Overlapping responsibilities may create the potential for power struggles among professionals. The potential for "turf wars" or power struggles can be minimized through synchronous or asynchronous team meetings or discussions that provide opportunities to specifically address any confusion over roles and responsibilities and clarify roles in the care situation. Such interactions serve as a forum where team members can develop a shared knowledge and expertise of another profession. Such recognition triggers the request for consultation from another provider to best fill the gap in providing optimal patient care.

RESEARCH HIGHLIGHT

Clarifying Interprofessional Roles in Clinical Education

Working together with other professional groups during a 2-week interprofessional clinical placement improved both students' understanding of their own role, as well as the roles of others (Hood et al., 2014). Opportunities to practice professional communication improved students' role confidence; students reported that the interprofessional clinical placement enabled them to learn how to work together more effectively than their previous experiences (Hood et al., 2014).

Interprofessional Consultation With Team Members

The clear understanding of the roles and responsibilities of diverse healthcare professionals will foster appropriate collaboration with other team members who complement your own expertise. Individual team members involved in a patient's care often identify additional problems that would benefit from the specialized knowledge and expertise of another professional. Such recognition should trigger the request for consultation with another healthcare provider to seek the additional expertise needed. In turn, consultation with other professionals on a patient case fosters the exchange of expertise and perspectives needed to determine an optimal patient-centered plan of care.

Consultation occurs through formal mechanisms as well as through informal exchanges. Healthcare professionals working in close proximity are likely to engage in synchronous communication; this communication can range from brief verbal interactions to formal team meetings. Close physical proximity promotes more team interactions, providing more opportunities for casual exchanges. On the other hand, team members working in different physical locations may face barriers to working collaboratively (MacNaughton et al., 2013). When working in varied community settings, for example, these barriers can be overcome through the use of routine routes of communication and requests for consultation that can happen asynchronously through electronic or paper processes. Although asynchronous communication can be as effective as synchronous communication, it tends to be slower, so it may not be appropriate for emergencies.

Team members may consult some colleagues more often than others, based on the perceived relevance of their professional knowledge, to assist in their routine patient care decisions (MacNaughton et al., 2013). For example, nurse practitioners routinely consult pharmacists to discuss specific patient medication issues. The specific healthcare setting may also influence the process of consultation with other professionals. For example, in the inpatient rehabilitation setting, formal team conferences to discuss the patient plan of care typically include physicians, nurses, social workers, therapists, the patient, and family who are generally present in that setting.

ADDITIONAL RESOURCES

The following resources are provided to assist you in fully understanding the roles and responsibilities of various healthcare professions. You are also encouraged to search for the websites of specific professional organizations, and to ask members of specific professions what they perceive their role is in different situations.

Educational Resources

Interprofessional Care: An Introductory Session on the Roles of Health Professionals. Durham, M., Lie, D., & Lohenry, K. (2014). MedEdPORTAL. 2014;10:9813. https://doi.org/10.15766/mep_2374-8265.9813

This is a curriculum for a one-session class to help students in the health professions to recognize professional roles in the context of team-based care.

Roles and Responsibilities. Adams Tufts, K. (2016). Norfolk, VA: ODU Monarch Center for Comprehensive Interprofessional Education and Collaborative Practice. https://online.odu.edu/bin/interprofessional_education/

This is an educational video (27:53 minutes) from Old Dominion University demonstrating the Core Competency of Roles/Responsibilities. The video starts with an explanation of Interprofessional Collaborative Practice. The video then focuses on an interprofessional team developing a plan of care for a patient.

Roles and Responsibilities: It Takes a Team! Kennedy, T. (2016). Y. Price, Designer. [Interactive video module]. Center for Advancing Interprofessional Practice, Education & Research, Arizona State University, Phoenix. http://www.asu.edu/courses/ipe000/fm3/story.html

Continued

📄 **ADDITIONAL RESOURCES—cont'd**

This resource is a module to introduce students to the Core Competency of Roles/Responsibilities. The self-paced, interactive module allows the student to read and hear the information provided. The module is divided into four sections and provides several links to supplemental content. This resource is free.

Assessment Tool
The Role Perception Questionnaire (RPQ). Mackay, S. (2004). The role perception questionnaire (RPQ): A tool for assessing undergraduate students' perceptions of the role of other professions. *Journal of Interprofessional Care, 18*(3), 289–302. http://informahealthcare.com/

This tool was developed to assess undergraduate healthcare students' perceptions about the role of other health professionals. Access to this tool requires a fee.

United States Government Resource
Occupational Outlook Handbook; Healthcare Occupations: 2015-16 Edition. Washington, DC: US Department of Labor. http://www.bls.gov/ooh/healthcare/home.htm

This is an excellent resource for employment outlook, salary information, and description of a variety of health-related occupation developed by the United States Bureau of Labor Statistics (BLS). It is updated frequently.

KEY POINTS

- The word *role* refers to a set of expected behaviors that fit together into a unified whole. Those behaviors characterize a person in a given context.
- A profession is a calling requiring specialized knowledge and often long and intensive academic preparation in an institution of higher learning. Educational preparation for each profession and regulatory requirements for practice vary among professionals and from state to state.
- Healthcare professionals become socialized to their roles in educational programs designed specifically to prepare them for their scope of practice and expected roles.
- The development of a professional identity is important in the formation of healthcare professionals.
- It is no longer enough for healthcare providers to simply be professional; healthcare workers also need to be prepared to practice as members of interprofessional collaborative teams.
- Interprofessional teams are made up of healthcare professionals from two or more healthcare disciplines or professions.
- An *interprofessional collaborative healthcare team* is defined as a team that engages in cooperation, coordination, and collaboration that is characterized by the relationships between the professionals involved in the delivery of patient-centered care.
- Interprofessional Collaborative Practice requires a clear and accurate understanding of all professional roles and responsibilities and a working knowledge related to how the roles of all healthcare professionals complement one another in the provision of optimal patient-centered care.
- Knowledge about the roles and responsibilities of others on the interprofessional team is essential in the identification of overlapping roles and responsibilities in a care situation.
- Interprofessional Collaborative Practice requires assigning overlapping skills and responsibilities within the team to avoid duplication and conflict of care.

REFERENCES

American Nurses Association (ANA). (2015). *What is nursing?* Retrieved from http://www.bls.gov/ooh/healthcare/nurse-anesthetists-nurse-midwives-and-nurse-practitioners.htm.

APHA (n.d.). *What is public health?* Author. Retrieved from https://www.apha.org/what-is-public-health.

Birden, H., Glass, N., Wilson, I., et al. (2014). Defining professionalism in medical education: A systematic review. *Medical Teacher, 36*, 47–61.

Bixler, G., & Bixler, R. (1945). The professional status of nursing. *The American Journal of Nursing*, 45(9), 730–735.

Bostock-Cox, B. (2015). Making sense of reflective practice. *Practice Nurse*, 45(10), HTML full text retrieved from EBSCO Host.

Brathovde, A., Bodine, J., Cagliostro, J., et al. (2013). Using reflective journaling to establish a holistic nursing practice council. *International Journal of Human Caring*, 17(2), 35–38.

Bulman, C., & Schutz, S. (2013). *Reflective practice in nursing* (5th ed.). West Sussex, UK: Wiley-Blackwell.

Bureau of Labor Statistics (BLS). (2015). *Occupational outlook handbook; Healthcare occupations* (16th ed.). Washington, DC: US Department of Labor. Retrieved from http://www.bls.gov/ooh/healthcare/home.htm.

Caldwell, L., & Grobbel, C. C. (2013). The importance of reflective practice in nursing. *International Journal of Caring Sciences*, 6(3), 319–326.

Chitty, K. (2011). Nursing's pathway to professionalism. In K. K. Chitty & B. Black (Eds.), *Professional nursing: concepts and challenges* (6th ed.). St. Louis: Saunders Elsevier.

Crisp, N., & Chen, L. (2014). Global supply of health professionals. *New England Journal of Medicine*, 370, 950–957. Retrieved from http://www.nejm.org/doi/full/10.1056/NEJMra1111610#t=article.

D'Amour, D., Ferrada-Videla, M., San Martin Rodriguez, L., et al. (2005). The conceptual basis for interprofessional collaboration: Core concepts and theoretical frameworks. *Journal of Interprofessional Care*, 5(S1), 116–131.

Deepa, E. (2016). A study on team cohesiveness. *International Journal of Applied Research*, 2(5), 302–305.

Dufour, S. P., & Lucy, S. D. (2010). Situating primary health care within the International Classification of Functioning, Disability and Health: Enabling the Canadian Family Health Team Initiative. *Journal of Interprofessional Care*, 24(6), 666–677.

Durgahee, T. (1997). Reflective practice: Nursing ethics through story telling. *Nursing Ethics*, 4(2), 135–146.

Enuku, C. A., & Evawoma-Enuku, U. (2015). Importance of reflective practice in nursing education. *West African Journal of Nursing*, 26(1), 52–59.

Flexner, A. (1915). *Is social work a profession?* General Session Presentation, May 17. Forty-Second Annual Session, National Conference of Charities and Correction: Baltimore, Maryland, May 12–19, 1915.

Forsyth, D. R. (2006). *Group dynamics* (4th ed.). Belmont, CA: Thomson Wadsworth.

Gibson, D. M., Dollarhide, C. T., & Moss, J. M. (2010). Professional identity development: A grounded theory of transformational tasks of new counselors. *Counselor Education & Supervision*, 50, 21–38.

Gouylet, M. H., Larue, C., & Alderson, M. (2015). Reflective practice: A comparative dimensional analysis of the concept in nursing and education studies. *Nursing Forum*, 51(2), 139–150.

Grumbach, K., & Bodenheimer, T. (2004). Can health care teams improve primary care practice? *Journal of the American Medical Association*, 291, 1246–1251.

Hannah, S., & Carpenter-Song, E. (2013). Patrolling your blind spots: Introspection and public catharsis in a medical school faculty development course to reduce unconscious bias in medicine. *Culture, Medicine and Psychiatry*, 37, 314–339.

Hood, K., Cant, R., Leech, M., et al. (2014). Trying on the professional self: Nursing students' perceptions of learning about roles, identity and teamwork in an interprofessional clinical placement. *Applied Nursing Research*, 27, 109–114.

Ibarra, H. (1999). Provisional selves: Experimenting with Image and Identity in professional adaptation. *Administrative Science Quarterly*, 44, 764–791.

Interprofessional Education Collaborative Expert Panel (IPEC). (2011). *Core competencies for interprofessional collaborative practice: Report of an expert panel*. Washington, DC: Interprofessional Education Collaborative.

Interprofessional Education Collaborative Expert Panel (IPEC). (2016). *Core competencies for interprofessional collaborative practice: 2016 update*. Washington, DC: Interprofessional Education Collaborative.

Johnson, M., Cowin, L. S., Wilson, I., et al. (2012). Professional identity and nursing: Contemporary theoretical developments and future research challenges. *International Nursing Review*, 59, 562–569.

Josephsen, J. M. (2013, January–February). Evidence-based reflective teaching practice: A preceptorship course example. *Nursing Education Perspectives*, 8–11.

Kim, L., Couden Hernandez, B., Lavery, A., et al. (2016). Stimulating reflective practice using collaborative reflective training in breaking ad news simulations. *Family, Systems, & Health*, 34(2), 83–91.

Lordly, D., & MacLellan, D. (2012). Dietetic students' identity and professional socialization. *Canadian Journal of Dietetic Practice and Research*, 73(1), 7–13.

MacNaughton, K., Chreim, S., & Bourgeault, I. (2013). Role construction and boundaries in interprofessional primary health care teams: A qualitative study. *BioMed Central Health Services Research*, 13, 486. Retrieved from http://www.biomedcentral.com/1472-6963/13/486B.

Maylone, M. M., Ranieri, L. A., Griffin, M. T. Q., et al. (2011). Collaboration and autonomy: Perceptions among nurse practitioners. *Journal of the American Academy of Nurse Practitioners*, 23, 51–57.

Merriam-Webster, Incorporated. (2015). *Merriam-Webster online dictionary*. Retrieved from http://www.merriam-webster.com/dictionary/autonomy Springfield, MA: Author.

Meyer, E. M., Zapatka, S., & Brienza, R. S. (2015). The development of professional identity and the formation of teams in the Veterans Affairs Connecticut Healthcare System's education program (CoEPCE). *Academic Medicine*, *90*(6), 802–809.

Mosby's Medical Dictionary. (2017). M. O'Toole (Ed.). Elsevier: St. Louis.

National Council of State Boards of Nursing (NCSBN). (2009). *Changes in healthcare professions' scope of practice: Legislative considerations*. Chicago, IL: Author.

Pavalko, R. M. (1971). *Sociology of occupations and professions*. Itasca, IL: F. E. Peacock.

Pololi, L., Frankel, R. M., Clay, M., et al. (2001). One year's experience with a program to facilitate personal and professional development in medical students using reflection groups. *Education for Health*, *14*(1), 36–49.

Schein, E. H. (1978). *Career dynamics: Matching individual and organizational needs*. Reading, MA: Addison-Wesley.

Shapiro, J., Kasman, D., & Shafer, A. (2006). Words and wards: A model of reflective writing and its uses in medical education. *Journal of Medical Humanity*, *27*, 231–244.

Sherwood, G., & Horton-Deutsch, S. (2012). *Transforming education and improving outcomes*. Indianapolis, IN: Sigma Theta Tau International.

Trede, F., Macklin, R., & Bridges, D. (2012). Professional identity development: A review of the higher education literature. *Studies in Higher Education*, *37*(3), 365–384.

Turner, H. (2015). Reflective practice for paramedics: A new approach. *Journal of Paramedic Practice*, *7*(3), 138–141.

Watts, G. W. (2012). The power of introspection for executive development. *The Psychologist-Manager Journal*, *15*, 149–157.

Willis, S. (2010). Becoming a reflective practitioner: Frameworks for the prehospital professional. *Journal of Paramedic Practice*, *2*(5), 212–216.

World Health Organization (WHO). (2010). *Framework for action on interprofessional education & collaborative practice*. Geneva: Author.

8

The Competency of Roles/ Responsibilities

LEARNING OUTCOMES

After studying this chapter, you will be able to:

1. Communicate your roles and responsibilities clearly to patients, families, community members, and other professionals.
2. Recognize your limitations in skills, knowledge, and abilities.
3. Engage diverse professionals who complement your own professional expertise, as well as associated resources, to develop strategies to meet patient specific health and healthcare needs of patients and populations.
4. Explain the roles and responsibilities of other care providers and how the team works together to provide care, promote health, and prevent disease.
5. Use the full scope of knowledge, skills, and abilities of available professionals from health and other fields to provide care that is safe, timely, efficient, effective, and equitable.
6. Communicate with team members to clarify each member's responsibility in executing components of a treatment plan or public health intervention.
7. Forge interdependent relationships with other professionals within and outside of the health system to improve care and advance learning.
8. Engage in continuous professional and interprofessional development to enhance team performance and collaboration.
9. Use the unique and complementary abilities of all members of the team to optimize health and patient care.
10. Describe how professionals in health and other fields can collaborate and integrate clinical care and public health interventions to optimize population health.

The interprofessional Core Competency of Roles/ Responsibilities, as defined by the Interprofessional Education Collaborative Expert Panel (IPEC, 2011; 2016), is explained and operationalized in this chapter. Remember that "common" or overlapping Core Competencies are those expected of all healthcare professionals. In considering the Core Competency of Roles/Responsibilities, it is important to clearly identify the roles and responsibilities within your own professional scope of practice for which you will be responsible in a given care situation and, further, to identify those that may overlap with those of one or more other healthcare professionals in a given care situation. For true collaboration to occur, each professional on the team must plan together with other professionals, with patients and families, with nonprofessionals and volunteers, within and between organizations, and within communities to clearly identify who will be responsible for overlapping roles and responsibilities (IPEC, 2011). The clear and deliberate illumination of these specific roles and responsibilities contributes to efficiency and safety while optimizing patient outcomes.

After the presentation of the Roles/Responsibilities Core Competency statement and specific Sub-competencies, case studies and caselets are used as appropriate to set the stage and illustrate each specific behavior. Not every possible profession or team member is involved in the provided patient care scenarios. Additional case studies are provided in Chapter 9. You are encouraged to apply each specific Sub-competency to examples in your own clinical practice and experience to determine any missed opportunities for Interprofessional Collaborative Practice.

THE ROLES/RESPONSIBILITIES CORE COMPETENCY STATEMENT

Use the knowledge of one's own role and those of other professions to appropriately assess and address the healthcare needs of patients and to promote and advance the health of populations served (IPEC, 2016, p. 12).

THE SUB-COMPETENCIES OF ROLES/ RESPONSIBILITIES

Recognizing the need for cooperation, coordination, and collaboration with other healthcare professionals begins the process of interprofessional teamwork that is essential to the achievement of optimal patient and population health outcomes (IPEC, 2011). Understanding your professional role and responsibilities, as well as those of other healthcare team members, is at the core of the Sub-competencies of Roles/Responsibilities (IPEC, 2011; 2016). It is the diversity of education, expertise, background, culture, and experience brought to the team by each member that provides essential team resources. These resources will lead to effective coordination and collaboration when they are used in a patient- and population-centered way (IPEC, 2011; 2016).

Each patient care situation is unique. To fully access and use team resources, you will need to first identify your own professional role and responsibilities in providing the needed care and then identify any limitations you may have in providing that care. Self-reflection is an essential tool for becoming competent in this domain. The process of self-reflection will help you to identify the boundaries of your own role and responsibilities within each care situation.

It is also important to identify areas in which your role and responsibilities may overlap with those of other team members. This information is crucial as you collaborate with team members to identify specific roles and responsibilities in the patient's care. It is through this process that the need for expertise from others who are not already on the team can be identified.

Whenever possible, involve the patient, family, and other significant carers in the plan of care; it is essential to acknowledge that professional healthcare providers are not the only members of the healthcare team who have roles and responsibilities. An early Institute of Medicine (IOM, 2003) report stressed that patients should participate in their own care through shared decision

making. Successful patient outcomes involve the active participation of patients, family members, and all other significant participants; the most perfect treatment plan means very little if the patient is not willing or able to engage in it.

Consider Case Study: The Case of Mr. Webb that presents what may be considered "routine" patient care. The discussion questions that follow will help you identify areas in which the application of the Sub-competencies associated with Roles/Responsibilities could transform Mr. Webb's "routine" care into a true example of Interprofessional Collaborative Practice and potentially improve his outcome.

After surgery, the physical therapy was consulted by Mr. Webb's physician and asked to begin mobility and gait training. Mr. Webb was evaluated by a physical therapist (PT), and a care plan was developed. He was non–weight bearing on his left lower limb. The case study is an account of the initial meeting of Mr. Webb and his assigned physical therapist (PT).

🌐 GLOBAL PERSPECTIVES ON ROLES AND RESPONSIBILITIES

The Canadian Interprofessional Health Collaborative (CHIC) National Interprofessional Competency Framework (2010) includes Role Clarification as one of their six competency domains. Their competency statement requires that practitioners understand their own role and the roles of those in other professions, and use this knowledge appropriately to establish and achieve patient/client/family and community goals.

RR1: Communicate One's Roles and Responsibilities Clearly to Patients, Families, Community Members, and Other Professionals

Always introduce yourself by name and identify your professional role when meeting the patient and family. In addition to that introduction, clearly identify your specific role and responsibilities in the provision of that specific patient's care (Fig. 8.1). Informing everyone involved in a case (the team, including the patient and family) of your roles and responsibilities in the care of the patient is essential. In many healthcare settings, patients, their families, and all those involved in the

CASE STUDY

The Case of Mr. Webb

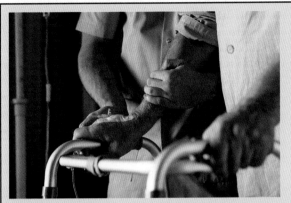

(Photo © KataryznaBialasiewicz/iStock/Thinkstock.)

Mr. Webb is a 50-year-old man admitted to the hospital through the Emergency Department after falling off of a ladder while trimming some tree branches. As a result of his accident he sustained a fracture of his left hip that required surgical pinning to repair. He was referred for physical therapy after surgery.

Paul Kane, the physical therapist (PT), entered Mr. Webb's room, introduced himself ("Hi, I'm Paul, your physical therapist"), and announced, "I'm going to work with you to get you out of bed and moving." During the initial examination, Mr. Webb began expressing concerns about his painful incision and difficulty moving; he seemed afraid. The PT emphasized to Mr. Webb that he was on "the schedule" for 11:00 a.m. physical therapy and stressed the importance of getting out of bed to prevent complications and restore mobility. The PT told Mr. Webb that he would

need his shoes for therapy, but Mr. Webb told him that his family took them home. He also informed the PT that his incision was too painful for him to put on his socks and shoes so he really didn't need them. The PT assisted Mr. Webb in putting on his slippers; they were worn and did not have nonskid soles, but he was able to easily slip his feet into them. By the end of this initial examination session, Mr. Webb was able to use a walker to ambulate 10 feet and maintain the non–weight-bearing restrictions for his left lower limb with considerable assistance from the PT.

The PT identified that this was a good start toward recovery but suggested that Mr. Webb ask his family to bring in a pair of sneakers or other sturdy shoes for tomorrow's therapy session. He also instructed Mr. Webb to ask his nurse to give him his pain medications with breakfast the next morning so that he would be ready for his next therapy session tomorrow at 11 a.m. The PT documented his session and recommendations in the patient's chart.

Discussion Questions

1. Can you identify any areas where there may be overlapping responsibilities among those caring for Mr. Webb?
2. With which members of the interprofessional team could the PT have communicated (and by what means) to improve the care provided to Mr. Webb? Please identify at least three.
3. Did the PT treat Mr. Webb as a decision-making participant in his own health care? Explain your answer.
4. What role do you think Mr. Webb could play in his PT care planning and how?

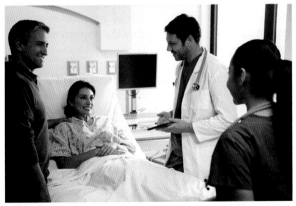

FIG. 8.1 A healthcare professional communicating his role and responsibilities to a patient and her family. (From © monkeybusinessimages/iStock/Thinkstock.)

provision of care encounter a stream of new faces continually throughout their care. For example, several different healthcare professionals from the same discipline (e.g., physicians, nurses) may care for the same patient at different times, and most patients interact with a significant number of healthcare professionals from different disciplines as well as with nonprofessional healthcare workers throughout their care. This makes it difficult for healthcare professionals, patients, and their families to keep track of who is responsible for what at any given time.

In Case Study: The Case of Mr. Webb, the PT did not demonstrate all elements of Sub-competency RR1. Although he did introduce himself by name and identify his profession, he did not communicate his role and responsibilities in Mr. Webb's care to the patient or to other team members involved in Mr. Webb's care. Instead, the PT suggested to Mr. Webb that he should be responsible for communicating his need for pain management to the nurse and suggest when pain medication should be provided in preparation for the next PT treatment. Direct communication and collaboration between the PT and nurse would have resulted in a more dependable and effective plan to administer Mr. Webb's pain medication daily, with breakfast, to control his pain and maximize his participation in his therapy. The collaboration between the PT, nurse, and patient would ensure a plan acceptable to all, thus contributing to its success. The ideal approach would have been for the PT to communicate his plan of care to the other members of the interprofessional team for adaptation and incorporation into the overall team plan of care for the patient.

Mutual understanding of the roles and responsibilities in a specific patient's care is essential. In each case, after you communicate your role and responsibilities to the patient and others, obtain confirmation that the information has been understood and agreed upon by asking team members, including the patient and family members, to share their understanding of who is responsible for what. This sharing provides everyone the opportunity to clarify any misunderstandings. Sub-competency RR1, "Communicate one's roles and responsibilities clearly to patients, families, and other professionals," requires the recipient of the communication (e.g., patient, nurse, family member) to listen attentively, to assimilate the information, and to react to it appropriately.

✳ ACTIVE LEARNING

To learn how to clearly communicate your professional role to patients and family members, as well as to other members of the healthcare team, try the following:
1. Explain your professional role in three sentences or fewer. Use your professional organization as a resource or reference.
2. Ask for feedback from a peer.

Self-Evaluation of RR1

Communicate your own roles and responsibilities clearly to patients, families, community members, and other

professionals. Identify an example from your own clinical experience that demonstrates that you have met Sub-competency RR1. If you can't identify an experience, prepare to engage in this competency by role playing with a person who is not in your discipline (e.g., a friend, a neighbor, an acquaintance):

1. Set the stage by telling them that you would like them to role play being a patient of yours. Explain a common reason you may be seeing a patient (i.e., if you are a physician's assistant, the common scenario might be that this is a patient coming in for a routine physical examination).
2. Communicate your name to the "patient" and explain your role and responsibilities in his or her care.
3. Answer any questions about your role and responsibilities that the patient may have.
4. Ask your patient to tell you his or her understanding of your role and responsibilities in his or her care.

When the patient can accurately describe your role and responsibilities to you, you have demonstrated Sub-competency RR1.

RR2: Recognize One's Limitations in Skills, Knowledge, and Abilities

The complexity of the healthcare system and the specialization of healthcare professions and professionals necessitates that healthcare professionals recognize their strengths and limitations and, more than ever, depend on each other's expertise. Sub-competency RR2 requires you to use self-reflection related to the roles and responsibilities for which you will be accountable in a given care situation. Self-aware healthcare professionals are able to recognize when the patient has needs that are outside of their own profession scope of practice or area of expertise. IPEC (2011) describes the importance of this competency as follows:

The need to address complex health promotion and illness problems, in the context of complex care delivery systems and community factors, calls for recognizing the limits of professional expertise, and the need for cooperation, coordination, and collaboration across the professions in order to promote health and treat illness. (IPEC, 2011, p. 20)

You will need to cultivate and maintain an accurate understanding related to the roles of the other healthcare professionals who are involved in a patient's care, or those who should be involved. This knowledge base is important in recognizing areas in which the roles and responsibilities of team members may overlap and deciding, within the context of the team, which team member will assume responsibility for those specific aspects of care.

Once you identify patient needs that fall outside of your own scope of practice or experience, expertise to fill that gap should be sought; the solution may range from simply seeking consultation from a colleague with more experience to adding a new healthcare professional to the care team. In Case Study: The Case of Mr. Webb, the PT could have acknowledged Mr. Webb's concern about his inability to put on his own shoes and recognized it as a self-care need that was outside of his role and responsibilities in this case. Recognition of this need may have indicated the need for another healthcare professional to become involved in the care of Mr. Webb. Collaboration between the PT, patient, and nurse may have led to the identification of a need for an occupational therapy (OT) consultation related to meeting Mr. Webb's needs (i.e., adaptation to physical limitations and learning self-care/ how to get dressed). To meet this need, the PT would have to acknowledge the role of the physician as the leader of Mr. Webb's care team; subsequent communication and collaboration with Mr. Webb's attending physician could have then made an OT consultation possible and added another essential member to the care team. As a result of identifying strengths and recognizing the limitations in the existing team members' specific skills, knowledge, and abilities, the team would now be better equipped to support Mr. Webb in achieving his goals.

Self-Evaluation of RR2

Recognize your own limitations in skills, knowledge, and abilities.
1. Choose a case study from Chapter 16, or consider an actual case that you have been involved with in clinical practice and found challenging.
2. Reflect on your own professional roles and responsibilities in the patient's care to identify strengths and limitations in your skills, knowledge, and abilities related to the patient's care.

When you have successfully identified your limitations in skills, knowledge, and abilities related to a specific patient's care, you have demonstrated Sub-competency RR2.

RR3: Engage Diverse Professionals Who Complement One's Own Professional Expertise, as Well as Associated Resources, to Develop Strategies to Meet Specific Health and Health Care Needs of Patients and Populations

The third specific Sub-competency (RR3) attempts to resolve the paradox between the way in which healthcare professionals are educated and how they are expected to practice. On the one hand, healthcare professionals tend to be educated in silos, with little interaction with other healthcare professionals. On the other hand, once healthcare professional students graduate, they are expected to practice collaboratively within healthcare teams. This Sub-competency demands movement away from a siloed approach to care planning and into a rich collaborative interprofessional approach that will enhance the professional practice of all team members while improving health outcomes for patients and populations.

The key word in this Sub-competency (RR3) is "engage." It means that each healthcare professional needs to be fully involved in the care of the patient. This care begins with mutual goal setting and the collaborative planning of appropriate strategies to meet the specific care needs of the patient. The process of engaged collaboration requires ongoing communication among all team members, including the patient. Collaboration uses the collective expertise, experience, and resources available within the team to enhance the individual work of each healthcare profession to better achieve quality patient outcomes. Collaboration within the healthcare team can take many forms. It can be synchronous, with team members communicating at the same point in time (e.g., team meetings, phone consultation, staffing cases, handing off patients, grand rounds), or asynchronous through a variety of electronic, written, oral, or verbal communication methods.

Engaged team members can observe and provide previously unknown information about the patient to the team. They can "pick up the slack" from an overwhelmed team member and remain alert to potential errors or mistakes in logic or practice. Engaged healthcare professionals can learn new strategies for addressing healthcare and population health issues from more experienced colleagues or those from different disciplines. The benefits of practicing collaboratively are rich and varied.

Self-Evaluation of RR3

Engage diverse professionals who complement your own professional expertise, as well as associated resources, to develop strategies to meet specific health and healthcare needs of patients and populations.

1. Refer back to the care situation you focused on for Self-Evaluation of RR2.
2. Identify other professionals who could be engaged to provide the specific aspects of care that fall outside of your own skills, knowledge, or abilities.
3. Choose one of the healthcare professionals that you identified as necessary to engage in that patient's care.
4. Describe the process that you would use to engage other professionals in meeting the healthcare needs of the patient.

When you have successfully identified a professional who can provide care in your area(s) of limitations and you can describe a process to engage that professional in the care of your patient, you have demonstrated an understanding of Sub-competency RR3.

🌐 **GLOBAL PERSPECTIVES ON ROLES AND RESPONSIBILITIES**

The education, titles, roles, and responsibilities of specific healthcare professionals vary from country to country. Do not assume that you know about roles and responsibilities based solely on the healthcare system of your own country. Healthcare systems vary greatly throughout the world. When involved in international practice, or when reading publications from other countries, it is necessary to explore and clarify the roles and responsibilities of the professionals involved.

RR4: Explain the Roles and Responsibilities of Other Care Providers and How the Team Works Together to Provide Care, Promote Health, and Prevent Disease

Whereas the Sub-competency RR1 is concerned with the need to communicate *your* role to others, Sub-competency RR4 involves the ability to explain the roles and responsibilities of the *other* care providers and how the team will work together to provide care to a specific patient, to promote the health of a population, or to prevent disease. Suter et al. (2009) identified being able to understand others' roles and responsibilities in relation to one's own role as a core competency domain

for collaborative practice. It is an extension of RR1 and is important for many of the same reasons. Consider Caselet 8.1.

Caselet 8.1 illustrates how each member of the healthcare team, from the clerk to the doctor, was able to explain to the patient and family the roles and responsibilities of other team members. There was no confusion or worry on the part of the patient and family because they knew who was who, how the team worked together to provide his care, and who would be doing what. Mr. Williams was not left wondering who anyone was, or what would happen next. This reduces anxiety and increases confidence in the team on the part of the patient and family. This caselet shows the importance of RR4: explaining the roles and responsibilities of other care providers and how they work together to provide care, promote health, and prevent disease. It is not enough just to communicate your role as a healthcare professional; you must be able to communicate the roles and responsibilities of everyone on the team. This demonstrates a planned, systematic, well-understood team approach to each patient's care.

Most professionals believe that they know the roles of other professions; however, they may be operating based on stereotypes rather than factual knowledge. Stereotypes can contribute to erroneous ideas about each profession's relative worth (Edmondson & Roloff, 2009); in turn, this may lead to the devaluing of certain team members and the erosion of the interprofessional team's ability to function. To fully understand, appreciate, and explain the contributions of each member of the interprofessional team to patient care, and to avoid assumptions based on stereotypes, professionals should be fully informed about one another's professional roles and responsibilities.

✳️ **ACTIVE LEARNING**

Explore your own assumptions.
1. Select any two healthcare professions and write down all the things you think these professionals do.
2. Then, go to the websites of the respective professional organizations or interview members of the professions to explore the role of each profession.
3. Compare your "assumptions" about the role with what you found in your research.
4. Identify where you may have inadvertently stereotyped that profession.

CASELET 8.1 Mr. Williams

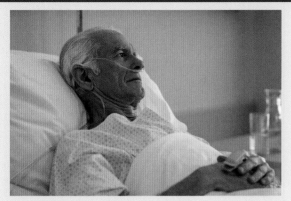

(Photo © Ridofranz/iStock/Thinkstock.)

Imagine taking your grandfather, Bill Williams, who has a high fever, to the emergency department of the local hospital. You are worried, and so is your loved one. A hospital worker takes Mr. Williams' insurance information and asks about the nature of his problem. She explains she is a clerk and that in a few minutes a triage nurse will take his medical history and vital signs. Next, he is called into another room where another worker introduces herself as June, the triage nurse. She explains she will record information about his problem to share with the emergency department team to decide who is best to care for him and how immediate the problem is. June asks questions related to the problem and measures blood pressure, pulse, respirations, and oxygen saturation (vital signs). This happens just as the clerk said it would. You are both sent out to the waiting room to wait some more. Finally, your grandfather's name is called and he is sent to a small cubicle, given a gown, and asked to change into it. That person says, "My name is Mary and I am a nursing assistant. I will ask you several questions about your health history, and record your information so the doctor and nurse can review it. Soon your nurse, George, will come in and take your vital signs. He will ask you some more questions about your health status. His job is to help carry out some of the doctor's orders, and he is in charge of giving you medication. Then Dr. Mason will examine you. If you need anything, press this call button and an assistant or nurse will answer and share your needs with your specific team." George comes in,

introduces himself, and explains that he and the doctor work closely together. In a few minutes, Dr. Mason examines your grandfather and says it may be pneumonia, but some laboratory tests and a chest x-ray are needed. She explains, "Your nurse will be back to draw the blood and to start an I.V. to give you some fluids which may help bring the fever down. He will bring you some Tylenol, which should also help reduce the fever. We will also start you on some oxygen." Dr. Mason explains that the x-ray results will be available on the computer and reminds you and your grandfather to tell the nurse if he feels any worse or needs anything. Everything occurs exactly as explained when George the nurse returns. He says that an assistant will come to take Mr. Williams to x-ray. Again, all goes as explained. Shortly Dr. Mason returns and says that the x-ray indicated pneumonia, and because of that and his fever, Mr. Williams will be admitted to the hospital. Later the nurse returns to check Mr. Williams' temperature and tells him it is going down, and that he will be sure the doctor is aware of that. George then explains that Mr. Williams will be moved to a hospital unit when a bed is available, and that all of his information will be available in his electronic record. George tells you that he will personally report all information to the nurse on the hospital unit, and a different physician who specializes in respiratory illnesses will be taking over Mr. Williams' case when he gets to the hospital unit. George explains that Dr. Mason just ordered respiratory therapy and that a respiratory therapist will be administering a treatment designed to help his breathing.

Discussion Questions

1. Do you think that the introductions and explanations provided by the various healthcare workers in this case helped to reduce the patient's and family's anxiety? Explain your answer.
2. Why it is important for each healthcare professional to understand and be able to explain the role and responsibilities of other healthcare workers to patients and families?
3. Consider how the patient outcome could be affected if each healthcare worker in Mr. Williams case had only explained his or her role and did not mention the roles of other members of the healthcare team.

Self-Evaluation of RR4

Explain the roles and responsibilities of other care providers and how the team works together to provide care, promote health, and prevent disease.

1. Use the same case study from Chapter 16 or the actual case that you have been involved with in clinical practice and identify all of the team members involved.
2. Describe the roles and responsibilities of all identified team members.
3. Prepare descriptions of each team member's role and responsibilities in three sentences or less: one to be shared with other professionals on the team, and another to be shared with the patient, family, and significant nonprofessionals.
4. Consult with a representative of at least two of the professions you included to see how accurate your descriptions were.

When you receive validation that you accurately described the roles and responsibilities of at least two professional team members who share roles and responsibilities within the team, you have successfully demonstrated an understanding of Sub-competency RR4.

⬛ RESEARCH HIGHLIGHT

Education Can Improve Understanding of Professional Roles

A study by Ateah et al. (2011) demonstrated that a brief but concentrated interdisciplinary educational experience involving preprofessional students can result in a more accurate understanding of professional roles and interdisciplinary collaboration. Stereotypes that students initially held about other professions were replaced with factual knowledge after the education.

RR5: Use the Full Scope of Knowledge, Skills, and Abilities of Professionals From Health and Other Fields to Provide Care That Is Safe, Timely, Efficient, Effective, and Equitable

To most efficiently and effectively achieve optimal patient outcomes each team member must be allowed to function using his or her full scope of practice as appropriate to the patient care situation. Lack of understanding of other professionals' roles can contribute to underutilizing their expertise, conflict, and role blurring (Suter et al., 2009). Consider Caselet 8.2.

CASELET 8.2   Carla Alvarez

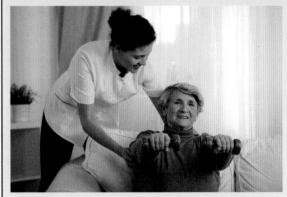

(Photo © KatarzynaBialasiewicz/iStock/Thinkstock.)

Carla Alvarez is an 82-year-old resident of Longview, a long-term care facility. She has limited mobility, and her healthcare team determined that daily passive range of motion (PROM) exercises are necessary to prevent contractures (i.e., a permanent shortening of a muscle or joint). The physical therapist (PT) comes to Longview three times a week. There are no physical therapy assistants employed at Longview.

Discussion Questions

1. Can Mrs. Alvarez only receive these PROM exercises when the PT is available on-site?
2. Besides the PT, are there others who can provide PROM exercises for Mrs. Alvarez?
3. Who might be able to provide them, and how could this be enabled?
4. Who is responsible for the effectiveness of the PROM plan?
5. How is the plan effectiveness evaluated and by whom?

It is the healthcare team's responsibility to find a solution that allows Mrs. Alvarez to get the recommended exercises as often as they are required. What specific PROM exercises are needed by this patient? How often should they be done and by which members of the team? In the case of Mrs. Alvarez, although it is clearly within the scope of practice for the PT to provide effective PROM exercises, it is also within the nursing staff's scope of practice to perform them. The most effective, timely, efficient, and equitable care for Mrs. Alvarez can be provided through the involvement of all appropriate team members in her care. This involves the PT teaching the nurses and certified nurse assistants (CNAs) involved in

Mrs. Alvarez's daily care how to perform the most appropriate range-of-motion exercises as a component of her care. If family members visit frequently and express a desire to be involved in the patient's care, they could also be taught how to help her with these exercises. However, it is not the family's responsibility to see that the exercises are performed while Mrs. Alvarez is in the Longview facility. Understanding the roles of PTs, nurses, and CNAs could lead to a relatively easy solution to the problem of how to ensure that Ms. Alvarez can receive effective daily PROM exercises. If the team did not use the full scope of knowledge and skills of the nursing staff as well as the PT to perform these exercises, the patient may have developed easily preventable complications.

Using the full scope of knowledge, skills, and abilities of all health professionals caring for Mrs. Alvarez ensures equitable, timely, and efficient care. This solution is equitable because it would not be fair to expect the PT, who is only at the facility 3 days per week, to provide all of the PROM exercises needed by Mrs. Alvarez. The care is timely because Mrs. Alvarez does not need to wait for the PT to perform her exercises; she can get them as frequently as needed to be at the appropriate standard of care. Her care will be efficient because with the nursing staff performing these routine exercises, the PT will be free to engage in the full scope of PT practice, assessing and planning interventions for other Longview residents with complex PT needs during this limited availability at the facility. There is no role blurring; the PT is clearly responsible for planning the PT aspects (PROM exercises) of Mrs. Alvarez's care, whereas qualified nursing staff will carry out and evaluate the plan on all shifts. Working together, the team can implement and evaluate the effectiveness of the plan and discuss any other needs that may arise.

✳ ACTIVE LEARNING

List at least five healthcare activities that more than one professional may be qualified to do and who can do them. For example—measuring blood pressure: nurses, physicians, physician assistants, etc.

Self-Evaluation of RR5

Use the full scope of knowledge, skills, and abilities of professionals from health and other fields to provide care that is safe, timely, efficient, effective, and equitable.

1. Use the same case study from Chapter 16 or the actual case that you have been involved with in clinical practice and identify overlapping areas of knowledge, skills, and abilities in the team members.
2. Designate who should be responsible for these areas of overlapping knowledge, skills, and abilities and provide your rationale.
3. Identify professionals from fields other than health care who could contribute to the care of a patient or population, and explain how you would collaborate with them.
4. Explain how this distribution of responsibilities will result in safe, timely, efficient, effective, and equitable care for the patient.

When you can clearly demonstrate the ability to complete this process, you have demonstrated an understanding of Sub-competency RR5.

RR6: Communicate With Team Members to Clarify Each Member's Responsibility in Executing Components of a Treatment Plan or Public Health Intervention

Sub-competency RR6 requires you to move beyond simply recognizing which team member should be responsible for performing the varied roles and responsibilities of a patient's care or public health intervention; this Sub-competency requires you to be able to clearly and accurately communicate those responsibilities within the team (Fig. 8.2). This involves respect for the roles, abilities,

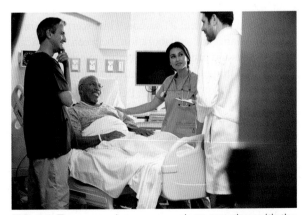

FIG. 8.2 Team members communicate together with the patient to clarify each member's responsibilities in the plan of care. (© monkeybusinessimages/iStock/Thinkstock.)

and contributions of each team member. After ascertaining who has the most appropriate knowledge and skills needed to address the identified needs, individual team members must understand their role and commit to taking responsibility for those aspects of the plan. You may think that once the roles of each member of the team executing the plan have been clarified, each team member can work independently to carry out the portion of the plan for which they are responsible. This is not true; this traditional approach to practice leads to fragmentation and may produce less than optimal patient outcomes. This Sub-competency, far from being static, requires continuing communication and coordination among team members throughout the care process because, although each team member is uniquely qualified to provide certain aspects of care, the practice of each member of the team invariably affects the practice of the others. Preventing duplication of services, and safe and effective care, this process promotes the appropriate use of individual practitioners' time and a fair and efficient distribution of work (CHIC, 2010).

Consider the following excerpt from Case Study: The Case of Mr. Webb, in which Mr. Webb "reports that his incision is too painful for him to put on his socks and shoes … Paul Kane (PT) suggests that Mr. Webb … ask his nurse for his pain medications with breakfast tomorrow so that he will be ready for his next therapy session." It was clear to the PT that he was in charge of the physical rehabilitation aspects of Mr. Webb's care. Similarly, it was clear to the nurse that she was in charge of the medication management of the patient. However, the fact that these healthcare professionals were clear about their roles in these two aspects of Mr. Webb's plan did not result in an efficient PT session. This excerpt illustrates the importance of collaboration between healthcare professionals and patients. Direct communication between the PT and nurse about the timing of pain medication could result in a more optimal patient outcome.

Pellatt (2005) interviewed healthcare team members in an attempt to identify why teams were not functioning well. He found the following themes: not knowing the roles of each discipline; doctor perceived as team leader; and the overlap of roles. Each team member believed he or she knew the others' roles, but each thought that his or her own role was not understood by others. A pilot study involving nurses, PTs, and OTs revealed that "understanding of each discipline's role, respect, trust, equal standing of each member, focusing on patient goals,

participation by each member, collaboration, and the difference in perspective of each member" were important factors in promoting interprofessional teamwork (White et al., 2013, p. 150).

Self-Evaluation of RR6

Communicate with team members to clarify each member's responsibility in executing components of a treatment plan or public health intervention.

1. Use the same case study from Chapter 16 or the actual case that you have been involved with in clinical practice, and select one area of overlap you previously identified in Sub-competency Self-Evaluation of RR5.
2. Find peers who can role play the team members involved in the area of overlap.
3. In the role play, demonstrate communicating the distribution of overlapping responsibilities within the interprofessional team.

When all team members can correctly verbalize their responsibility for areas of overlap and come to an understanding of who is executing what, you have demonstrated an understanding of Sub-competency RR6.

🌐 GLOBAL PERSPECTIVES ON ROLES AND RESPONSIBILITIES

Many global rescue organizations send teams of professionals to disaster areas or to areas experiencing a health crisis. These teams are often multinational as well as multidisciplinary. Collaboration across global rescue organizations is complex but essential for success. Understanding team members' roles and responsibilities in the context of country of origin is essential to successful teamwork, especially in stressful working conditions.

RR7: Forge Interdependent Relationships With Other Professions Within and Outside of the Health System to Improve Care and Advance Learning

Roles/Responsibilities' Sub-competencies RR3, RR5, and RR9 require healthcare professionals to use each other's "knowledge, skills, and abilities" to enhance their own professional practice at all appropriate times. Interdependent relationships require dependence on the expertise of all team members, at all times, to achieve optimal care outcomes. Professional interdependent relationships need to be purposefully cultivated; you will need to develop a shared language, learn to anticipate one another's needs, enhance understanding related to one another's roles and scopes of practice, and strategize to prevent conflicts that might interfere with professional practice in the delivery of optimal patient-centered care. Effective collegial relationships develop over time; they require mutual trust, respect, and open communication. Caselet 8.3 illustrates the importance of such relationships in achieving optimal patient outcomes.

CASELET 8.3 Baby Winter

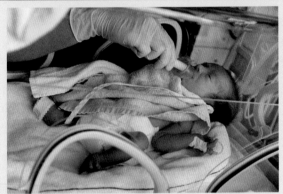

(Photo © metinkiyak/iStock/Thinkstock.)

The goal of the interprofessional team caring for Baby Winter is that he will be able to suck adequately and retain at least 1 oz of breast milk every 2 hours by June 1. Baby Winter was born prematurely and was admitted to the neonatal intensive care unit (NICU). He had a low birth weight, and it was essential that he gain weight. After his first week he exhibited sucking ability, and the neonatologist and nurse decided it was time to begin oral feeding. The speech–language pathologist (SLP) assigned to the unit was not present and was not consulted. The neonatologist ordered a thickening agent to be added to the mother's expressed breast milk. The pharmacist provided the thickening agent as ordered, and the nurse added the agent to the breast milk. The initial feeding was administered to the neonate by his mother under the supervision of the nurse. The feeding was unsuccessful. It was later determined, after consultation with the SLP, that there was a more effective thickening agent for use in Baby Winter's feeding.

Discussion Question

1. How could an interdependent relationship between the neonatal unit professionals and the SLP contribute to a better patient outcome in this case?

The failure of care in this case suggests the lack of a close interdependent relationship among team members. Assessment, diagnosis, and treatment of swallowing disorders in children are part of the role of a speech–language pathologist (SLP; ASHA, n.d.a). In an interdependent healthcare team that had forged close collaborative team relationships, one or more team members might have suggested that they obtain an asynchronous consultation with their missing team member, the SLP. The absence of this team member's input demonstrated the team's lack of dependence on this team member's professional input, yet working with this additional team member would clearly have strengthened the existing team by adding to their individual areas of specialized expertise in dealing with this neonate's swallowing difficulty.

Interdependence can be used as an asset to strengthen the team. The team could have assessed the feeding outcome and recognized their need for input from all team members in similar care decisions. The team could collaborate to develop evidence-based methods and procedures for evaluating the sucking ability of neonates and their readiness for oral feedings. The pharmacist and SLP could work collaboratively to develop a list of recommended thickening agents and identify specific indications for the use of each. Feeding protocols could be developed collaboratively with guidelines for their application and evaluation of their effectiveness. Together the team could plan and deliver education for the entire staff. Working together collaboratively strengthens interprofessional relationships; the more interprofessional team members work together, the more they learn from one another. The more they learn from one another, the more they trust and respect one another. This trust fosters more collaboration and interdependence in the provision of care. When patient outcomes improve as a result of collaboration, professionals rely on one another more and more.

✴ ACTIVE LEARNING

Building your own interdependent relationships.
1. Name at least three things that you currently do to promote interdependent relationships with your professional peers within and outside of the health system.
2. Identify at least three things that you can do in the future to increase the number and strength of your interdependent relationships with professional colleagues within and outside of the health system.

Self-Evaluation of RR7

Forge interdependent relationships with other professions within and outside of the health system to improve care and advance learning.

1. Reflect on your own clinical practice. Identify professionals outside of the healthcare system with whom you could collaborate to improve care and advance learning. Explain.
2. How could these professionals contribute to patient care or population health in this situation?

If you were able to identify professionals outside of the health system and explained how these professionals could improve care and advance learning in the care of patients or promote population health and quality of care, you have demonstrated your understanding of Sub-competency RR7.

RR8: Engage in Continuous Professional and Interprofessional Development to Enhance Team Performance and Collaboration

According to IPEC (2011), "Team members' individual expertise can limit productive teamwork across the professions. Collaborative practice depends on maintaining expertise through continued learning and through refining and improving the roles and responsibilities of those working together" (p. 20). To be a valued member of the healthcare team, professionals have a responsibility to maintain and improve their knowledge, skills, and practice within their individual disciplines and specialties. This includes obtaining and maintaining certifications, participating in continuing education activities, and keeping abreast of new developments in their respective fields to maintain and increase competency in their own areas of practice. Continuous professional development within one's discipline is consistent with expectations for evidence-based practice.

Additionally, all healthcare professionals need to participate in Interprofessional Education (IPE) experiences to enhance their ability to function as members of an interprofessional patient care team. Such activities include participation in interdisciplinary continuing education activities such as in simulation experiences, attending formal IPE programs and interprofessional conferences, and educating other professionals regarding one's own discipline. Interprofessional learning is a continual process (IPEC, 2011). Although it may begin in the preprofessional stage, it continues throughout one's professional career. There are several levels of interprofessional skill

development (Fig. 8.3). A pre-licensure student is expected to develop baseline knowledge and novice-level skills in the Interprofessional Core Competencies. Graduate education should also include opportunities for Interprofessional Education. As one gains clinical skills and practice experience, Continuing Interprofessional Education (CIPE in Fig. 8.3) will foster increased proficiency in interprofessional collaboration. Engaging in interprofessional development to enhance team collaboration and performance within the unique circumstances of each organization and each care situation will benefit both the providers and recipients of healthcare services.

Self-Evaluation of RR8

Engage in continuous professional and interprofessional development to enhance team performance and collaboration.

1. Identify three opportunities for professional development (e.g., conferences, continuing education) in your discipline that would enhance interprofessional collaboration.
2. Identify three opportunities for interprofessional development (e.g., conferences, continuing education).

When you engage in continuous professional and interprofessional development, you have demonstrated an understanding of Sub-competency RR8.

 GLOBAL PERSPECTIVES ON ROLES AND RESPONSIBILITIES

The World Health Organization (2011) listed Roles and Responsibilities as an essential outcome of Interprofessional Education. They define this as "understanding one's own roles, responsibilities and expertise, and those of other types of health workers" (p. 26).

RR9: Use the Unique and Complementary Abilities of All Team Members to Optimize Health and Patient Care

Sub-competencies RR1 to RR8 were designed as behavioral learning objectives to be completed by the end of your prelicensure or precertification education (IPEC 2011, p. 26). Sub-competency RR9 assumes your ability to implement Sub-competencies RR1 through RR8 in an interprofessional team context to obtain optimal patient care outcomes. Using all of the Sub-competencies of Roles/Responsibilities in your own professional practice will allow you to work effectively and collaboratively with

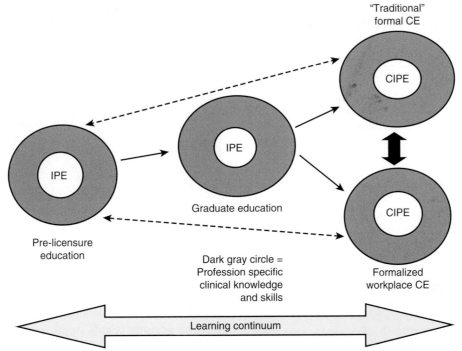

FIG. 8.3 Continuum of Interprofessional Education (IPE). *CE,* Continuing education; *CIPE,* continuing Interprofessional Education. (From Owen, John A. EdD, MSc; Schmitt, Madeline H. PhD, RN. Integrating Interprofessional Education into Continuing Education: A Planning Process for Continuing Interprofessional Education Programs. Journal of Continuing Education in the Health Professions: April 2013, 33(2), 109–117.)

others to provide comprehensive health and patient care, improve overall quality of care, and improve your own experience of care.

ACTIVE LEARNING

Refer to Box 8.1.
1. Review each competency statement and reflect upon your level of achievement based on self-evaluation strategies.
2. For those you have not fully achieved, reflect on how you might improve.
3. Enlist appropriate support to reach your goals.

Self-Evaluation of RR9

Use the unique and complementary abilities of all team members to optimize health and patient care.

When you have demonstrated Sub-competencies RR1 through RR8 consistently, you have demonstrated Sub-competency RR9.

RR10: Describe How Professionals in Health and Other Fields Can Collaborate and Integrate Clinical Care and Public Health Interventions to Optimize Population Health

This Sub-competency was added to the Roles/Responsibilities Core Competency in the IPEC 2016 update to reflect the emphasis on population health as well as individual health. It is important for healthcare professionals to recognize that they can play a part in optimizing the health of the population through collaboration and integration of care with other professionals within and outside of the healthcare system and community agencies. The first and easiest way to accomplish this is for healthcare professionals to become aware of community resources accessible to the patient populations they serve and to include referral to such programs in the clinical care of patients as appropriate (Fig. 8.4). For example, what exercise programs are available in your own community at senior centers, schools, and community

> **BOX 8.1   Specific Sub-Competencies of Roles/Responsibilities**
>
> RR1. Communicate one's roles and responsibilities clearly to patients, families, community members, and other professionals.
> RR2. Recognize one's limitations in skills, knowledge, and abilities.
> RR3. Engage diverse professionals who complement one's own professional expertise, as well as associated resources, to develop strategies to meet specific health and healthcare needs of patients and populations.
> RR4. Explain the roles and responsibilities of other providers and how the team works together to provide care, promote health, and prevent disease.
> RR5. Use the full scope of knowledge, skills, and abilities of professionals from health and other fields to provide care that is safe, timely, efficient, effective, and equitable.
> RR6. Communicate with team members to clarify each member's responsibility in executing components of a treatment plan or public health intervention.
> RR7. Forge interdependent relationships with other professions within and outside of the health system to improve care and advance learning.
> RR8. Engage in continuous professional and interprofessional development to enhance team performance and collaboration.
> RR9. Use unique and complementary abilities of all members of the team to optimize health and patient care.
> RR10. Describe how professionals in health and other fields can collaborate and integrate clinical care and public health interventions to optimize population health.

From Interprofessional Education Collaborative Expert Panel (IPEC). (2016). *Core competencies for interprofessional collaborative practice: 2016 update*. Washington, DC: Interprofessional Education Collaborative.

centers? Many such programs are available at no charge or for a modest fee. Referring patients to such programs has a twofold benefit. First, patients may be more likely to exercise regularly if they participate with others, rather than alone. Second, referring patients to such programs supports these programs and may help the programs continue. Encouraging patients to use community resources may also reduce the cost of care. Healthcare professionals can encourage patients to participate in local health fairs and screenings, public health immunization clinics, and other services.

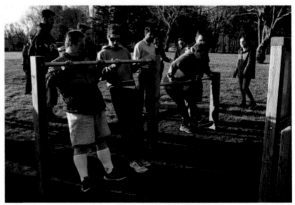

FIG. 8.4. Stockton University's Get FIT program fitness trail.

Healthcare professionals can play a role in the development of community health promotion initiatives by calling attention to the need for such services. Another way you, as a healthcare professional, can collaborate to optimize population health is to volunteer your services at clinics, serve on advisory boards, or get involved in healthcare policy making.

Self-Evaluation of RR10

Describe how professionals in health and other fields can collaborate and integrate clinical care and public health interventions to optimize population health.

1. List some ways that you could collaborate to integrate clinical care with public health interventions in your own practice. Think about an individual patient, and identify public health resources that may benefit him or her.
2. Are there community or public health programs that are available or need to be developed that would promote the health of the community that you serve?
3. What can you do to improve the health of the population you serve?

When you can identify several ways in which you can collaborate and integrate clinical care and public health interventions to optimize population health, you have demonstrated an understanding of Sub-competency RR10.

DEMONSTRATING THE SUB-COMPETENCIES OF ROLES/RESPONSIBILITIES

Exemplar Case Study: The Sub-competencies of Roles/Responsibilities (Part 1) and Exemplar Case Study: The

◎ EXEMPLAR CASE STUDY

The Sub-competencies of Roles/Responsibilities (Part 1)

Mr. Charles Webb is a 50-year-old male admitted to the hospital through the emergency department after falling off of a ladder while trimming some tree branches. He sustained a fracture of his left hip, which required surgery and pinning to repair. The physician consulted physical therapy to begin mobility and gait training [RR5] At this time he is non–weight bearing on his left lower extremity.

Paul Kane, the physical therapist (PT), entered Mr. Webb's room for his initial examination and said, "I'm Paul from physical therapy. I'm a member of the team caring for you. My role is to work with you while you are in the hospital to be able to get you out of bed and start walking again now that your surgery is complete" [RR1]. Mr. Webb smiled and said, "Yes, the doctor said we would be working together. Great! But, I'm not sure this will work today, my incision is pretty painful and it really hurts to move (grimacing)." After assessing his level of pain, the PT and Mr. Webb agreed to consult with the nurse about Mr. Webb's pain management needs [RR2, RR3]. The nurse stated that Mr. Webb could have his pain medication at that time. Together, the PT, the nurse, and Mr. Webb agreed to hold off on beginning therapy immediately; they planned for Mr. Webb to receive his pain medication first and give it time to become effective [RR6]. The PT agreed that he would see another patient on the PT schedule first and then begin Mr. Webb's session after the pain medication took effect [RR9].

Later that morning, the PT returned. He confirmed that Mr. Webb had received his pain medication and was comfortable enough to participate in therapy. After examining his strength and range of motion in bed, the PT asked if Mr. Webb had shoes and determined that the family had taken them home. Mr. Webb said that he was not able to put on his own socks and shoes anyway because of his painful incision, and would just use his slippers. The PT noticed that the slippers were worn and did not have non-skid soles. The PT explained his concerns to Mr. Webb, and they both agreed that Mr. Webb would use non-skid socks today to ensure safe out of bed activity and that Mr. Webb would ask his partner to bring in his sneakers the next time he visits. The PT asked the nurse for non-skid socks and assisted Mr. Webb in putting them on. He suggested to Mr. Webb that it might be helpful to involve an occupational therapist (OT) in his care. He explained that an OT could help him with dressing and other activities of daily living and offered to contact the doctor for permission to arrange that if Mr. Webb and the nurse agreed [RR2, RR4, RR5, RR9].

The PT determined that Mr. Webb was able to use a walker to ambulate 10 feet with considerable assistance to maintain the non-weight bearing restrictions for his left lower leg. Based on his assessment, the PT communicated directly to the nurse about how much assistance Mr. Webb would need for out of bed activities [RR3, RR5]. He also discussed with the nurse Mr. Webb's difficulty with putting on his shoes and dressing, and the nurse agreed with his suggestion to involve an OT to help with dressing needs. The nurse agreed to contact the physician to discuss an OT consultation related to restoring Mr. Webb's self-care activities and for recommending adaptive devices to foster his independence in those activities [RR2, RR3, RR6, RR7, RR9]. The PT documented the activities conducted during Mr. Webb's physical therapy session and his recommendations and communication with other team members. The nurse documented her activities in the patient's electronic health record and shared the information with the nursing staff during the change of shift report [RR6].

Sub-competencies of Roles/Responsibilities (Part 2) demonstrate the application of the Sub-competencies of Roles/Responsibilities in the provision of optimal interprofessional collaborative care. The presence of specific Sub-competencies is indicated throughout the case studies.

The interactions described in Exemplar Case Study: The Sub-competencies of Roles/Responsibilities (Part 1) provide examples of using the unique and complementary abilities of all team members, including the patient and his family, to enhance the quality of patient-centered care.

The professionals moved beyond minimal expectations of providing discipline-specific care and recognized the interdependence of all team members in planning care. The planning and provision of collaborative interprofessional care does not sacrifice the autonomy of individual team members; professional autonomy is needed in the identification of the specific roles and responsibilities you will assume for a patient's care and in the identification and assignment of overlapping roles and responsibilities within the interprofessional healthcare team. Exemplar Case Study: The Sub-competencies of

◎ EXEMPLAR CASE STUDY

The Sub-competencies of Roles/Responsibilities (Part 2)

The interprofessional team continued to work together to provide effective, safe, and efficient care throughout Mr. Webb's hospital stay. Ongoing collaboration across professions continued as a key element of achieving optimal patient outcomes and satisfaction. Synchronous and asynchronous communication continued as the team worked with Mr. Webb and his partner to develop a discharge plan [RR6, RR7].

The social worker met with Mr. Webb and his partner to explore options for postacute care services, outlining his insurance coverage for inpatient rehabilitation versus outpatient therapies [RR3, RR9]. Although many patients with similar injuries are discharged from the hospital to inpatient rehabilitation, Mr. Webb and his partner expressed a strong preference for him to return home and receive outpatient follow-up care. They had questions about the provision of transportation to outpatient therapies until Mr. Webb would be cleared to resume driving. The social worker agreed to communicate Mr. Webb's preference to the other team members and seek their recommendations as well [RR6]. In addition, the social worker noted that Mr. Webb lives on the third floor of a high-rise condominium with elevator access.

After reading the social worker's note, the occupational therapist (OT) contacted the physical therapist (PT) to discuss Mr. Webb's progress and options for discharge [RR5, RR7]. To date, Mr. Webb had made significant improvement and was able to safely use a walker for up to 150 feet. Together they discussed the equipment that would be needed for discharge to home: a tub bench for bathing, a walker, adaptive aids for dressing, and the short-term rental of a wheelchair for longer distances, including community mobility [RR3, RR5, RR9]. After their discussion, the OT called the social worker to inquire about insurance coverage and provided equipment recommendations so that the social worker could order it [RR7].

To discharge Mr. Webb to home with his partner, the team members clarified each member's responsibilities as follows [RR4, RR6, RR7, RR9]. The physician would provide written instructions for postoperative restrictions: non–weight bearing, follow-up in 2 weeks for removal of staples, and no driving until cleared by the physician. The nurse would instruct the patient and his partner regarding the purpose, administration, and potential side effects of his medications and the care of his incisional site and signs of infection to be reported. She would verify through a return demonstration that both Mr. Webb and his partner could perform incisional care properly and that they could accurately verbalize understanding of his medications. Furthermore, she would verify that they understand the written physician instructions and would answer any questions they have. Mr. Webb, his partner, and the OT would review the use of adaptive aids for lower body dressing. In addition, they would demonstrate the safe use of the tub bench in the hospital and discuss the optimal setup of the equipment that would be delivered to their home. The PT would instruct Mr. Webb's partner in supervising mobility with the walker (including the non–weight-bearing restrictions) and the home exercise program. The PT would confirm that Mr. Webb and his partner understand and perform the activities correctly. Together they would develop a plan for using the walker at home for short distances, using the wheelchair for longer distances and in the community such as for outpatient therapy and follow-up visits. The social worker would provide contact information for transportation services to the outpatient rehabilitation center. Each team member would document his or her discharge activities to communicate the plan accurately to the discharge coordinator, who would follow up with a phone call to Mr. Webb after he was home [RR6, RR9].

Roles/Responsibilities (Part 2) demonstrates the application of the Sub-competencies of Roles/Responsibilities in the provision of optimal interprofessional collaboration in discharge planning.

These exemplar case studies focusing on Mr. Webb provide just one example of the type of high-quality patient-centered care that results from the operationalization and incorporation of the Sub-competencies of Roles/Responsibilities. Every patient care scenario you encounter will be unique, with specific details varying based on factors such as the patient's own care needs, the setting, the organizational structure, the professionals involved, the care resources, and regional scope of practice guidelines, but regardless of case-specific factors, moving beyond the traditional fragmented delivery of services by individual providers to Interprofessional Collaborative Practice will enhance and improve patient care outcomes.

KEY POINTS

- The patient, family, and all who participate it the provision of care, in all settings, have meaningful roles within the healthcare team.
- Through self-reflection, all healthcare professionals must assess their own skills, roles, and responsibilities to identify what role they will play in a given care situation.
- Most professionals believe that they know the roles of other healthcare professions; however, they may be operating based on stereotypes rather than actual knowledge. Stereotypes can contribute to false ideas about each profession's relative worth.
- An accurate understanding of the roles and responsibilities of other team members is necessary to identify the team members with whom to collaborate to provide the best possible care to an individual patient.
- Each team member must be allowed to function using his or her full legal scope of practice as appropriate to the patient care situation to most efficiently and effectively achieve optimal patient outcomes.
- There are many ways in which you, as a healthcare professional, can collaborate and integrate clinical care and public health interventions to optimize population health.

REFERENCES

Ateah, C. A., Snow, W., Wener, P., et al. (2011). Stereotyping as a barrier to collaboration: Does interprofessional education make a difference? *Nurse Education Today*, *31*, 208–213.

Canadian Interprofessional Health Collaborative (CHIC). (2010). *A national interprofessional competency framework*. Vancouver, Canada: Author.

Edmondson, A. C., & Roloff, K. S. (2009). Overcoming barriers to collaboration: Psychological safety and learning in diverse teams. In E. Salas, G. F. Goodwin, & C. S. Burke (Eds.), *Team effectiveness in complex organizations* (pp. 183–208). New York: Psychology Press.

Institute of Medicine (IOM). (2003). *Keeping patients safe: Transforming the work environment of nurses*. Washington, DC: National Academies Press.

Interprofessional Education Collaborative Expert Panel (IPEC). (2011). *Core competencies for interprofessional collaborative practice: Report of an expert panel*. Washington, DC: Interprofessional Education Collaborative.

Interprofessional Education Collaborative Expert Panel (IPEC). (2016). *Core competencies for interprofessional collaborative practice: 2016 update*. Washington, DC: Interprofessional Education Collaborative.

Pellatt, G. C. (2005). Perceptions of interprofessional roles within the spinal cord injury rehabilitation team. *International Journal of Therapy and Rehabilitation*, *12*(4), 143–150.

Suter, E., Arndt, J., Arthur, N., et al. (2009). Role understanding and effective communication as core competencies for collaborative practice. *Journal of Interprofessional Care*, *23*, 41–51.

White, M. J., Gutierrez, A., McLaughlin, C., et al. (2013). A pilot for understanding interdisciplinary teams in rehabilitation practice. *Rehabilitation Nursing*, *38*, 142–152.

World Health Organization (WHO). (2011). *Framework for action on interprofessional education & collaborative practice*. Geneva: Author.

9

Roles/Responsibilities Case Studies

LEARNING OUTCOMES

After successfully working through the case studies in this chapter, you will be able to:

1. Demonstrate the ability to apply the Roles/Responsibilities Sub-competencies to problem-based case studies in this chapter.

2. Identify the importance of Interprofessional Collaboration as it applies to each case in this chapter.

3. Operationalize the behaviors of Roles/Responsibilities through case study application.

This chapter presents patient- and population-based case studies designed to highlight the application of the Core Competency of Roles/Responsibilities to interprofessional practice (IPEC, 2011; 2016). Case studies are intended for use in group discussions or debates, as role playing exercises, or as individual learning exercises. The authors acknowledge that all four Core Competencies may apply in each case; however, learning in this chapter is purposefully focused on the Roles/Responsibilities Sub-competencies. Carefully crafted discussion questions will provide direction for learners and faculty facilitators.

CASE STUDY ACTIVITY GUIDELINES

For each practice case study, you will be directed to consider and apply specific Sub-competencies of Roles/Responsibilities. These will be clearly indicated to you

before you begin to read the case study. The Sub-competencies of Roles/Responsibilities are provided for your reference in Box 9.1.

Case studies can be used as individual problem-based learning activities or incorporated as part of a variety of group learning activities. You can independently determine how each case study will be used after considering your specific learning needs and educational setting. Discussion questions and/or suggested learning activities are provided after each case study. You are encouraged to modify these questions and activities, or pose your own, to meet specific learning needs. Chapter 7 of this text provides foundational theory related to Roles/Responsibilities. Chapter 8 provides examples to help readers operationalize specific Sub-competencies. Both chapters will be useful in considering the case studies that follow.

BOX 9.1   Roles/Responsibilities Core Competency and Related Sub-competencies (IPEC, 2016, p. 12)

Statement: General Core Competency of Roles/Responsibilities
Use the knowledge of one's own role and those of other professions to appropriately assess and address the healthcare needs of patients and to promote and advance the health of populations.

RR1. Communicate one's roles and responsibilities clearly to patients, families, and other professionals.
RR2. Recognize one's limitations in skills, knowledge, and abilities.
RR3. Engage diverse healthcare professionals who complement one's own professional expertise, as well as

---

BOX 9.1   **Roles/Responsibilities Core Competency and Related Sub-competencies (IPEC, 2016, p. 12)—cont'd**

associated resources, to develop strategies to meet specific patient care needs.

RR4. Explain the roles and responsibilities of other care providers and how the team works together to provide care.

RR5. Use the full scope of knowledge, skills, and abilities of available health professionals and healthcare workers to provide care that is safe, timely, efficient, effective, and equitable.

RR6. Communicate with team members to clarify each member's responsibility in executing components of a treatment plan or public health intervention.

RR7. Forge interdependent relationships with other professions to improve care and advance learning.

RR8. Engage in continuous professional and interprofessional development to enhance team performance.

RR9. Use unique and complementary abilities of all members of the team to optimize patient care.

RR10. Describe how professionals in health and other fields can collaborate and integrate clinical care and public health interventions to optimize population health.

CASE STUDY: CO-TREATMENT AT THE BEDSIDE

Specific Sub-competencies to consider and apply: RR1, RR3, RR6.

Mrs. Denise Watkins is hospitalized after a stroke that has impaired her swallowing ability. She demonstrates right-sided weakness. A speech–language pathologist (SLP) is addressing her swallowing dysfunction, and an occupational therapist (OT) is helping her learn to use her left hand to perform self-care activities. The OT and SLP on this unit work together frequently, maximizing their complementary abilities to provide optimal patient outcomes. Today the OT and SLP are meeting for a planned cotreatment session with Mrs. Watkins and her family, at her bedside. The goal of the session is to develop strategies to support Mrs. Watkins in self-feeding while avoiding choking. The SLP plans to evaluate Mrs. Watkins' ability to swallow and assess readiness for progression of her modified diet to pureed food consistencies. They enter Mrs. Watkins' room and explain their goal and their roles for the session. The SLP focuses on the alignment of Mrs. Watkins' head and neck that will facilitate her ability to swallow small amounts at a time. The OT focuses on optimal positioning of Mrs. Watkins' trunk and upper limbs to facilitate self-care activities. The OT instructs Mrs. Watkins in the use of an adaptive spoon to provide better control in bringing food toward her mouth. They alternate activities throughout the session. At the end of the session, they acknowledge the progress that Mrs. Watkins has made and determine that Mrs.

Watkins needs more practice before she can attempt self-feeding. They share this with the patient and the family. The OT agrees to communicate their plan to the nurse caring for Mrs. Watkins.

Discussion Questions

1. Imagine that you are the SLP caring for Mrs. Watkins. How would you communicate your role and responsibilities for Mrs. Watkins to the patient and to the family? Repeat this exercise assuming you are the OT caring for Mrs. Watkins.

2. Explain how engaging another team member in a co-treatment session was more effective than providing discipline-specific care.

3. Explain how the roles and responsibilities of the patient, family members, OT, SLP, dietary, and nursing staff members are interrelated in providing nutrition to Mrs. Watkins.

CASE STUDY: ENGAGING DIVERSE PROFESSIONALS IN THE PLAN OF CARE

Specific Sub-competencies to consider and apply: RR3, RR4.

Joseph Kane is a 78-year-old widowed male who lives alone. Two weeks ago, his adult son and daughter-in-law became alarmed when he didn't come to their home for Sunday brunch as was his routine. His son, Jeff, called Mr. Kane on the phone and got no answer, so he went to Mr. Kane's home. Jeff found Mr. Kane lying on the floor in the kitchen. Mr. Kane did not seem to understand what was happening and was soaked in urine. Because there were no lights on in the home and because Mr. Kane's car keys, unopened mail, and a bag of groceries were on the table, it was estimated that he had been lying there for more than 20 hours. Mr. Kane was transported to the trauma center via ambulance, where he was diagnosed as having an acute left-sided cerebrovascular accident (CVA), or stroke.

Mr. Kane was admitted to the stroke unit. As a result of his CVA, he is unable to move the right side of his body and has difficulty understanding and expressing verbal communication. He appears confused and frightened at times but is able to cooperate during care. He follows simple commands. His movements are slow and cautious.

Mr. Kane does not appear to be in pain. His skin is warm and dry. He has bruises on his left forehead, shoulder, and hip areas, probably as a result of falling. He was dehydrated on admission and has an intravenous line in place. Mr. Kane demonstrated dysphagia (difficulty swallowing). A swallow function test (lateral video fluoroscopic observation) revealed abnormalities in swallowing.

The unit's interprofessional stroke care team meet to plan a comprehensive care plan for Mr. Kane. In addition to the professionals on the team, Mr. Kane's son, his daughter-in-law, and their two college-aged children come to visit each day and want to be involved in his care. The team's goal is to return Mr. Kane to his maximum level of independent functioning.

Discussion Questions

1. List the members of the group of professionals and others, including Mr. Kane and his family, who should be represented on the stroke care team.
2. Identify at least one specific team goal for Mr. Kane's care. Explain how team members will use their complementary roles and responsibilities, collaboratively, to achieve this goal.

Role Play Activities

1. Form groups of two to three. Have each person assume the role of a different professional or of a family member caring for Mr. Kane.
2. Role play explaining each member's role to other members of the interprofessional team caring for Mr. Kane.

CASE STUDY: OPTIMIZING WELLNESS IN A REFUGEE POPULATION

Specific Sub-competencies to consider and apply: RR3, RR7, RR9, RR10.

The resettlement of refugees to the United States is a process that can take months or even years. In one city, community leaders formed an interprofessional, multidisciplinary community coalition with an identified goal of forming a Refugee Healthcare Program to treat the unique needs of the immigrant and refugee populations living there. Approximately 10% of the city's residents are refugees with needs that include inadequate past medical and dental care, exposure to untreated diseases, and experiences that include torture and terrorism.

The Refugee Healthcare Program is being formed with shared resources from many partners, including the area's primary refugee resettlement agency, the Department of Human Services, and the Department of Public Health. The Refugee Healthcare Program is being designed to provide primary healthcare services in a culturally appropriate and sensitive way, including the use of "cultural health navigators." These cultural health navigators will be drawn from resettled refugees who work with the interprofessional team to offer interpretation and promote care coordination. Services will be provided in two ways: at a storefront clinic location in the downtown area and, remotely, via a mobile health van visiting schools, retirement communities, shelters, and public housing complexes.

Discussion Questions

1. List the professionals in health care and other fields whom you would expect to be members of the interprofessional and multidisciplinary community coalition mentioned in this case study who are planning the Refugee Healthcare Program. Identify the specific needs of the refugee population that each professional would be expected to address.
2. Describe at least two distinct healthcare services that might be offered through the Refugee Healthcare Program (i.e., mental health, well-child care, women's health, dental), and identify which members of the interprofessional team might collaborate to provide those services comprehensively.
3. What do you see as the specific roles and responsibilities of "cultural health navigators"?

4. Describe the anticipated effects of the "cultural health navigators" on patient outcomes and on the cultural competency of those professionals in health care and other fields who are associated with the Refugee Healthcare Program.

CASE STUDY: TRAUMA PATIENT

Specific Sub-competencies to consider and apply: RR1, RR3, RR4, RR9.

Mary Nelson is a 30-year-old divorced female who lives in the suburbs with her 7-year-old son, Robert, and her 60-year-old widowed mother. She is employed full time as a legal secretary.

She was driving home from work one evening when a car crossed into her lane and hit her car head-on. Ms. Nelson was taken by helicopter to the nearest trauma center, where she was stabilized and treated for multiple injuries. Her mother, Mrs. Richards, was listed as her emergency contact and was contacted. Diagnostic tests confirmed fractures of her left ulna (arm) and left femur (leg). Her jaw was severely fractured, she lost most of her teeth, and her left hand was crushed. She also experienced a concussion.

Ms. Nelson was admitted to the hospital's trauma unit. She underwent multiple surgical procedures to repair her many fractures. She has been in the trauma unit for several weeks. Her fractures are healing well, and her condition is stable. Her pain control is good on oral pain medication.

Ms. Nelson has lost weight since admission. Her jaw is wired shut to promote healing, and, although she is receiving high-calorie liquid supplements by mouth, she does not like their taste. Her mother often brings milkshakes, which she enjoys; however, she does not have much of an appetite.

Mary Nelson has limited mobility due to her fractured femur. She also has difficulty moving her left arm and hand, with limited fine motor coordination and movement. The extent and permanency of these limitations are not yet known.

Ms. Nelson has a verbal communication impairment related to her jaw being wired shut. She occasionally gets frustrated when people cannot understand her. She is left-handed and cannot write due to the injury to her left hand.

Ms. Nelson hopes that she will return to full functioning. She actively participates in decision making about her care. Her cognition is intact. She is experiencing some shortness of temper and occasional mood swings since her accident and states she has no patience anymore.

Ms. Nelson's mother, Mrs. Richards, is caring for her son, Robert. Mrs. Richards and Robert visit frequently. Robert is worried about his mother, and his schoolwork is suffering.

Discussion Questions

1. List the members of the interprofessional team, including family members, who could be engaged in Mary Nelson's case to provide comprehensive care and meet her many needs.
2. Explain the roles and responsibilities of each team member in providing Mary Nelson's care.
3. Identify overlapping skills, and develop a strategy to clarify and assign responsibilities so that there is no duplication of services.
4. Using the same strategy as in question 2, explain how the team works together to provide care.
5. How does each professional's expertise contribute to the team to optimize Mary Nelson's care?

Role Play Activities

1. Form groups of two to three. Have each person assume the role of a different professional, Ms. Nelson, or a family member on the interprofessional team.
2. Role play each person explaining their role to other members of the interprofessional team. (Explain these roles both as a professional to a professional and as a professional to Ms. Nelson, her mother, and her son.)
3. Continue to role play until the recipient demonstrates an understanding of the role explanation by reflecting it back in his or her own words.

CASE STUDY: HEAD AND NECK CANCER

Specific Sub-competencies to consider and apply: RR3, RR5, RR7, RR8.

Alfred Dixon is a 55-year-old male who is being treated for laryngeal cancer. Mr. Dixon is unmarried and lives alone in a second-floor apartment. Mr. Dixon is 5 foot, 11 inches tall, and before diagnosis his weight was 185 pounds. This is the first major health problem he has experienced. His interprofessional healthcare team at the cancer center consists of an oncologist, radiation therapist, social worker, nurse, pharmacist, and nutrition specialist.

Mr. Dixon is on week 3 of a 7-week course of external beam radiation to the neck. He is experiencing a variety of side effects, including severe irritation around his neck, throat, and lower jaw. This has made bathing and dressing difficult because the skin is beginning to blister and peel and is very sensitive to the touch. His voice is hoarse and raspy. He also notes a significant loss in his ability to taste food and difficulty swallowing. He has lost about 10 pounds since beginning treatment. Mr. Dixon is experiencing extreme fatigue, although he continues to work. This is becoming increasingly more difficult for him, as is the daily commute by car. He is embarrassed by the way he looks and sounds and has communicated very little with his co-workers. He is becoming increasingly concerned that the changes to his physical appearance and vocal sound will be permanent and frequently feels depressed and frustrated with his current situation.

Discussion Questions

1. What other professionals and associated resources might be available to assist Mr. Dixon and his interprofessional team in his treatment and recovery?
2. How can the existing team forge interdependent relationships with other professionals within and outside of the healthcare system to provide safe, effective, and comprehensive care to meet all of Mr. Dixon's needs on an outpatient basis?
3. Discuss how Mr. Dixon's interprofessional team might provide a professional development activity for the healthcare professional and others in Mr. Dixon's work environment to enhance team performance and collaboration.

CASE STUDY: OVERLAPPING ROLES

Specific Sub-competencies to consider and apply: RR1, RR2, RR3, RR9.

The interprofessional team is meeting to determine the best plan for the after-discharge care of Judith Hansen, a 75-year-old patient in a rehabilitation facility who fractured her left hip after a fall at home, where she lives alone. She wants to go home, but her family is not comfortable with her being alone, fearing for her safety and ability to care for herself. The family prefers that she is transferred to a nursing home after discharge. The family requests that the interprofessional team evaluate the situation and offer their recommendations. The team

consists of a physician specializing in physical medicine and rehabilitation, a physical therapist, an occupational therapist, a registered nurse, a social worker, the patient, Mrs. Hansen, and her family.

When the team meets, the patient and family are not present. The professionals begin by discussing aspects of Mrs. Hansen's care. The occupational therapist (OT) states that Mrs. Hansen is able to dress herself and prepare simple meals and therefore should be able to go home. The physical therapist (PT) states that the patient is able to ambulate independently using a walker. The nurse has concerns about the patient's transportation needs, but the physician says the social worker should deal with that. Several team members think that a home visit will help in determining whether discharge to home is safe. This leads to discussion and uncertainty about who will to do the home visit. The PT planned to go to see whether the home is safe for using a walker, the nurse intended to have a member of the nursing staff go to determine environmental hazards, the OT expected to observe whether the kitchen is set up so that the patient can prepare meals, and the social worker says it is his job to make home visits. The team must determine who will do the home visit because the roles of several team members seem to overlap; making a home visit for the purpose each described is within each professional's legal scope of practice. The physician points out that the patient should be the one to decide where she wants to live, provided she is competent to do so, and suggests a psychiatric consult to evaluate the patient's competency to decide where she will go after discharge before proceeding further.

Discussion Questions

1. Explain how each team member's understanding of the roles and responsibilities of the other team members could help the team to work together effectively in providing comprehensive care to Mrs. Hansen.
2. For each team member mentioned in this case study, describe an interdependent team relationship that could improve Mrs. Hansen's discharge plan and health outcomes.
3. Explain how the interprofessional team might best decide whose role and responsibility it is to evaluate Mrs. Hansen's home environment.
4. Imagine you are the social worker for Mrs. Hansen. How would you describe your role and responsibilities

to the patient, family, and professionals on the team? How would you be able to assess their understanding of your explanation?

Role Play Activities

1. Role play an interaction between yourself (as one professional team member) and a peer (who can assume another team member's role) to communicate your individual perspectives of whether Mrs. Hansen should be discharged to her own home or to a nursing home.
2. Collaborate together to agree on a comprehensive and safe plan of care after discharge for Mrs. Hansen.
3. Together, plan to engage other members of the team who will complement your own expertise in better meeting Mrs. Hansen's discharge needs.

CASE STUDY: DISASTER PREPAREDNESS

Specific Sub-competencies to consider: RR7, RR8, RR10.

Emergency management officials and numerous agencies across multiple jurisdictions cooperate in staging disaster preparedness drills every other year. One year they simulated a collision between two aircraft at the airport. Other drills included a simulated explosion in the subway, a nuclear power plant emergency, and mass exposure to a highly contagious biological agent. This year they are planning to simulate a major flood disaster. Participants include (but are not limited to) first responders such as police, firefighters, and ambulance crews; area hospital systems, public health agencies, colleges, and universities; schools, mosques, churches, and other facilities that could be used as temporary shelters or staging areas; city officials; mass transportation agencies; heavy equipment companies; and communication specialists. The planning for each drill is extensive. Areas of concern that must be addressed include gaining access to the disaster site and victims; providing immediate emergency medical care; transport of people in need of hospital care; providing temporary shelter for displaced persons; and provision of food, water, medications, and other necessities. Communication between agencies and professionals is essential, as is communicating information to the public. These are just a few of the issues that need to be addressed. Collaboration between agencies and personnel is a key factor so duplication of services is avoided and use of available resources is maximized.

Discussion Questions

1. How can disaster preparedness drills help to forge interdependent relationships with other professions, including those outside of health care, to improve and advance learning?
2. Describe ways in which participation in large-scale community preparedness drills can provide opportunities for professional and interprofessional development.
3. Describe how professionals in health care and other fields can collaborate and integrate clinical care and public health interventions in a flood preparedness drill.

CASE STUDY: MORE THAN CLEANING PRODUCTS, IT'S MY JOB

Specific Sub-competencies to consider: RR2, RR3, RR6, RR7.

Mr. Simpson is a very dynamic young licensed practical nurse (LPN) at a large hospital. Frequently, when there is a spill of food or biological fluids, he takes it upon himself to clean it up. It is not uncommon for him to go to the housekeeping closet and get a bottle of cleaner to use for this purpose. This bothered the environmental services staff because they frequently found their cleaning supplies misplaced. They were also concerned that Mr. Simpson may be using the wrong products to clean the spills.

The head of environmental services decides to talk to Mr. Simpson's supervisor, Ms. Dean, about the matter. It was not clear Mr. Simpson was following the correct procedures to clean the spills. The head of environmental services reminded Ms. Dean that there are specific cleaners and procedures for each type of spill and that these procedures are available in the Material Safety Data Sheet (MSDS) manual on the unit. Ms. Dean replied that for small spills of harmless substances it makes sense for the nursing staff to attend to a spill so that it does not become a hazard. The head of environmental services suggests that she and Ms. Dean develop a review class for the nursing staff regarding the institutional policies and procedures for cleaning spills.

Discussion Questions

1. What are the issues around Roles/Responsibilities in this case?

2. Which Sub-competencies in Roles/Responsibilities were used in this case study? Which ones were not used, but still would have applied to the case study?

3. Was the main issue in Roles/Responsibilities resolved? If so, how?

CASE STUDY: QUICK REACTION IN THE EMERGENCY ROOM

Specific Sub-competencies to consider and apply: RR3, RR5, RR6.

Ms. Chen is a 53-year-old woman who arrived at the emergency room complaining of abdominal pain, sharp pain in the chest, and difficulty breathing. The licensed practical nurse (LPN) takes Ms. Chen's vital signs and becomes concerned. The LPN alerts the registered nurse (RN), who then assesses Ms. Chen more fully. The RN shares the findings with the emergency physician, who immediately orders oxygen for Ms. Chen. The doctor also requests that the patient be evaluated by the respiratory therapist and that an electrocardiogram (ECG) be obtained. The RN immediately contacts the respiratory therapist and the ECG technician. Once the results of the respiratory evaluation and the ECG come back, the RN and the physician meet to discuss next steps.

Discussion Questions

1. Who are the members of the interprofessional team in this case?

2. Because it is an emergency, which Sub-competencies of Roles/Responsibilities are most important in this case?

REFERENCES

Interprofessional Education Collaborative Expert Panel (IPEC). (2011). *Core competencies for interprofessional collaborative practice: Report of an expert panel.* Washington, DC: Interprofessional Education Collaborative.

Interprofessional Education Collaborative Expert Panel (IPEC). (2016). *Core competencies for interprofessional collaborative practice: 2016 update.* Washington, DC: Interprofessional Education Collaborative.

10

Foundations of Interprofessional Communication

LEARNING OUTCOMES

After studying this chapter, you will be able to:

1. Explain the essential components of interprofessional communication.
2. Identify appropriate communication tools and techniques to enhance team function.
3. Communicate with team members, patients, families, and community members with respect and clarity.
4. Demonstrate active listening skills in communication with others.
5. Explain the importance of using respectful language in difficult/crucial conversations.
6. Plan and participate in difficult conversations.
7. Communicate the importance of teamwork to others involved in patient-centered care, population health programs, or health-related policy development.
8. Provide timely, sensitive, and instructive feedback to others related to their performance on the team.

Developing competency in interprofessional communication requires moving beyond the basic principles of personal, professional, and therapeutic communication that are fundamental in every healthcare professional's basic role preparation. Competency in interprofessional communication involves specific behaviors and communication skills needed for interprofessional collaboration—those skills that are essential for the accurate, appropriate, and timely sharing of information between those who are involved in a specific healthcare situation. This chapter introduces the basic concepts associated with the Core Competency of Interprofessional Communication (IPEC, 2011; 2016).

Interprofessional communication is an essential component of Interprofessional Collaborative Practice (IPCP), and it is key to team relationships and patient safety. Communication failures have been cited as the leading root cause for medical errors, delays in treatment, and wrong-site surgeries, and the second most frequently cited root cause for operative and postoperative events and fatal falls (The Joint Commission, 2005). Communication breakdown was identified as one of the top three causes in 60% of the healthcare events resulting in unexpected death or permanent loss of function (known as sentinel events) between January 2013 and September 2015 (The Joint Commission, 2015). Clear, accurate, and timely communication positively influences team interactions, organization, and functioning (Essens et al., 2009, as cited by IPEC, 2011, p. 23). Healthcare professionals communicate with a wide variety of people each day, from patients and families to colleagues from their own and other disciplines, to staff and team members with varied educational levels, and to their own family and friends. Each encounter requires adaptation in the type and style of communication used. Professionals need to move fluidly from formal to informal, from professional to laypersons, and from simple to complex communication styles. In each encounter, there is a high potential for unclear or poor communication that may result in misunderstanding. There is clear evidence that both threats to patient safety and lawsuits against healthcare professionals are primarily related to failures of communication (Thistlethwaite, 2012).

To develop competency in interprofessional communication it is necessary to recognize and understand that in interprofessional healthcare teams "communication phenomena are surface manifestations of complex configurations of deeply felt beliefs, values, and attitudes" (Brown & Starkey, 1994, p. 808). This chapter provides foundational content designed to help you understand interprofessional communication within the culture of health care and healthcare teams. Common beliefs, values, and assumptions held by various team members are examined and considered as they affect attitudes toward communication and the interprofessional communication processes and systems in patient care. Other topics covered in this chapter include appropriate communication tools and techniques, guidelines for using respectful language in communicating, and considerations related to having difficult conversations.

✳ ACTIVE LEARNING

Interprofessional Communication

Think about a patient care or population health situation in which you recently participated that involved more than one other healthcare provider, caregiver, or colleague in the wider circle of the situation.

1. Write down at least two areas of shared concerns for team members involved. How did you know these were shared concerns?
2. Did you communicate with any of the other team members about these concerns? If so, which ones? What method(s) did you use to communicate with them?
3. Were there any barriers to this interprofessional communication? If so, what were they?
4. Could the overall outcome(s) of the care situation have been improved by better interprofessional communication? How?

BASICS OF INTERPROFESSIONAL COMMUNICATION

The ability to communicate clearly and respectfully is essential to interprofessional collaboration. This section provides an overview of some of the most critical communication skills you will need to participate fully in interprofessional collaboration.

Overview of the Communication Process

To understand the Competency of Interprofessional Communication and its Sub-competencies (IPEC, 2011; 2016), it is necessary to review the basic process of communication. All that ever was or will be accomplished involves communication with others (Adler & Towne, 1978). Communication is an interactive process (Adler & Towne, 1978; Halter, 2014) that begins with a stimulus. This can be a desire to give or receive information or to express a need or emotion on the part of the sender. The sender must translate the stimulus into a message that is verbal, nonverbal, or both. The basic communication process is operationalized in Fig. 10.1.

The next step in the communication process is to send the desired message to the intended receiver. There are several ways to send a message. Verbal communication is communication in words. It can be spoken or written. For example, a verbal message can be sent electronically as a text, email, voice recording, or an entry in the electronic health record. It can be spoken via telephone or in person. Nonverbal communication consists of body language such as position, gestures, eye contact, or touch. We also communicate using symbols such as pictures, graphics, or manual signs as used in American Sign Language (ASL).

Once a message is sent, the receiver must interpret its meaning and respond by acting and/or providing feedback to the sender. The sender will then convey feedback to the receiver and so on. Communication is effective when the sender's meaning is accurately interpreted by the receiver (Adler & Towne, 1978; Halter, 2014). This does not always occur. The process of communication within the wide circle of healthcare team collaborators can go wrong during any step of the process, and each method of communication requires specific skills and safeguards (Thistlethwaite, 2012). For this reason, it is important to think about exactly what you want to communicate, to whom, and in what manner. It is essential to get feedback from the receiver to make sure that your message was understood in the way in which you intended. This is true regardless of the person, or people, with whom you want to communicate.

There are many factors that affect communication. Some of these factors can obstruct or distort communication at any point in the process by causing inaccurate formulation of the message, inaccurate or improper transmission, or

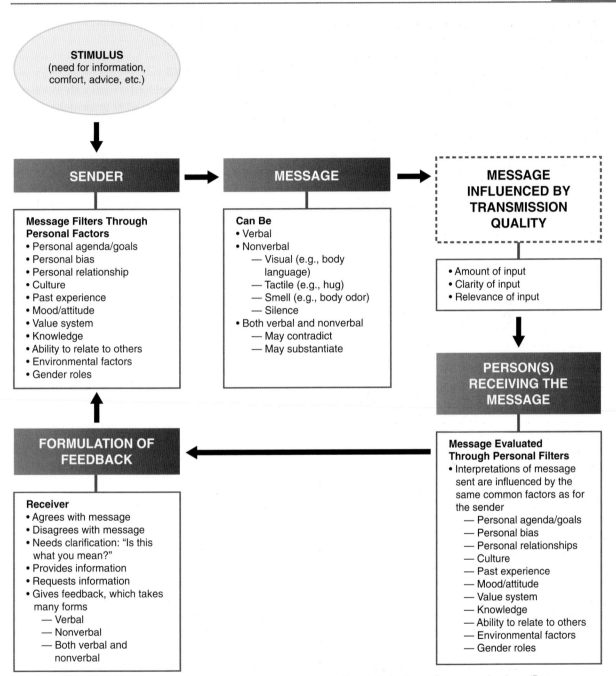

FIG. 10.1 The communication process source: operational definition of communication. (Data from Ellis, R., & McClintock, A. [1990]. *If you take my meaning.* London: Arnold. In Halter, M. [2018]. *Varcarolis' foundations of psychiatric-mental health nursing* [8th ed.]. St. Louis, MO: Saunders Elsevier.)

inaccurate interpretation by the receiver. These factors include personal, environmental, and relationship factors (Halter, 2014). Cultural differences must also be taken into consideration. An example of inaccurate interpretation by the receiver occurring is when two healthcare professionals are communicating. The first professional uses his or her professional culture (e.g., jargon) to formulate the message, and the second professional uses his or her professional culture as a filter through which to interpret the message. Without a common ground of understanding, the message may be misinterpreted.

After any communication exchange, it is important to make sure your message was clearly received and understood. A simple tool that can be used for confirming that you have explained things in an understandable manner to patients or others is the teach-back method. To use this method, simply ask the person to state, in his or her own words, his or her understanding of what you have explained to the person. If this process uncovers any misunderstandings, you will have the opportunity to clarify your message and recheck the person's understanding again. In instances when you have large amounts of information to convey, you can use the chunk-and-check method. Using this method, you can "chunk" out the information you need to provide in small segments and have the person "teach" it back at shorter intervals to ensure his or her understanding (AHRQ, n.d.).

Personal Factors

Personal factors that can affect communication include the sender's and receiver's emotional state, mood, or response to stress (Halter, 2014). For example, increased anxiety makes it difficult to process information. If a healthcare professional is having a stressful day, he or she may find it difficult to listen respectfully to a patient's or team member's minor complaints. Developmental level is another personal factor to consider. Consider the age and developmental levels of the patients with whom you communicate; for example, if your patient is a child you will communicate very differently from how you would with an adult. Generational differences within the interprofessional team itself may interfere with clear communication if they are not recognized.

Cognitive factors, such as ability to process information quickly, neurologic impairment, or level of problem-solving ability can also affect communication. Physical factors should also be considered. When a person feels too warm or too cold; is in pain; or has uncorrected visual, hearing, or speech impairments, accurate communication may be difficult.

Relationship Factors

Communication is affected by the relationship or status of the sender and receiver. Social or professional factors such as level of experience, perceived power status of the receiver or the sender, hierarchy within the organization, socioeconomic status, educational level, and people's expectations can also affect communication. The nature of the relationship between the sender and the receiver has a significant effect on communication. Consider how you speak to your close friends and family. Then consider how you speak with your professional colleagues or instructors (Halter, 2014). There is a different level of formality or intimacy within the communication, depending on your relationship. Cultural differences related to the professional–patient relationship sometimes exist and may negatively affect communication. For example, in some cultures it is considered disrespectful to question a healthcare provider.

Many healthcare environments are characterized by a hierarchical culture with physicians or dentists at the top of that hierarchy. Physicians, for example, often believe that the environment is collaborative and that communication is open, whereas nurses and other direct care providers perceive communication problems (O'Daniel & Rosenstein, 2008). Hierarchical differences can interfere with the interprofessional collaboration needed to ensure optimal care outcomes because those on the lower end of the hierarchy may be uncomfortable speaking up about problems and concerns. Lack of respect for other team roles and intimidating behaviors by those at the top of the hierarchy will prevent dynamic and free exchange of information within the team. Communication may be distorted or withheld when there are hierarchical differences between two communicators, especially when one person is concerned about appearing incompetent, does not want to offend the other, or perceives that the other person is not open to the communication (O'Daniel & Rosenstein, 2008). A significant barrier to interprofessional communication and collaboration is the perception of power imbalances between team members. Recognizing the value of contributions from all team members is essential; role clarification, role valuing, and power sharing within the interprofessional team are important for effective communication and collaboration (Dufour et al., 2010).

✦ **ACTIVE LEARNING**

Communication Methods

1. Make a list of all the possible ways that you might send a verbal message.
2. Imagine that you need to communicate a change in a patient's condition to another member of the interprofessional healthcare team. What factors might influence your decision regarding the best way to communicate this message?

Environmental Factors

The effect of environmental factors on communication may be overlooked by healthcare professionals because they are used to working in an environment that may be noisy and probably have developed the ability to "tune out" extraneous sounds such as the beeping of an empty intravenous (IV) pump or the sound of a dental drill. On the other hand, patients may find these sounds distressing and distracting and may not be able to fully focus on hearing information given by professionals. Other environmental factors that negatively affect communication may include a lack of privacy, the presence of others (Halter, 2014), unfamiliar or uncomfortable surroundings, and unfamiliar smells. There may also be other environmental factors depending on the specific situation.

TYPES OF COMMUNICATION

Verbal Communication

Verbal communication is communication using written or spoken words. There are several factors that can affect the interpretation of spoken verbal communication. Vocabulary and language can affect the receiver's understanding of the message. An example is a healthcare professional using words or technical language that are unfamiliar to patients or a patient with limited understanding of English. Pacing of speech is an important factor. Pacing is the speed, flow, pauses, rate, and rhythm of speech. Speech that is too fast may be difficult to understand, and speech that is too slow may cause the listener's attention to wander. Intonation includes tone of voice and placing emphasis on certain words. Think of the tone of voice you use when you are angry, sad, or happy. This affects the way your words are interpreted. Volume is important. Speaking too loudly or too softly can hamper communication. Clarity and brevity are also important factors. The shorter and

clearer the message, the more likely it is to be accurately understood. Avoid long drawn-out explanations; instead keep your communication simple. Another important factor in communication is the credibility or believability of the speaker. As a healthcare professional, you need to speak with confidence and authority when communicating with patients and colleagues. Timing and relevance are considerations when communicating with patients and other professionals. The best time to discuss a topic is when the person expresses interest or when it pertains to the current situation. The person should be in optimal condition to receive the message. For example, educating patients or obtaining informed consent should wait until they are comfortable and not in pain or extremely anxious. In urgent or emergent situations, this may not be possible. However, every attempt should be made to plan communications for when patients are best able to receive them.

Nonverbal Communication

Nonverbal communication includes such things as body language, eye contact, and gestures. Other aspects of nonverbal communication include personal appearance, body posture, movement, gait and stance, facial expression, and sounds such as sighs or groans. Nonverbal communication is heavily influenced by culture and is usually less controlled or planned than verbal communication (Halter, 2014) and may even occur outside of your awareness. However, nonverbal elements have a powerful effect on communication, often greater than the effect of the content or words that are spoken. It is important that your nonverbal communication is congruent with your verbal communication (Halter, 2014). This takes effort and requires self-awareness and monitoring. Achieving congruence between verbal and nonverbal communication may be learned through self-reflection (see Chapter 7).

Personal appearance can affect credibility. For example, an obese healthcare professional giving advice about diet and exercise may not be as believable as someone who appears fit. A professional appearance can facilitate the development of trust and a therapeutic relationship. On the other hand, inappropriate dress, heavy makeup, facial piercings and/or tattoos, unpleasant body odor, or lack of personal hygiene can detract from professional credibility. Although the importance of personal appearance may seem unfair, it is important to remember that the patient is the center of care, and every effort must be taken to establish a trusting relationship. This is true when working with other professionals. Therefore, presenting a professional appearance at work is helpful.

Body Language

Body language, also known as *kinesics,* is defined as a type of nonverbal communication in which physical behavior, gestures, movements, and mannerisms, as opposed to words, are used to express or convey information. Often, the emotional components of the message can be inferred by observing body language. Examples are slumped body posture and bowing the head in response to sad news. Posture and rhythm of movement are both forms of body language (Arnold & Boggs, 2016). A closed body posture, with arms or legs folded, can be interpreted as unwillingness to accept the message or not being "open" to what the other person is saying. On the other hand, leaning slightly forward with an open body posture can indicate interest in what the other person must say (Halter, 2014); this is the recommended posture for healthcare professionals to assume when speaking with patients, families, or colleagues.

Facial Expressions

Facial expressions are important in signaling feelings or emotions (Arnold & Boggs, 2016). They are almost universal in meaning across cultures, with a smile indicating happiness and a frown indicating displeasure. Facial expressions can reinforce spoken communications by connecting the message with the internal dialogue of the speaker (Arnold & Boggs, 2016). It is important that your facial expression matches the message you intend to convey. Otherwise, confusion can occur. For example, if a healthcare professional smiles while delivering bad news, it may appear that he or she does not care or may even be pleased. When the facial expression and message are inconsistent, the facial expression outweighs the content of the words (Arnold & Boggs, 2016). Lack of facial expression can be misconstrued as an indication of not caring. As a healthcare professional, do not be afraid to use facial expressions to reinforce your meaning, and make sure that you are aware of your expression when speaking with others.

Gestures

Gestures are often used to accentuate or reinforce verbal communication, or they may be used alone to communicate a message. An example is people who "talk with their hands." Overuse of gestures can be distracting and can cause the listener to lose focus. Gestures have different meanings in different cultures and should be used carefully to avoid unintentionally confusing or insulting people from cultures other than your own. For example, it is important to "understand the correct greetings (e.g., if a form of touch such as a handshake is permissible), what gestures mean, and the interpretation of eye contact" (Spector, 2017, p. 30). It is best to use gestures minimally and only when you are sure they will enhance your communication, such as pointing to a body area or demonstrating a movement.

Symbols

Symbols are representations of an event, action, object, person, or place that can be used to communicate about it. Examples of symbols used to communicate in healthcare settings include line drawings, graphic representations, and photographs. The variety of symbols used in health care range from concrete to abstract. The more a symbol resembles what it represents, the more concrete the symbol is. Fig. 10.2 depicts some familiar concrete symbols used to indicate "No Smoking" areas, parking areas for individuals with disabilities, and the universal symbol for female and male restrooms.

Less-concrete symbols include manual signs made with one or two hands and include a specific hand shape, position in space, and movement. Manual signs can be a visual or tactile way to communicate, borrowing vocabulary from ASL. Most of these signs do not clearly resemble their referent and are considered less concrete, or abstract. For examples, see Fig. 10.3.

Touch

Many professionals believe that the use of touch, as in holding a patient's hand, can convey caring. However, this type of touch may be unwelcomed or misinterpreted by some patients or families. If you feel the desire to touch or even hug a patient, first reflect on whether the touch has therapeutic value. It is always best to ask your patient for permission before touching to convey caring. Although some people may find it calming to be touched, others may consider it an invasion of privacy (Halter, 2014). It may be taboo in certain cultures. Some facilities, especially mental health facilities or those caring for children, have "no touch" policies (Halter, 2014). Make sure you know your facility's policy regarding the use of touch in non–direct care situations.

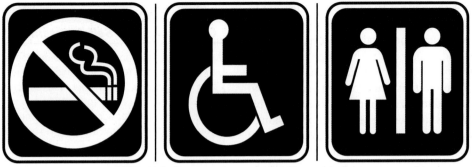

FIG. 10.2 Concrete communication symbols.

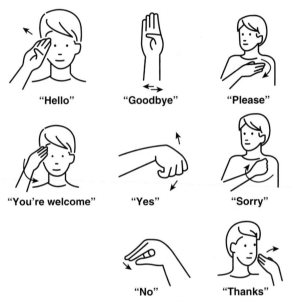

FIG. 10.3 Less concrete communication symbols, borrowed from American Sign Language. (From National Institute on Deafness and Other Communication Disorders. [2017, May 19]. *American Sign Language.* Retrieved from https://www.nidcd.nih.gov/health/american-sign-language.)

Much of what we do as healthcare professionals involves touching patients. In all situations, it is best to tell the patient you will need to touch him or her, where, and for what purpose before doing so. It is also good technique to tell patients what they can expect to feel, if this is known. For example, some IV medications may sting or burn while being injected, so warning patients that they may experience a burning sensation, and that this is normal, can help prevent anxiety.

Eye Contact

The level of comfort one has with direct eye contact and its social meaning and appropriateness is often culturally determined (Halter, 2014). Using direct eye contact while communicating with another can create a sense of confidence and credibility, whereas downcast or averted eyes can indicate shame, weakness, or submission. If the eyes wander during a conversation, it may be interpreted as a sign of dishonesty (Arnold & Boggs, 2016). On the other hand, in some cultures, direct eye contact may be considered a sign of disrespect. It is generally recommended to use direct eye contact (without staring) during professional discussions. Before making a clinical judgment of a patient's attentiveness or honesty based on eye contact, determine whether there is a cultural aspect operating.

It is always best to verify any interpretation you make of a patient's eye contact directly with the patient or the family. For example, a 24-year-old outpatient mental health patient who was Hispanic would not look directly at the nurse practitioner (NP) during the assessment interview. The NP attempted to determine the reason for the lack of eye contact, stating, "I notice you seem to be avoiding looking directly at me. Tell me about that." The patient leaned over and whispered something to his mother, who then said to the NP, "Juan said he can't look at you because he sees skeletons when he looks at people's faces." If the NP had assumed that the patient was avoiding eye contact out of a cultural norm of respect, and not asked about it, she may have missed the fact that the patient was experiencing visual hallucinations.

Improving Nonverbal Communication

The first step in improving nonverbal communication is to relax, then take a few deep breaths and clear your mind. Focus on the issue at hand and pay attention to your body. Lean slightly forward with an open body posture, arms and legs uncrossed. Use facial, hand, and body gestures judiciously and with thought. Watch the people with whom you are communicating to detect their nonverbal communication, which may be in response to yours. One method to use in improving your nonverbal communication is to observe effective professionals interacting with others. Another strategy is to ask a trusted colleague for feedback on your nonverbal communication. Videotaping interactions (with permission) can also be helpful in analyzing your nonverbal communication. You should consciously practice improving your identified areas of weakness and practice active listening, which is detailed later in this chapter.

CULTURAL CONSIDERATIONS IN COMMUNICATION

How people communicate and what constitutes "appropriate" communication vary among cultures. The United States is one of the most ethnically and culturally diverse countries in the world; therefore, many patients and clinicians come from a variety of cultural backgrounds. A person's culture includes membership in any number of subcultures, such as people with disabilities or certain sexual identification. Ideally, to promote culturally competent health care, settings should provide a culturally diverse staff that reflects the communities they serve. However, this is usually not the case.

When interacting with patients or colleagues, it is important to determine the degree to which their communication is affected by culture-specific practices and beliefs. Ask your patient if there are any cultural considerations related to care, communication, or touch that you should be aware of (Hook, Davis, Owen, Worthington, & Utsey, 2013). If time permits, perform a cultural assessment (as discussed in Chapter 5). Do not assume you know your patient's preferences based on your ideas of his or her cultural background, or even worse, based on physical features. See Caselet 10.1 for an example.

Language Barriers

Language differences may be a significant obstacle to providing multicultural health care (Spector, 2017). It may be difficult to understand patients and colleagues who are nonnative English speakers or those with a different regional accent than yours. Healthcare professionals who

 ACTIVE LEARNING

Communication Self-Assessment

Answer the following true-or-false questions as honestly as possible; then review your answers and draw at least two conclusions about your habitual communication patterns that you need to work on to improve. Check your conclusions for accuracy with a friend who knows your style of communicating well. Then score yourself using the following key.

1. I find it easier to start conversations by talking about myself.
2. I usually listen about as much as I talk.
3. I tend to be long-winded.
4. I rarely interrupt others.
5. When people hesitate or speak slowly, I try to complete their sentences for them.
6. I pay close attention to what others say, as well as to bodily cues.
7. I find it difficult to make eye contact with the person I am talking with.
8. I can usually tell if someone is angry or upset.
9. I find it difficult to express myself assertively.
10. I expect others to read my mind.
11. I hesitate to interrupt someone to ask for clarification.
12. People often tell me personal things about themselves.
13. I find it is best to change the subject if someone gets too emotional.
14. If I cannot "make things better" for a friend with a problem, I feel uncomfortable.
15. I am comfortable talking with people much older or much younger than I am.
16. I have difficulty saying no.
17. I speak to others the way I like to be spoken to.
18. I get irritated easily.
19. I tend to withdraw from conflict or remain silent.
20. I try to evaluate when someone will be most receptive to my message.

Key: If you answered True to questions 2, 4, 6, 8, 12, 15, 17, and 20, you are on your way to becoming an effective communicator. If you answered True to other questions, select several to improve. Set a realistic goal and seek help from a trusted friend or faculty member.

From Black, B. (2012). *Professional nursing: Concepts & challenges* (8th ed.). St. Louis: Saunders.

CASELET 10.1 Antonia Di'Giovanni

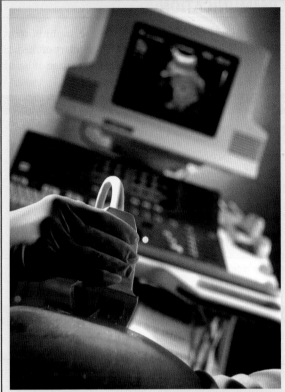

(Photo © Ingram Publishing/Thinkstock.)

Antonia Di'Giovanni was a patient in the prenatal clinic. She was getting an ultrasound and has expressed her desire to know the gender of her unborn child if possible because she really wanted a boy. When the sonographer determined that it was a boy and announced it to Ms. Di'Giovanni she impulsively hugged Ms. Di'Giovanni, who became very upset, stiffened, and told the sonographer, "Get your hands off me!" This confused the sonographer because she thought that Italian people liked to be touched. She asked Ms. Di'Giovanni if she wanted her cell phone to call her family, and made a gesture meant to convey talking on the phone. Ms. Di'Giovanni became even more upset and yelled at the sonographer, "Get out of here right now and get my mother!" The sonographer did so, and asked someone else to attend to Ms. Di'Giovanni but was very confused regarding the patient's behavior.

It was determined that Ms. Di'Giovanni was uncomfortable with being touched because of childhood trauma. When the sonographer hugged her, it brought uncomfortable feelings and caused anxiety for Ms. Di'Giovanni. The gesture meant to convey talking on the phone was interpreted by Ms. Di'Giovanni as a gesture that means "giving the evil eye," and she thought that the sonographer was placing a curse on the unborn child. This example demonstrates the danger of using touch and gestures without knowledge of the patient's preferences or cultural meanings.

Discussion Questions

1. What should the sonographer have done to avoid upsetting the patient?
2. Can you see evidence of stereotyping in this caselet? Explain.

---

want to improve their communication skills can learn to change their speech pronunciation with the help of a qualified speech–language pathologist (SLP). The process of changing an accent is known as "accent modification" or "accent reduction" (ASHA, n.d.).

When communicating with non-English speaking patients or family members, or those who do not speak English fluently, you should obtain the services of a trained medical interpreter. See Box 10.1 for guidelines concerning the use of interpreters.

In addition to accents, language usage and colloquialisms also vary. For example, in some parts of the United States, sweet carbonated beverages are called "soda," and in others, "pop." It is always a good idea to clarify terms. Certain expressions, phrases, or "sayings" may be specific to one's culture and not understood by those from other cultures. For example, the phrase "a stitch in time saves nine" is meant to indicate the value of prevention or early intervention. However, to someone unfamiliar with this adage, it may be misinterpreted to mean that sutures are needed. Avoid using such phrases, unless you are sure the person with whom you are speaking will understand.

ACTIVE LISTENING

How well do you listen to patients, to other healthcare providers, or to others in general? In an iconic study by Beckman and Frankel (1984), it was found that physicians interrupted patients' initial statements 77% of the time and that the average time to interruption by the physician was only 18 seconds. In a more recent study, Rhoades, McFarland, Finch, and Johnson (2001) reported that patients spoke, uninterrupted, an average of only 12 seconds after a resident entered the room. See Research Highlight: Speaking and Interruptions During Primary Care Office Visits.

VOCABULARY AND INTERPROFESSIONAL COMMUNICATION

The actual words that we choose to use are important. Healthcare professionals have a large vocabulary of medical terminology and technical terms. This "language of health

---

BOX 10.1 Guidelines for the Use of Interpreters

- Use trained interpreters whenever possible.
- Avoid using family members as interpreters, except in a life-threatening emergency.
- Obtain the patient's permission to use an interpreter.
- Explain that the interpreter is required to keep all information confidential.
- Many healthcare facilities have a "language line" with which you can call a trained interpreter in one of many available languages to communicate with your patient.

- Allow extra time for communication.
- Speak directly to the patient, not to the interpreter.
- Be sure the interpreter is interpreting verbatim, not summarizing or explaining.
- Clarify with both the patient and interpreter if something is unclear.
- Make sure you allow the patient opportunity to ask questions or add information.

Adapted from Arnold, E., & Boggs, K. (2016). *Interpersonal relationships: Professional communication skills for nurses.* St. Louis: Saunders Elsevier.

RESEARCH HIGHLIGHT

Speaking and Interruptions During Primary Care Office Visits

One study examined physician–patient communication patterns and interruptions in communication during patient visits with family practice and internal medicine. The results revealed that patients spoke, uninterrupted, an average of 12 seconds after the resident entered the room. One-fourth of the time, residents interrupted patients before they finished speaking. Residents averaged interrupting patients twice during a visit. The time spent with patients averaged only 11 minutes, with the patient speaking for about 4 minutes. Verbal interruptions, a knock on the door, pager interruptions, and computer use all interfered with communication. Computer use during the office visit accounted for more interruptions than pagers. The frequency of interruptions was associated with the patient's less-favorable perceptions of the office visit. Female residents interrupted their patients less often than did male residents. All residents interrupted female patients more often than male patients. Early and increased interruptions were associated with patients' perceptions that they should have talked more. Third-year residents interrupted patients less frequently than did first-year residents (Rhoades, McFarland, Finch, & Johnson, 2001).

Not listening is the most common problem in communication. Poor listening skills prevent the receiver from correctly understanding the content of the sender's message. Many people have developed what is known as *selective listening.*

Because healthcare professionals are asked to absorb so much information in a given encounter, they often become selective listeners. Selective listening means filtering out sounds and details that are believed to be of no interest or concern to them. One physician explained it this way: "It is not that we don't hear our patients; we are very good at practicing 'selective listening,' in which we pick out those patients' words that align best with our own clinical interpretation" (Buist, 2016, pp. 286–287). Unfortunately, selective listening often results in inadvertently filtering out valuable information.

Often, listening is passive. The use of standardized assessment questions often contributes to this problem. A healthcare professional, for example, may be focused on a standardized assessment format of questions and not listening attentively to the answers received; most often they are distracted, half listening, or half thinking about something else. In addition, the interviewer may be focused on the patient's words, or on the form or the computer screen, and not be at all aware of the patient's nonverbal communication as the exchange occurs. Sometimes, even before the patient provides the complete information needed, the healthcare provider is busy formulating a response to what he or she already decided the problem is. Although practitioners have limited time for patient interactions and this approach often seems the

Speaking and Interruptions During Primary Care Office Visits—cont'd

most efficient, it is commonly ineffective in gathering robust and pertinent assessment data. In contrast, posing open-ended questions to the patient such as "What can I do for you today?" has been shown to be far more effective to gather the necessary information. Asking open-ended question provides the opportunity for the practitioner to be quiet and listen. However, regardless of the types of questions that we ask our patients or our colleagues, *actively* listening (to their responses) is the key to clear communication and mutual understanding. Active listening encourages people to be more open and provide more complete information.

Active listening is a structured form of listening and responding in which the listener focuses on the speaker's message with all senses (Fig. 10.4). Active listening requires skill and practice; it requires that you focus and give your undivided attention to the speaker. You need to pay attention to both verbal and nonverbal communication while observing for congruence. Active listening requires that you relate what you hear to what you already know and to analyze the speaker's entire message for a deeper understanding (Davis & Brantley, 2005). You must convey sincere interest and caring as you listen. Do not interrupt the speaker, but instead give him or her the deliberate opportunity to complete his or her message. Be aware of your body language; make eye contact and assume an open, engaged posture. Use nonverbal cues to show that

you are listening (changing head position, nodding, smiling, etc.). The speaker is the focus of your attention, so take notes and record information only as needed during the interaction. You should use open-ended questions and prompts such as, "Go on" or "Can you tell me more about that?" to encourage more information and further signal that you are actively listening. Seek clarification as needed. It is most important to be silent and listen intently. Withhold your comments and judgment until you have heard and processed the entire message.

To make sure that you correctly understand the sender's message, briefly summarize what the sender has told you and reflect it back to him or her for confirmation after the interaction. This provides the speaker with the opportunity to clarify unclear points and to be sure that you understood the intended message. If you did not, he or she can explain further. You should also take this opportunity to interpret the speaker's words in terms of feelings. Instead of simply interpreting the verbal communication, you might summarize your interpretation of his or her emotion or psychological response to the matter at hand (e.g., "You seem afraid," or "That was really hard for you, wasn't it?"). Active listening is key to avoiding misunderstandings because the process allows you to confirm that you actually do understand what the speaker has tried to communicate to you. Some of the most common active listening techniques are illustrated in Table 10.1.

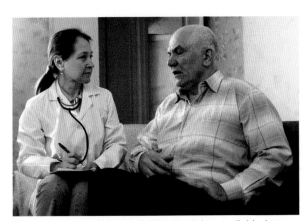

FIG. 10.4 Active listening requires giving undivided attention to the speaker. (© JackF/iStock/Thinkstock.)

care" is often foreign to those unfamiliar with medical terminology. In fact, sometimes the use of discipline-specific terminology is not understood by our professional colleagues. The use of this unfamiliar language, or jargon, may lead to misunderstanding and intimidation in our patients and our colleagues. Both patients and professionals sometimes fail to seek clarification and hesitate to ask questions for various reasons (being embarrassed at not knowing, feeling "less than," feeling "stupid"); therefore, it becomes imperative that we avoid jargon and choose words that can be clearly understood by most people. Lack of a common language can result in diagnostic errors and inappropriate treatment. Use terms that provide clear, objective, and specific information and that are not open for interpretation. When it is necessary to use unfamiliar words and terms, it is our responsibility to clearly explain them and make sure that our patient or colleague understands our message. For example, a

TABLE 10.1   Active Listening Techniques

Technique	Description	Example
Using silence	Refrain from speaking. Give the person time to think and organize and share their thoughts without interruption. A healthcare professional may express interest nonverbally through body language.	Healthcare professional is silent and waits for patient to respond.
Offering general leads	The use of short phrases to encourage the person to continue talking.	"Go on." "Anything else?" "And then what?"
Accepting	A nonjudgmental attitude and response that indicates understanding (but not necessarily agreement).	"I understand that you think this amputation is the worst thing that could happen to you." Eye contact; nodding.
Restating	Healthcare professionals use their own words to repeat the main idea expressed by the person. This gives the person the opportunity to correct inaccuracies.	Patient: "I don't believe in taking medication." Physician: "You don't want to take medication."
Reflecting	Questions are reflected back to the person so that he or she can process his or her own answers. The healthcare professional verbalizes the implied feelings in the person's comment.	Patient: "Do you think I should have the radiation?" Nurse: "What do you think you should do?" Patient: "I'm not ready to be discharged." Social Worker: "It sounds like you are afraid to go home tomorrow."
Focusing	Call attention to certain points, words, or events of importance; this is especially useful when the person moves rapidly from subject to subject.	"You are describing many problems with your illness. Let's focus on the sleep problem you mentioned."
Exploring	Examining certain ideas, experiences, or relationships further.	"Tell me more about that." "Can you describe that experience a bit more?"
Seeking clarification	An attempt to clearly understand the meaning of the person's statements by asking for further information.	"I'm not sure I understand exactly what upset you during your daughter's visit. Can you explain that to me again, please?"
Verbalizing the implied	Put into words what the person has only said indirectly. This allows the person to agree or disagree.	Patient: "It's a waste of time for me to be here." Physical therapist: "Are you feeling like no one is helping you?"
Summarizing	The healthcare professional highlights the main idea expressed during the interaction.	"You had two main concerns tonight. The first one was..."

statement like "You should take your Lisinopril once a day" is not clear; the healthcare professional giving this instruction should say clearly, "You will need to take Lisinopril, which is your blood pressure medication, once a day. It is best to take it in the morning when you first get up so it will work throughout the day."

Respectful Language

The way we use language affects others. Healthcare professionals are expected to demonstrate respectfulness in all communications by using words that respect the strengths, skills, talents, and individuality of others. The principles that follow will be useful in acknowledging all

✳ ACTIVE LEARNING

Listening Exercise

This exercise requires you to have a partner to complete it. It will provide you with an opportunity to practice and experience active listening. One person will be the "speaker," and one person will be the "listener." Roles may be switched after completion of the exercise, if desired, so that both participants will have a chance to practice and experience active listening.

Instructions for the Experience

1. The speaker is instructed to describe a loss he or she has experienced in his or her own life. It can be loss of a significant person, loss of a pet, loss of some aspect of health, loss of an object, or any other significant loss in the person's life.
2. The speaker is to talk about the loss for 5 minutes.
3. The second person is the listener. The listener needs to listen silently for 5 minutes. The listener may not speak at all during the 5 minutes.

Discussion Questions

1. For the speaker:
   What did it feel like to describe your loss?
   How did the listener respond to you?
   Did you feel that they were being attentive?
   Was there any particular thing that made you feel that they were in fact listening to you?
2. For the listener:
   How did it feel for you to listen in silence for 5 minutes?
   Did the 5 minutes seem short or long?
   What aspects of the telling of the story of loss were most significant to you?
   What did you learn from this experience of attentive listening?

Hospice Education Network. (2013). *ELNEC Core Module 6: Communication—Listening Exercise.* Washington, DC: American Association of Colleges of Nursing.

people on an equal basis through the language that you use (Law Society of British Columbia, n.d.). They are useful in helping to avoid unintended offence through increasing our awareness of many common assumptions and prejudices used in everyday language.

These principles are useful for ensuring respectful language usage; the first two principles are closely related. The first principle is *Avoid mentioning personal characteristics unless they are relevant.* Personal characteristics, such as race, sexuality, diagnosis, or disability should be used only when they are relevant to the specific communication. When a person's personal characteristics are relevant to the communication, follow the second principle of *inclusive language and person-first construction.* Inclusive language doesn't demean or stereotype people based on personal characteristics like gender, race, ethnicity, disability, religion, or sexual orientation. Inclusive language avoids the use of certain words that might be considered to exclude particular groups or people, especially gender-specific words, such as "man" or "mankind," and masculine pronouns, such as "his," the use of which might be considered to exclude women (Collins English Dictionary, n.d.). It is equally important to avoid terms that exclude, marginalize, diminish, or lower the status of any individual group (e.g., "us and them" constructions). Person-first construction places the person ahead of personal characteristics (e.g., "a person with schizophrenia" instead of "a schizophrenic"). *Person-first communication* focuses respectful attention on the individual's personhood rather than on characteristics such as their disease, disability, culture, or ethnicity (Law Society of British Columbia, n.d.).

The third principle relates to specific terms that you might use when referring to groups or individuals. Do not make assumptions about how an individual may want to be addressed; it is most important to respect the preferences of the person being addressed (Law Society of British Columbia, n.d.). One example can be found in Chapter 1 in the discussion related to which term should be used when referring to the consumer of care (patient, client, consumer, or service-user). The solution to this dilemma is if in doubt, it is best to simply ask what the person wishes to be called. The same holds true for the dilemma of what "name" to call a person. So, when deciding whether to call a person (colleague or patient) by a formal title or simply by his or her first name, it is generally best to ask. This same principle applies to groups we may work with in our communities; for example, a group for teens overcoming issues related to an experienced sexual assault may prefer to be called a "survivors" group rather than a "victims" group. Another example is the use of gender-specific pronouns with transgender patients. Sometimes, especially at the beginning of the transition process, transgender individuals may adopt a gender identity different from their gender presentation. In these cases, it is best to ask for the gender-specific pronoun preference of the individual, instead of making an assumption about how the person would like to be addressed.

The fourth principle focuses on the use of *gender-neutral language*. Avoid the use of biased or stereotyped terms that may be demeaning. Generics are nouns and pronouns that are intended to be used for both men and women. However, linguistically, some terms once considered generic are now seen as male-specific. For example, the word "man" was generically used to mean "human being" or "person," but over the years it has come to mean only "male persons," and the term "chairman," originally intended to be gender neutral, has been replaced by the term "chairperson" as a more appropriate generic term. Be careful that the generics you choose to use are indeed gender neutral. In addition, avoid using gendered adjectives where gender is not relevant (e.g., "male nurse," "lady doctor") (Law Society of British Columbia, n.d.).

The use of respectful language is incredibly powerful in healthcare communication. Consider the way that colleagues and patients speak to you; consider how the words that they use to describe you can create pride, identity, and purpose. On the other hand, consider how the use of negative, incorrect, or demeaning language can be detrimental to your sense of self-worth and well-being. It is important that we consistently incorporate all of the principles of respectful communication in creating and nurturing a sense of partnership with those we care for.

INTERPROFESSIONAL COMMUNICATION TOOLS

Accurate and complex information needs to be communicated within the context of the interprofessional team, sometimes within a short period. As part of an effort to reduce errors in healthcare settings, The Joint Commission analyzed more than 4800 sentinel events and identified communication as the top contributing factor to medical error, with handoffs playing a "role in an estimated 80% of serious preventable adverse events" (The Joint Commission, 2010, as cited in Popovich, 2011, p. 55). Preventable adverse events, such as injuries related to medical errors, are a major cause of death in the United States. Failures of communication, including miscommunication during transfer of patient care from one clinician to another, are a leading cause of these errors.

The phrase *patient handoff* is used to indicate "a transfer of care involving a transfer of information, responsibility, and authority between clinicians" (Abraham, Kannampallil, & Patel, 2014, p. 154). The handoff process involves a "sender," the caregiver transmitting the patient information and care of the patient to the next clinician, and a "receiver," the caregiver who accepts patient information and the care of the patient. The intent of the handoff is to clearly and accurately communicate patient information in the provision of safe and continuous high-quality care. Handoffs happen when accountability and responsibility for a patient are transferred from one team member to another (e.g., shift-to-shift report), from one service program to another (e.g., from an inpatient unit to a diagnostic service area), or from one organization to another (e.g., from inpatient rehabilitation to a community rehabilitation program).

Standardized Communication Tools

The commercial aviation industry had significant success preventing flight accidents related to communication failures using standardized communication tools (Nemeth, 2012). These tools have been instrumental in the creation of strategies to enhance teamwork and reduce risk in healthcare settings (Leonard, Graham, & Bonacum, 2004). Because of the complexity of care, coupled with the inherent limitations of human performance, it is critically important that clinicians have standardized communication tools to ensure accuracy during patient handoffs (Leonard, Graham, & Bonacum, 2004). The adoption of standardized communication tools is proposed to be an effective strategy in enhancing teamwork and reducing risks; standardized communication techniques can serve the same purpose that clinical practice guidelines do in assisting practitioners to make decisions and take action (O'Daniel & Rosenstein, 2008). To meet this need, a wide variety of handoff strategies and tools were developed and implemented.

Simple guidelines are best for managing complex environments. One example is SBAR (situation, background, assessment, recommendation), an easy-to-remember situational briefing model for communication, which has been found to be very effective in briefing the entire care team. It quickly ensures that all team members are "on the same page" and that all relevant clinical issues are being addressed (Leonard, Graham, & Bonacum, 2004). More information about SBAR can be found in the Additional Resources box at the end of this chapter. The quality of a handoff process "is adversely affected by many factors, including the lack of standardized handoff tools; information omissions and inaccuracies; communication breakdowns related to language, social, and skill issues; lack of training; and contextual constraints" (Abraham, Kannampallil, & Patel, 2014, p. 154). Although many quality improvement projects on patient handoffs have been conducted, the search for the ideal standardized tool continues (Patterson & Wears, 2010). Each healthcare institution should identify standardized communication tools that are best suited to their own needs and environments. Information related to some of the most common handoff tools can be found in the Additional Resources box at the end of this chapter.

DIFFICULT CONVERSATIONS WITHIN THE INTERPROFESSIONAL TEAM

Difficult conversations in the workplace are challenging to everyone. These include conversations with patients or colleagues in which we have to deliver unpleasant news, discuss a safety concern, address a delicate personal subject, or talk about something that needs to change or has gone wrong. These conversations can be uncomfortable, and therefore they are often avoided. The problem with avoidance is that it blocks interprofessional communication, it is an obstacle to achieving optimal care outcomes, and it may contribute to inadvertent patient harm. When considering whether to have a difficult conversation, it is important to consider that best practices dictate effective communication, even when difficult (Polito, 2013). There are published guidelines and recommendations available to assist healthcare professionals in this area (Kersun, Guy, & Morrison, 2009). The following section presents discussion and guidelines for having difficult conversations.

Effective teams share a common purpose and intent, trust, respect, and collaboration; they value familiarity over formality and watch out for one another so that mistakes are not made (O'Daniel & Rosenstein, 2008). Creating a safe environment for such familiarity to occur is a prerequisite and requires flattening the hierarchy, or power distance, between team members to make it safe to speak up, express concerns, and alert team members to unsafe situations (Leonard, Graham, & Bonacum, 2004). Knowing how to speak up and communicate concerns is an important skill to acquire. Although we can sometimes take time to plan for a difficult conversation, that is not always possible, so it is crucial to be prepared.

General Guidelines for Having Difficult Conversations

Concerns, problems, and issues should be handled quickly and at the level at which they arise. The first step in the process is to approach the interaction with openness and an interest in problem solving, rather than a need to blame or to be right. Use direct statements (i.e., "I see a problem and I need to talk to you about that now"). Address the person involved calmly and directly in a "matter-of-fact" manner; state the problem clearly and objectively and with respect for the person you are addressing. Ask that you be allowed to share your concern fully, without interruption, with the promise that you will listen to what the other person must say afterward. Stay on point; be focused. Focus on the problem without value judgment; avoid value-laden terms (e.g., "good," "bad," "wrong"). Avoid words like "always" and "never," they overgeneralize and are generally inaccurate. Do not just focus on the problem; propose what you think is a safe and realistic solution. After you have shared your concern and proposed a solution, actively listen to the other person's response; do not interrupt. Make sure you understand what he or she said before you respond. Ask for clarification if needed. Continue the process illustrated by the assertion cycle (Fig. 10.5) until you agree on a solution.

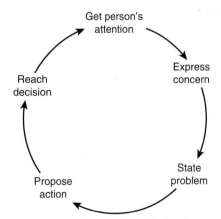

FIG. 10.5 The assertion cycle. (From Leonard, M., Graham, S., & Bonacum, D. [2004]. The human factor: The critical importance of effective teamwork and communication in providing safe care. *Quality and Safety in Health Care, 13*[suppl 1], i85–i90.)

These guidelines can be adapted to talk about interpersonal issues between you and a peer or another team member. When discussing the issue, focus on how it specifically affects you, be clear and calm, be respectful, and use "I" statements (for information on "I" statements, see the section on "I" statements that follows). Ask how the situation affected the other person. Give the person the opportunity to share his or her perspective. Use active listening. Acknowledge your contribution to the situation, see your part, and invite the other person to work with you to make things better.

Tempering Emotion

The expression of strong feelings, or emotions, interferes with problem-solving communication. It is important to own your own feelings, rather than blaming other people. There will be differences in how you and others see things. One communication strategy that is effective in preventing blame and shame related to others is the use of "I" statements. "I" statements allow you to be assertive in telling another how you feel and state your case without arousing the defenses of the other person. Be clear and specific about what the other person may have done that contributed to your reaction, but frame it carefully. "I" statements allow you to say how the situation makes you feel or what you would do in that situation instead of telling the other person what he or she should or should not do. Consider, for example, that you are angry and becoming resentful because your peer frequently comes back from lunch late, causing you to miss having lunch with your friends at a prearranged time. Using an "I" statement you might say, "Tom, I feel pretty angry because I missed having lunch with my friends. This is the second time this week you came back late; can we talk about that?" Addressing the issue of your anger in this way, instead of avoiding it, represents clear, respectful communication that can lead to a problem-solving conversation instead of growing resentment. In another example, consider observing a team member preparing to remove a surgical dressing and inspect an incision on a patient, without first washing hands and donning gloves. Rather than saying, "Wash your hands. You can cause an infection by not washing your hands and wearing gloves!" you can focus calmly on the other person's actual behaviors. You can say something like, "I know you are really busy. I'll get you some gloves while you wash your hands." In this way, you focus on resolving your fear that the patient will get

an infection as well as providing the solution to the identified problem.

Critical Language: Using the CUS Strategy

The use of critical language is a strategy that identifies agreed-upon communication signals (short phrases) within the culture of a specific interprofessional team to indicate the need to stop and communicate a significant care concern. To do this the team agrees on several short phrases that they will adopt. The adoption of critical language was derived from the CUS Program at United Airlines; CUS stands for the following short phrases: "I'm *concerned,* I'm *uncomfortable,* this is *unsafe,* or I'm *scared*" (Leonard, Graham, & Bonacum, 2004, p. i87). When any of these phrases are used, all team members know that "we have a serious problem here, stop and listen to me." The use of critical language creates the needed environment to get everyone to stop, listen, and problem solve. It creates the expectation that the issue at hand will be communicated clearly and directly.

Crisis Communication

Leadership and clear communication are critical in an emergency or crisis situation. Those present must work together smoothly as an effective team. Because most clinical and community emergencies don't allow for precise preplanning, a leader must quickly emerge at the scene who will provide clear direction. The leader in an emergency or crisis situation is usually the professional at the scene who has the education, training, and the team expectation of being in charge before the emergency occurred. The leader "must be able to rapidly analyze a complex environment, assess where and what sort of help is required, assemble an effective, multidisciplinary staff of care providers, and communicate effectively among staff and population in need" (Hershkovich, Gilad, Zimlichman, & Kreiss, 2016, p. 1). There can be only one leader. The leader is in charge during the emergency and responsible for navigating stressful and frequently changing, circumstances. The leader must be able to make informed decisions rapidly and be capable of ongoing self-assessment and adaptation to unfamiliar and rapidly changing conditions, thus ensuring the seamless provision of optimal care (Hershkovich, Gilad, Zimlichman, & Kreiss, 2016).

Efficient communication is a crucial aspect of leadership during an emergency situation. Team discussions and consensus have no place during an emergency; to

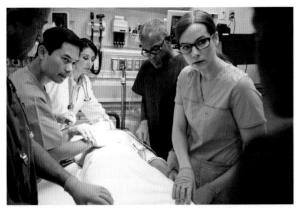

FIG. 10.6 In emergency situations, verbal communication is handled by a designated team member.

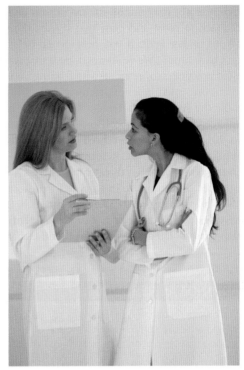

FIG. 10.7 Resistance in confronting performance issues is common.

avoid confusion, errors, and omissions the leader is the only one who gives directions and/or delegates to the team. Effective leaders are decisive and able to communicate clearly (Fig. 10.6). There is no debate about directions given by the leader in an emergency. To provide both efficient and effective direct communication the leader should address team members by name to make it clear who they are speaking to; no one on the team is named *somebody*, so saying "Somebody call a Code!" may not get immediate results. A form of physical contact, such as placing a hand on a person's shoulder, can be used to get someone's needed attention, and in all cases, the leader should make eye contact with the person he or she is communicating with to further confirm who he or she is speaking to. When giving directions to the team it is important that the leader "tell, don't ask." Although it is considerate to say "please," saying "Will you…?" or "Could you…?" leaves some question about what is expected.

Throughout any crisis situation, the leader is constantly processing verbal and nonverbal communication from the team and from the emergency situation. If something is not working, the leader must demonstrate the confidence and flexibility to change direction and clearly communicate changes to the interprofessional team.

Giving and Receiving Performance Feedback

Giving timely, sensitive, instructive feedback to someone related to workplace performance can be challenging. Responding to someone's response to your evaluation of their performance or responding to feedback on your own performance can be equally challenging. When faced with performance issues that have the potential for negative patient or population outcomes, it is best to deal with them promptly. Many healthcare professionals feel poorly equipped to handle such conversations, and resistance to confronting performance issues is common (Fig. 10.7). Effective team members must be able to tackle, rather than avoid, such conversations. Guidelines vary, but generally it is always best to provide performance feedback in an appropriate space, preferably one that is quiet and private. Maintaining confidentiality is important. It is important to set a positive tone and be empathetic, respectful, and open-minded. Always project willingness to understand the other person's point of view. People do not always understand how their behaviors affect others around them; they do not want to be told they are failing or making mistakes. Come to the discussion prepared for an open dialogue with facts and data to support your case, but allow the other person to offer a plan for improved performance and remediation of the situation.

Stay positive. Focus on the issue, not the person. Do more active listening than talking. Explore the issue together. It is not uncommon for the person receiving the feedback to resist and deny that it (i.e., the situation) is his or her fault. If you hear denial or excuses ("I don't have time," "We've always done it that way"), a suggested practice is to "respond with fogging"; a partial agreement presented in a nondefensive and caring way to handle the resistance statement ("That may be, yet you still need to follow protocol," or "Perhaps so, yet…") (Polito, 2013, p. 142). Do not dwell on the negative. Be respectful, calm, and clear. Research shows that these conversations are made less threatening and less difficult if the parties communicate in ways that "protect" and "give face to" each other (Bradley & Campbell, 2016). This involves downplaying or not drawing attention to the other person's failings; giving the other the chance to

rationalize or justify his or her actions; and supporting and enhancing the other's status through complements, affirmations, and indications of group inclusion. These acts show respect for the other person and help him or her to feel competent, liked, and valued (Bradley & Campbell, 2016).

Work toward what is expected next. Ask for the individual's suggestions on how he or she might improve performance; consider alternatives. Be clear with what is expected. The goal is that the team member will leave the conversation knowing he or she can do better and what the expectation is. The person should know and acknowledge that he or she is accountable for self-improvement. Plan to follow up in a reasonable amount of time to see how things are improving.

ADDITIONAL RESOURCES

The following resources are provided to assist you in identifying effective communication tools and techniques to facilitate discussions and interactions enhancing interprofessional collaboration. These resources are especially useful during transition periods and emergencies, when mistakes due to miscommunication are more likely to happen.

Foundational Resource

The Transitions of Care Portal. https://www.jointcommission.org/toc.aspx

This portal is a valuable source of information from The Joint Commission and other healthcare organizations related to the topic of transitions of care (the movement of patients between various healthcare settings).

Patient Handoff Resources

A *hand-off* is a real-time process of passing patient-specific information from one caregiver to another to ensure the continuity and safety of the patient's care (The Joint Commission, 2014). This process results in the transfer and acceptance of patient care responsibility and is achieved through effective communication. Some of the most common hand-off tools are presented here.

CLINIC SAFE Handoffs Pocket Card. http://www.beckersasc.com/asc-quality-infection-control/patient-safety-tool-clinic-safe-handoffs-pocket-card.html

The Picker Institute offers a free pocket card that was developed by University of Chicago Medical Center researchers to guide safe end-of-year patient handoffs in an internal medicine residency clinic. The CLINIC SAFE

pocket card is part of a University of Chicago project called Engineering Patient Oriented Clinic Handoffs, or EPOCH.

Hand-off Communications Targeted Solutions Tool™ (TST). http://www.centerfortransforminghealthcare.org/tst_hoc.aspx

The Joint Commission's Center for Transforming Healthcare offers this tool to organizations working to improve their hand-off process. The TST® for Hand-off Communications:

- Facilitates the examination of the current hand-off communication process
- Provides a measurement system that produces data that support the need for improving the current hand-off communication processes
- Identifies areas of focus, such as the specific information needed for the transition that is being measured
- Provides customizable forms for data collection
- Provides guidelines for most appropriate hand-off communication processes

Medical Transitions and Clinical Handoffs Toolkit. https://www.ahrq.gov/professionals/quality-patient-safety/patient-safety-resources/resources/match/index.html

The Agency for Healthcare Research and Quality released a toolkit designed to help hospitals improve medication safety. This toolkit addresses *medication reconciliation*, a complex process that impacts all patients as they move through healthcare settings. The process involves comparison of a patient's current medication regime against a physician's admission transfer or discharge orders to identify discrepancies. Although this toolkit is based on processes developed in acute-care settings, the core

ADDITIONAL RESOURCES—cont'd

processes, tools, and resources can be adapted for use in nonacute facilities. The toolkit includes a workbook designed to help users implement it.

Safer Sign Out Toolkit. http://safersignout.com/safer-sign-tool-kit/

The Emergency Medicine Patient Safety Foundation offers a free Safer Sign Out form to improve the safety of patient handoffs at the end of a shift. Safer Sign Out is a patient-centered, team-based innovation that was developed by emergency physicians to improve the safety and reliability of end of shift patient handoffs.

Situation, Background, Assessment, Recommendation (SBAR). http://www.ihi.org/resources/Pages/Tools/sbar-toolkit.aspx

SBAR is a widely recognized standardized communication format used to share nonemergent situational information about a patient within the healthcare team; it provides a common and predictable structure for communication. SBAR can be used to organize relevant patient information when preparing to contact another team member and serves as a framework for presenting that information, appropriate assessments, and recommendations.

The Team Strategies and Tools to Enhance Performance and Patient Safety (TeamSTEPPS). https://www.ahrq.gov/sites/default/files/wysiwyg/professionals/education/curriculum-tools/teamstepps/instructor/essentials/pocketguide.pdf

The TeamSTEPPS communication training model is widely used to train healthcare teams to communicate effectively with each other in a team context. Communication tools include SBAR, Call-Out, Check-Back, and "I PASS THE BATON."

KEY POINTS

- The basic communication process begins with a stimulus, which is then translated into a message. The message is then transmitted by various means to a receiver, who then must interpret the message. The potential exists for communication to be misinterpreted at any step in the process.
- Verbal communication is communication using written or spoken words. There are several factors that can affect the interpretation of spoken verbal communication. These include vocabulary and language, pacing of speech, clarity and brevity, credibility or believability of the speaker, and timing and relevance.
- There are many factors that can affect communication. Among these are personal factors, relationship factors, environmental factors, and cultural differences.
- Active listening is a structured form of listening and responding in which the listener focuses on the speaker's message with all senses. Active listening requires skill and practice; it requires that you focus and give your undivided attention to the speaker.
- The "language of health care" is often foreign to those unfamiliar with medical terminology. Sometimes our use of discipline-specific terminology is not understood by our professional colleagues. The use of this unfamiliar language, or jargon, may lead to misunderstanding by and intimidation of patients and colleagues.

- Healthcare professionals are expected to demonstrate respectfulness in all communications by using words that respect the strengths, skills, talents, and individuality of others.
- A significant barrier to interprofessional communication and collaboration is the perception of power imbalances among team members. Recognizing the value of contributions from all team members is essential; role clarification, role valuing, and power sharing within the interprofessional team is important for effective communication and collaboration (Dufour et al., 2010).
- Hierarchy differences within an interprofessional team can interfere with the interprofessional collaboration needed to ensure optimal care outcomes, because those on the lower end of the hierarchy may be uncomfortable speaking up about problems and concerns.
- The phrase *patient handoff* is used to indicate "a transfer of care involving a transfer of information, responsibility, and authority between clinicians" (Abraham, Kannampallil, & Patel, 2014, p. 154). The intent of the handoff is to clearly and accurately communicate patient information in the provision of safe and continuous high-quality care.
- SBAR (situation, background, assessment, recommendation) is an easy-to-remember situational briefing

model for clear team communication. It has been found to be very effective in briefing the entire care team quickly to ensure that they are all "on the same page" and that all relevant clinical issues are being addressed.

- Difficult conversations include conversations with patients or colleagues in which we have to deliver unpleasant news, discuss a safety concern, address a delicate personal subject, or talk about something that needs to change or has gone wrong.
- When involved in a difficult conversation, address the person involved calmly and directly in a "matter-of-fact" manner; state the problem clearly and objectively, and with respect for the person you are addressing. Ask that you be allowed to share your concern fully, without interruption, with the promise that you will listen to what the other person must say after that. Stay on point; be focused.
- The use of "I" statements is effective in preventing blame related to others during a difficult conversation. "I" statements allow you to be assertive in telling another how you feel without arousing the defenses of the other person. "I" statements allow you to say how it appears for you instead of telling others what they should or should not do.
- The use of critical language is a strategy that identifies agreed-upon communication signals (short phrases) within the culture of a specific interprofessional team to indicate the need to stop and communicate a significant care concern. An example of a critical language strategy is CUS. CUS stands for the following short phrases: "I'm *concerned,* I'm *uncomfortable,* this is *unsafe,* or I'm *scared.*"
- Team discussions and consensus have no place during an emergency; to avoid confusion, errors, and omissions the leader is the only one who gives directions and delegates to the team.
- Effective teams share a common purpose and intent, trust, respect, and collaboration; they value familiarity over formality and watch out for each other so that mistakes are not made.
- Concerns, problems, and issues related to performance should be handled quickly and at the lowest hierarchical level.

REFERENCES

Abraham, J., Kannampallil, T., & Patel, V. L. (2014). A systematic review of the literature on the evaluation of handoff tools: Implications for research and practice. *Journal of the American Medical Informatics Association,* 21(1), 154–162.

Adler, R., & Towne, N. (1978). *Looking out/looking in* (2nd ed.). New York: Holt, Rinehart, & Winston.

Agency for Healthcare Research and Quality (AHRQ). (n.d.). *Use the teach-back method tool #5. Health Literacy Universal Precautions Toolkit (2nd ed.).* Retrieved from https://www.ahrq.gov/professionals/ quality-patient-safety/quality-resources/tools/ literacy-toolkit/healthlittoolkit2-tool5.html.

American Speech-Language-Hearing Association (ASHA). (n.d.). *Accent modification.* Retrieved from http://www.asha.org/public/speech/development/ accent-modification/.

Arnold, E., & Boggs, K. (2016). *Interpersonal relationships: Professional communication skills for nurses* (7th ed.). St. Louis: Saunders Elsevier.

Beckman, H., & Frankel, R. (1984). The effect of physician behavior on the collection of data. *Annals of Internal Medicine,* 101(5), 692–696.

Bradley, G. L., & Campbell, A. C. (2016). Managing difficult workplace conversations: Goals, strategies, and outcomes. *International Journal of Business Communication,* 53(4), 443–464.

Brown, A., & Starkey, K. (1994). The effects of organizational culture on communication and information. *Journal of Management Studies,* 31, 807–828.

Buist, M. (2016). Patient-centered care: Just ask a thoughtful question and listen. *Joint Commission Journal on Quality and Patient Safety,* 42(6), 286–287.

Davis, B. J., & Brantley, C. P. (2005). *Listening: The forgotten skill. Communication for a global society.* Reston, VA: National Business Education Association.

Dufour, S. P., & Lucy, S. D. (2010). Situating primary health care within the International Classification of Functioning, Disability and Health: Enabling the Canadian Family Health Team Initiative. *Journal of Interprofessional Care,* 24(6), 666–677.

Halter, M. (2014). *Varcarolis' foundations of mental health nursing* (7th ed.). St. Louis: Saunders Elsevier.

Hershkovich, O., Gilad, D., Zimlichman, E., et al. (2016). Effective medical leadership in times of emergency: A perspective. *Disaster and Military Medicine,* 2(1), 4.

Hook, J. N., Davis, D. E., Owen, J., et al. (2013). Cultural humility: Measuring openness to culturally diverse clients. *Journal of Counseling Psychology, 60*(3), 353–366.

Hospice Education Network. (2013). *ELNEC core module 6: Communication-listening exercise.* Washington, DC: American Association of Colleges of Nursing.

Inclusive language. (n.d.). *Collins English Dictionary— Complete & Unabridged (10th ed.).* Retrieved from http://www.dictionary.com/browse/inclusive-language.

Interprofessional Education Collaborative Expert Panel (IPEC). (2011). *Core competencies for interprofessional collaborative practice: Report of an expert panel.* Washington, DC: Interprofessional Education Collaborative.

Interprofessional Education Collaborative Expert Panel (IPEC). (2016). *Core competencies for interprofessional collaborative practice: 2016 update.* Washington, DC: Interprofessional Education Collaborative.

Kersun, L., Gyi, L., & Morrison, W. E. (2009). Training in difficult conversations: A national survey of pediatric hematology–oncology and pediatric critical care physicians. *Journal of Palliative Medicine, 12*(6), 525–530.

Law Society of British Columbia. (n.d.). *Practice resource: Guideline for respectful language.* Retrieved from https://www.lawsociety.bc.ca/docs/practice/resources/Policy-Language1.pdf.

Leonard, M., Graham, S., & Bonacum, D. (2004). The human factor: The critical importance of effective teamwork and communication in providing safe care. *Quality and Safety in Health Care, 13*(Suppl. 1), i85–i90.

Nemeth, C. P. (Ed.). (2012). *Improving healthcare team communication: Building on lessons from aviation and aerospace.* Burlington, VT: Ashgate Publishing, Ltd.

O'Daniel, M., & Rosenstein, A. H. (2008). Professional communication and team collaboration. In R. G. Hughes (Ed.), *Patient safety and quality: An evidence-based handbook for nurses.* Rockville, MD: Agency for Healthcare Research and Quality. Retrieved from https://www.ncbi.nlm.nih.gov/books/NBK2681/.

Patterson, E. S., & Wears, R. L. (2010). Patient handoffs: Standardized and reliable measurement tools remain elusive. *Joint Commission Journal on Quality and Patient Safety, 36*(2), 52–61.

Polito, J. M. (2013). Effective communication during difficult conversations. *The Neurodiagnostic Journal, 53*(2), 142–152.

Popovich, D. (2011). 30-second head-to-toe tool in pediatric nursing: Cultivating safety in handoff communication. *Pediatric Nursing, 37*(2), 55.

Rhoades, D. R., McFarland, K. F., Finch, W. H., et al. (2001). Speaking and interruptions during primary care office visits. *Family Medicine, 33*(7), 528–532.

Spector, R. (2017). *Cultural diversity in health and illness.* New York: Pearson.

The Joint Commission. (2005). *The Joint Commission guide to improving staff communication.* Oakbrook Terrace, IL: Joint Commission Resources.

The Joint Commission. (2015). *Sentinel event data, 2004-3Q.* Retrieved from http://www.jointcommission.org/assets/1/18/General-Information_1995-3Q-2015.pdf.

Thistlethwaite, J. E. (2012). *Values-based interprofessional collaborative practice: Working together in health care.* Cambridge, UK: Cambridge University Press.

11

The Competency of Interprofessional Communication

LEARNING OUTCOMES

After studying this chapter, you will be able to:

1. Choose effective communication tools and techniques, including information systems and communication technologies, to facilitate discussions and interactions that enhance team function.

2. Communicate information with patients, families, community members, and health team members in a form that is understandable, avoiding discipline-specific terminology when possible.

3. Express your knowledge and opinions to team members involved in patient care and population health improvement with confidence, clarity, and respect, working to ensure common understanding of information, treatment, care decisions, and population health programs and policies.

4. Listen actively, and encourage ideas and opinions of other team members.

5. Give timely, sensitive, instructive feedback to others about their performance on the team, responding respectfully as a team member to feedback from others.

6. Use respectful language appropriate for a given difficult situation, crucial conversation, or interprofessional conflict.

7. Recognize how your own uniqueness (experience level, expertise, culture, power, and hierarchy within the health team) contributes to effective communication, conflict resolution, and positive interprofessional working relationships (University of Toronto, 2008, as cited in IPEC, 2016).

8. Communicate the importance of teamwork in patient-centered care and population health programs and policies.

This chapter will help you move beyond basic communication skills and focus on developing the higher competencies you will need for effective interprofessional communication. For true collaboration to occur, each member of the healthcare team must communicate clearly when planning care with other professionals, with patients and families, and with nonprofessionals and volunteers. Communication is also key when working within and between organizations in our communities to clearly identify who is responsible for essential aspects of care and to share the outcomes of that care. Conscious attention to the message that is communicated and how best to communicate it promotes strategic and clear interprofessional collaboration within the healthcare team. The Core Competency of Interprofessional Communication (IPEC, 2011; 2016) is explained and operationalized in this chapter.

After the presentation of the Interprofessional Communication Core Competency Statement and specific Sub-competencies, practice case studies and caselets are used to set the stage and illustrate each specific Competency or behavior. Not every possible profession or team member is involved in the provided patient care scenarios. Additional practice case studies are provided in Chapter 12. You are encouraged to apply each specific Sub-competency to examples in your own clinical practice and experience to determine any missed opportunities for Interprofessional Collaborative Practice that you may discover.

THE INTERPROFESSIONAL COMMUNICATION CORE COMPETENCY STATEMENT

Communicate with patients, families, communities, and professionals in health and other fields in a responsive and responsible manner that supports a team approach to the promotion and maintenance of health and the prevention and treatment of disease (IPEC, 2016, p. 10).

THE SUB-COMPETENCIES OF INTERPROFESSIONAL COMMUNICATION

Although basic and therapeutic communication skills are taught in some profession-specific educational environments, students in the healthcare professions often have little practical knowledge or actual experience with interprofessional communication (IPEC, 2011). The ability to appropriately share information within the healthcare team, with patients and families, and with those in wide-reaching networks involving the patient is essential for interprofessional collaboration.

Each patient care situation is unique. It is necessary to have a wide variety of well-developed communication strategies and skills that you can use as you collaborate with colleagues, patients, families, and other significant participants in the plan of care. Consider Case Study: The Case of Kendra Kea, Part 1. Mrs. Kea, a 38-year-old woman, was celebrating with friends and family at a local restaurant when she suddenly became symptomatic and a family member called 911. This case study presents what you may consider to be a "typical" chain of events. The discussions that follow are designed to help you identify areas where mastery of the Sub-competencies associated with Interprofessional Communication might have made a significant difference in Kendra's care.

Case Study: The Case of Kendra Kea, Part 1 demonstrates communication that is fragmented and not inclusive of everyone involved in this patient's care. Examples from this case study will be used several times within this chapter to explain and illustrate some of the Sub-competencies associated with the Interprofessional Communication Core Competency (Box 11.1).

> **BOX 11.1 Interprofessional Communication Sub-competencies (IPEC, 2016, p. 13)**
>
> CC1. Choose effective communication tools and techniques, including information systems and communication technologies, to facilitate discussions and interactions that enhance team function.
> CC2. Communicate information with patients, families, community members, and health team members in a form that is understandable, avoiding discipline-specific terminology when possible.
> CC3. Express one's knowledge and opinions to team members involved in patient care and population health improvement with confidence, clarity, and respect, working to ensure common understanding of information, treatment, care decisions, and population health programs and policies.
> CC4. Listen actively, and encourage ideas and opinions of other team members.
> CC5. Give timely, sensitive, instructive feedback to others about their performance on the team, responding respectfully as a team member to feedback from others.
> CC6. Use respectful language appropriate for a given difficult situation, crucial conversation, or conflict.
> CC7. Recognize how one's uniqueness (experience level, expertise, culture, power, and hierarchy within the health team) contributes to effective communication, conflict resolution, and positive interprofessional working relationships (University of Toronto, 2008).
> CC8. Communicate the importance of teamwork in patient-centered care and population health programs and policies.

CC1: Choose Effective Communication Tools and Techniques, Including Information Systems and Communication Technologies, to Facilitate Discussions and Interactions That Enhance Team Function

In all settings, critical information must be shared accurately. The care of just one patient requires interaction with many different team members who have varying levels of education and training; some may have no formal health-related education at all. For all team members, including nonprofessional members, this Sub-competency requires a conscious choice of the tools and techniques

CASE STUDY

The Case of Kendra Kea, Part 1

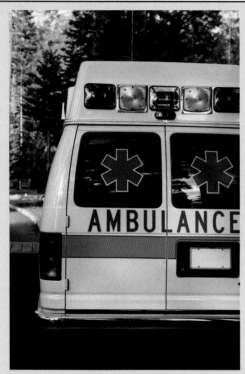

(Photo © Jupiterimages/PHOTOS.com/Thinkstock.)

Kendra Kea, her husband Clint, and their 4-year-old daughter, Karli, were celebrating the retirement of a favorite uncle with friends and family at a local restaurant when Mrs. Kea suddenly had some chest discomfort, became dizzy, and felt as if she might faint. She attempted to get up from the table, became weak, and was eased to the floor by her husband. Her sister called 911 and told the dispatcher that Mrs. Kea got weak and was going to "pass out." She shared information with the operator about Mrs.

Kea's age and state of consciousness and stated that Mrs. Kea was a "bad" diabetic. A paramedic unit was dispatched to the restaurant for a "diabetic emergency."

There was a flurry of activity as the first responders arrived at the restaurant and began their assessment protocol. This included obtaining vital signs and a blood sugar level, as well as initiating cardiac monitoring. The paramedics evaluated Mrs. Kea's level of consciousness and asked her to describe her symptoms and pain level. They determined that her blood sugar was within normal limits but recognized that her cardiac assessment indicated a possible myocardial infarction (heart attack). One of the emergency team members kept everyone away from Mrs. Kea by using hand motions and establishing a perimeter around her. There were hushed, hurried communications between the first responders that included "looks of urgency" as they prepared Mrs. Kea for transport. The paramedics informed Mrs. Kea that she was going to be transported to the hospital for further assessment. Throughout the assessment and interventions at the scene, there was no direct communication with Mrs. Kea's family members except to tell them nonverbally to "stay clear" of the assessment area.

On the way to the hospital emergency department (ED), the paramedic reported assessment data in SBAR format (see discussion in Chapter 10) to the nurse in medical command. The family followed the ambulance to the ED.

Discussion Questions

1. Who would you identify as key members of the interprofessional team in this situation?
2. What was communicated in this example and to whom? Include verbal and nonverbal communication.
3. Identify positive and negative aspects of the communication you identified.
4. How effective was the communication?

used to communicate essential information within the team. This Sub-competency requires you to take the time to consider the entire team and the needs of the individual members before you choose how to communicate. Interprofessional communication is a deliberate process that involves communicating clearly to all members of the team. You must attend to the entire communication process; always be aware of the listener's response to ensure that both your verbal and nonverbal communication was accurately understood.

It is important to look carefully at how we communicate with others in the patient care setting, recognizing our verbal and nonverbal communication styles. You are communicating with everyone around you by your mere presence. The goal of this Sub-competency is to communicate with all members of the team in a way that will meet their need for information and that will support optimal team functioning. In Case Study: The Case of Kendra Kea, Part 1, essential assessment data related to the patient's status were shared between Kendra's sister and the 911 operator, the 911 operator and the response team, the first responders at the scene—both verbally and nonverbally (e.g., gesturing to the crowd to stay clear of the assessment area)—and between the first responders and the emergency department (ED) nurse (e.g., using the SBAR format). The tools and technology chosen by the medical personnel to communicate with one another may seem appropriate; however, the tools and techniques used did not facilitate helpful discussion or interactions between the healthcare providers and the family members, who are also essential members of the team. What was communicated to the family verbally and nonverbally was that they should "stand back"; that they were peripheral to what was happening to the patient; and that they were not members of the team. The communication process probably created fear and anxiety for the family and possibly for Mrs. Kea herself (the patient). Even though this was an emergent situation, providing support and encouragement was important and could have decreased their emotional distress and enhanced team function; having a role in what is going on helps people have a sense of control and may serve as a distraction to decrease stress.

Information must be communicated objectively and clearly both verbally and electronically. Planning the communication requires thought and logical decision making; first, you need to determine the specific message that you intend to communicate and identify those team members who need the information. The method and content that you choose to use to communicate depends on the role of the team member with whom you intend to communicate and the feedback you need from them to work collaboratively. For example, in Case Study: The Case of Kendra Kea, Part 1, one message that needed to be communicated by the paramedic was related to the assessment of the patient's condition. This same message needed to be communicated to several different team members, but each team member needed to be considered separately. For example, because a diabetic emergency was ruled out and a more serious cardiac event was suspected, this information needed to be shared appropriately with each individual team member: the paramedic performing the assessment needed to communicate to the rest of the first response team that they must switch protocols from diabetic emergency to suspected cardiac event; the first responders needed to inform the family that their loved one needed to be transported to the hospital; and the paramedics needed to communicate

---

✳ ACTIVE LEARNING

Think about your last significant patient care encounter. What was the purpose of that encounter?

1. Did you seek out or facilitate interactions with other members of the team related to the care that was needed?
2. If you did, what communication tools and techniques were used?

    Did you take time to consider which communication methods were best or did you just act?

    Did these tools and techniques facilitate discussions and interactions within the team?

    Was team function enhanced?

    What was the outcome of that encounter?
3. If you did not facilitate any interactions with other members of the team, why not?
4. What was the outcome of that encounter?
5. Identify effective communication tools and techniques, including information systems and communication technologies, that could have been used to facilitate discussions and interactions that might have enhanced team function related to this patient's care.
6. Discuss this exercise with a peer and ask for feedback.

---

the status of the patient to the ED nurse at medical command so that her arrival was anticipated. A single situation required communication with different content, tone, and method for each team member.

Self-Evaluation of CC1

Choose effective communication tools and techniques, including information systems and communication technologies, to facilitate discussions and interactions that enhance team function.

1. Evaluate how well you meet this competency by doing the following:
    a. Think about a task in a clinical setting that you perform frequently and that involves more than one healthcare professional.
    b. Identify all the team members, including the patient, that you will need to communicate with to complete the task.
    c. Create a plan of action by identifying the appropriate and effective communication tools and techniques, for each member of the team, that will facilitate discussions and interactions to enhance team collaboration.

2. The next time that you engage in this patient care activity, activate your plan and evaluate the outcome.

When you can choose effective communication tools and techniques, including information systems and communication technologies, to facilitate discussions and interactions that enhance team function, you have demonstrated the CC1 Sub-competency.

CC2: Communicate Information With Patients, Families, Community Members, and Health Team Members in a Form That Is Understandable, Avoiding Discipline-Specific Terminology When Possible

Health care is complex and is addressed from many different professional perspectives. Each profession has its own discipline-specific terminology, or jargon, that is used and can be easily misunderstood or misinterpreted by others. Sub-competency CC2 requires that you avoid the use of all unnecessary discipline-specific terminology and jargon, which includes the use of abbreviations and special words or expressions that are used by one particular profession but that may be difficult for others (i.e., those not in that profession) to understand (Fig. 11.1). If you are unable to avoid the use of such words or phrases, they must be thoroughly and clearly explained. This Sub-competency may also require the team to be proactive and agree beforehand on the use of terminology

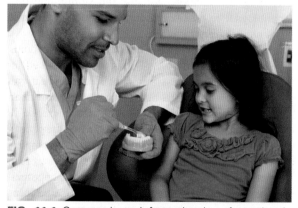

FIG. 11.1 Communicate information in a form that is understandable, and avoid discipline-specific terminology. (Photo © bowdenimages/iStock/Thinkstock.)

to prevent confusion and misunderstanding, especially during an emergency.

Information shared within the team should be simple, direct, and free of jargon. Caselet 11.1 illustrates a patient's misunderstanding of the common abbreviation that some healthcare providers use to indicate shortness of breath (SOB). Although this interaction may seem humorous at first, it could have caused significant damage to the provider–patient relationship. It is also possible that the distraction caused by this unintended use of a common abbreviation interfered with the flow of information and the quality of the information exchanged. The physician's assistant (PA) in this scenario did not explain the meaning of the accepted abbreviation (jargon), which left the issue unresolved.

One of the major problems associated with unclear communication between colleagues, and between medical professionals and patients and families, is that the recipient of the unclear message may not be comfortable asking for clarification. This often occurs because patients, and even colleagues, may be afraid to appear "dumb" or "less than" in the eyes of the professional.

Miscommunication related to the use of jargon can result in a wide variety of poor patient outcomes ranging from simple misunderstandings to fatal medical errors. To prevent such misunderstandings professionals must be aware of nonverbal feedback such as confused facial expressions or hesitancy during an information exchange. In addition to paying attention to nonverbal feedback, it is essential that you ask for verbal confirmation from your colleagues and your patients to ensure that your message has been received as intended. Seeking clear confirmation from colleagues that they understand is as important as using the teach-back method, described in Chapter 10, with patients and their families. It is equally important for you to ask for clarification from patients and colleagues if you are not clear on the message they intended to convey.

Self-Evaluation of CC2

Communicate information with patients, families, community members, and healthcare team members in a form that is understandable, avoiding discipline-specific terminology when possible.
1. Think about a routine patient care scenario in which you are frequently involved, one that requires avoiding discipline-specific terminology or jargon in the sharing of information with a patient, family member, or colleague from a different discipline.

CASELET 11.1 **What Did She Call Me?**

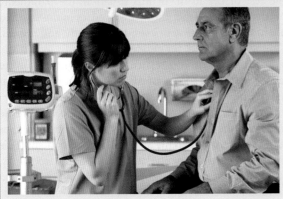

(Photo © monkeybusiness/iStock/Thinkstock.)

Mr. Walsh was visiting his primary care provider for treatment of an upper respiratory infection. While he was being assessed in the treatment room by the physician's assistant (PA) the following exchange occurred:

Exchange With Use of Jargon

PA: How are you feeling Mr. Walsh? How's your SOB?

Mr. Walsh: (confused and defensive) Who are you calling an SOB?

PA: Oh, I'm sorry. Your breathing. How's your breathing?

Mr. Walsh: Okay.

Exchange Without the Use of Jargon

PA: How are you feeling Mr. Walsh? How's your breathing been?

Mr. Walsh: It's not good when I get these coughing spells.

PA: Okay, I'm going to listen to your chest now and then we can talk about that.

Discussion Questions

1. Think about a recent exchange you have had with a colleague on your interprofessional team regarding an issue with a specific patient or a community project.
2. Make some notes about the discipline-specific terms or jargon used in that exchange.
3. Plan to share the outcome of your interaction with the patient or community group involved in the form of information sharing or patient teaching. Do not use any unnecessary discipline-specific terms or jargon.
4. How will you evaluate the recipient's understanding of your message?

2. Think about and plan the clearest and simplest way to communicate that information. Consider both your verbal and nonverbal communication in the plan.
3. Implement your plan the next time you are in that particular patient care situation.
4. Ask your patient, his or her family member, or a colleague to explain, in his or her own words, what you have just shared to make sure that you have clearly communicated the necessary information.

When your patient, his or her family member, or your colleague has clearly communicated back to you what you intended to communicate, you have demonstrated the use of the CC2 Sub-competency.

CC3: Express One's Knowledge and Opinions to Team Members Involved in Patient Care and Population Health Improvement With Confidence, Clarity, and Respect, Working to Ensure Common Understanding of Information and Treatment, Care Decisions, and Population Health Programs and Policies

The third communication Sub-competency (CC3) emphasizes how team members should communicate their knowledge and opinions within the interprofessional team. Emphasis is placed on three elements—confidence, clarity, and respect—as being necessary for ensuring common understanding of communications related to patient care and population health improvement. This Sub-competency suggests that members of the team must express their knowledge and opinions with confidence in their expertise, free of distractions, and with appreciation for each team member.

All members of the interprofessional collaborative team may have knowledge and opinions to share related to a given care situation. All members have the right and obligation to communicate pertinent information related to the patient care or population health situation in which they are involved. For example, in cases of disagreements within the team, each team member has the responsibility to express his or her expert knowledge and opinion. When disagreement occurs, it is especially important that the team member communicates with confidence, clarity, and respect so that his or her contribution can be heard by the rest of the team. Reestablishing team consensus is important so that patient outcomes are not

CASE STUDY

The Case of Kendra Kea, Part 2

Kendra Kea was transported by ambulance with continuous cardiac monitoring, a peripheral intravenous line, and nasal oxygen in place. En route, the paramedics continued to communicate to the emergency department (ED) staff regarding her vital signs, blood sugar level, and cardiac rhythm. Upon arrival in the ED, the ED staff quickly took over the patient care and transferred Kendra to a patient cubicle, where the ED resident on duty promptly examined her. Kendra was alert and expressed some mild chest discomfort. The resident reassured her that she was "in good hands" and, turning to the paramedic, who was still in the area, the resident said, "Thanks, we'll run some tests, but it looks like it's just gastric reflux." The paramedic was surprised because she was reasonably sure, based on her observations, that Kendra showed signs of a cardiac event. Furthermore, she thought that the assessment data that she provided supported this conclusion.

Discussion Questions

1. What barriers to communication do you identify within this team?
2. Reflect on the way that the resident presented his knowledge to the paramedic in terms of the three elements required by this Sub-competency: confidence, clarity, and respect.
3. Considering the same three elements (confidence, clarity, and respect):
   a. What action(s) should the paramedic take to contribute her knowledge and opinion related to the patient to the resident on the team?
   b. Give at least two options and the pros and cons of each.

compromised. Consider the event in Case Study: The Case of Kendra Kea, Part 2.

This example illustrates the traditional power imbalance within a healthcare team. By virtue of role alone, the physician (resident) is the traditional and actual leader of the team in this setting. Not only does the resident suggest a diagnosis based solely on his own assessment, but he first ignores, then verbally dismisses, the paramedic. The paramedic is a member of the interprofessional team involved in Mrs. Kea's care. Her paramedic education and her experience caring for Mrs. Kea give her the right and obligation to share her expert knowledge and

professional opinion related to Kendra's condition with the rest of the team. In this situation, the paramedic needed to assert the knowledge and opinion she had about Kendra's case with confidence, clarity, and respect. On the other hand, the resident confidently and clearly stated his supposition related to the diagnosis, but he lacked respect for the paramedic's knowledge and opinion as a member of the team.

The resident should have acknowledged the paramedic as part of the team and shown respect by requesting her input to contribute to the assessment of the patient. This exchange of assessment data, clearly and respectfully, would demonstrate this competency and would promote a common understanding of the treatment and care decisions within the team. Sub-competency CC3 demands movement away from a siloed, and sometimes "egotistical," approach to patient care and into a respectful and rich collaborative interprofessional approach that will enhance the professional practice of all team members while improving health outcomes for the patient or population.

Self-Evaluation of CC3

Express your knowledge and opinions to team members involved in patient care and population health improvement with confidence, clarity, and respect, working to ensure common understanding of information and treatment, care decisions, and population health programs and policies.

1. Think about a patient or population care situation in which you did not feel confident expressing your own knowledge or opinion.
   a. Try to identify a reason why you did not express your knowledge or opinion.
   b. Reflect on how you might have responded with confidence, clarity, and respect.
   c. Role play this situation with a peer.

When you have successfully demonstrated the ability to express your knowledge and opinions to team members involved in patient care and population health improvement with confidence, clarity, and respect, you have demonstrated the CC3 Sub-competency.

CC4: Listen Actively, and Encourage Ideas and Opinions of Other Team Members

Sub-competency CC4 emphasizes the importance of active listening as a necessary skill to practice collaboratively as well as in the creation of an environment conducive to the free expression of the ideas and opinions of all team members. Active listening is a communication tool that should not be underestimated. Recall from Chapter 10 that for you to actively listen you need to intentionally focus on who you are listening to and what he or she is trying to say. You must give the speaker your full attention and make a determined effort to understand what is being communicated to you without being judgmental or argumentative. Interrupting, by interjecting your own thoughts and opinions, is not a part of active listening. Instead, demonstrating behaviors that communicate your interest, openness, and understanding by using verbal and nonverbal cues is actively listening. It is important to recognize that this Sub-competency requires an environment in which ideas and opinions are encouraged. If the team has not created an environment that is welcoming of the ideas and opinions from all members, then the skill of active listening will not be useful. Consider Case Study: The Case of Kendra Kea, Part 3.

CASE STUDY

The Case of Kendra Kea, Part 3

In the emergency department (ED), after examining Mrs. Kea, the resident turned toward the paramedic and said, "Thanks, we'll run some tests, but it looks like it's just gastric reflux." The paramedic looked questioningly at the resident. The resident, responding to the paramedic's nonverbal response, said, "Oh, I'm sorry, let me slow down here and take a look at your assessment data while the nurse gets her settled in. Let's step outside for a minute and talk." To the patient, he said, "You are doing alright now and you're in good hands here. I'll be back in a few minutes to discuss a plan with you. I'll ask your husband to join us here too." Mrs. Kea thanked him, and the nurse reassured Mrs. Kea as she continued the admission assessment protocol.

Once outside the room, the resident asked the paramedic for her input, saying, "What is your assessment?" The paramedic summarized her assessment using the SBAR format, which included her recommendation to continue assessment of a cardiac event.

Discussion Questions
1. Identify the aspects of active listening that are presented in this excerpt from the case.
2. How do you think that resident's use of active listening skills contributed to Mrs. Kea's health outcomes?
3. What impact do you think this exchange had on Mrs. Kea?

This example illustrates the importance of using active listening in an environment that is receptive to the opinions of all team members. Because the resident respected and was focused on the paramedic's response as he was speaking to her, he could see the nonverbal response that his words elicited. He continued to demonstrate active listening skills through his use of an open-ended question and giving the paramedic his undivided attention as she responded. The patient's emotional needs were also considered and supported throughout the interaction. In this way, the process of interprofessional communication was supported and these team members could continue the assessment process in support of optimal patient outcomes.

Self-Evaluation of CC4

Listen actively, and encourage ideas and opinions of other team members.

1. This is a Sub-competency that is always in development. Make an effort to attend fully (actively listen) to all members of the team whom you come into contact with each day.
2. Critically reflect on each interaction during your day to evaluate your active listening skills.
   a. Were you able to give the interaction your full attention? If not, what were some obstacles you encountered?
   b. Can you identify ways that can help you improve your ability to listen actively?
   c. Were you able to encourage your team member to provide ideas and opinions related to the care situation?
3. Plan to improve your active listening skills during your next opportunity.
4. Implement your plan and reflect once more using a, b, and c.

When you are able to consistently practice this reflective process in your clinical practice, you are demonstrating an awareness of the importance of the CC4 Sub-competency.

CC5: Give Timely, Sensitive, Instructive Feedback to Others About Their Performance on the Team, Responding Respectfully as a Team Member to Feedback from Others

During your routine practice "day," you probably observe many issues and challenges with patients, colleagues, or other team members that need to be addressed. What do you generally do about those issues? For example, have you ever watched someone beginning an element of patient care without washing his or her hands? What did you do? Did you let the person proceed without any comment from you? It is not unusual for healthcare professionals to ignore such incidents because they are uncomfortable and do not know how to intervene; however, this problem can be addressed by having a plan in place. Sub-competency CC5, though it sounds simple, is not easy to practice. The first part of the Sub-competency requires that you give timely, sensitive, and instructive feedback to others when you have a reason to do so. *Timely* often means immediate, and *sensitive* means with tact, caring, and respect. *Instructive* means that the feedback has to lead to a solution to the problem. The second part of this Sub-competency, responding respectfully as a team member to feedback from others, requires, first, that all feedback be respectfully and objectively given to individual team members within the context of interprofessional collaboration. In response, each team member is expected to consider the feedback objectively and respond appropriately and respectfully (Fig. 11.2).

The *timely and sensitive* part of this Sub-competency requires that you be prepared to have what might be a difficult conversation, whenever necessary. As a member of the healthcare team, your goal is to provide high-level care that is safe and efficient. If you believe that care is being compromised by the actions or omissions of others, you have a responsibility to provide immediate and

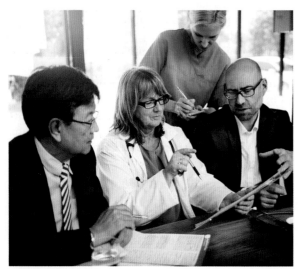

FIG. 11.2 Planning to provide performance feedback. (© Rawpixel Ltd/iStock/Thinkstock.)

objective feedback (instructive), always with the intention of correcting the problem observed. This Sub-competency requires practice and experience, as well as moral courage. It requires respect and understanding. Refer to Chapter 10 to review the material related to having a difficult conversation.

The second part of Sub-competency CC5 refers to the feedback you may receive from others related to your own performance on the team. This Sub-competency requires openness on your part and a degree of humility. It requires that you pause and actively listen to what is being communicated to you by others. Use self-reflection to fully and honestly consider and interpret the feedback you receive and then respond respectfully. Mutual respect is important in such interactions because that allows the interaction to continue in a positive direction toward optimal patient or population outcomes.

The ground rules for practicing this Sub-competency should be discussed and agreed upon within the interprofessional team. A collaborative team that is performing optimally will have in place a plan to address these kinds of situations. It is best to adopt a nonpunitive approach with the intention of correcting the problem in the name of providing optimal care for the patient or population. Trying to avoid hurting people's feelings will not solve the problem and will interfere with the performance of the team in this Sub-competency. Consider Case Study: Mrs. Martino's Confusion, Part 1, which features an interaction in an ED setting.

This case study illustrates a clear need for immediate (timely), sensitive, and instructive communication to the registered nurse and other team members. The continued absence of interprofessional collaboration in this situation would lead to the application of patient restraint with a subsequent negative impact on overall patient outcomes. To promote safe and effective care, the first nurse needed to advocate for this patient and interrupt the restraint. It is important for the nurse to share her own perspective and professional opinion in a way that will inform her colleagues of the situation and elicit their input in formulating a safe plan of care that will support positive patient outcomes. Now consider Case Study: Mrs. Martino's Confusion, Part 2.

Once the crisis was stabilized, Maria, the first nurse, took the opportunity to respectfully discuss her concerns with her teammate. They collaborated to identify the problem and develop a safe plan of care for Mrs. Martino. The interaction resulted in helping the second nurse to

CASE STUDY

Mrs. Martino's Confusion, Part 1

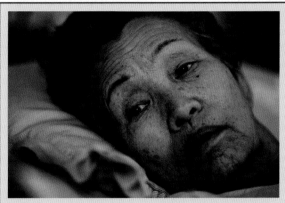

(Photo © bee32/iStock/Thinkstock.)

Mrs. Rose Martino is an 81-year-old woman with a history of Alzheimer's disease. At home, with environmental adaptation and close supervision by her daughter and son-in-law, she is safe, cooperative, and content. Her daughter became concerned about Mrs. Martino's persistent temperature elevation, worsening cough, and increasing periods of agitation and restlessness and called Mrs. Martino's primary care provider. She was instructed by the primary care provider to take her mother to the emergency department (ED) for treatment. The ED physician who saw Mrs. Martino diagnosed her as having pneumonia and decided to admit her; he ordered further diagnostic studies, intravenous (IV) antibiotics, and intensive respiratory therapy treatments. Mrs. Martino's daughter was sent to the admissions office to complete the necessary paperwork.

In the ED, Mrs. Martino appears frightened and agitated. She does not know where she is and is calling for her daughter. A registered nurse, a nursing assistant, and a laboratory technician, who just completed drawing blood, are present as another nurse hurriedly enters to insert a peripheral IV line. The second nurse goes directly to Mrs. Martino and, tourniquet in hand, reaches for her left arm. Mrs. Martino pulls her arm away and begins to shout loudly, "No, no, stop, get away!" The second nurse turns to the nursing assistant and says, "I'm going to need some help here. Can one of you hold her arm for me so I can get this IV started? We're going to need to restrain this one."

You (the original nurse) realize that Mrs. Martino's confusion is probably being exacerbated by the physical environment of the ED with its unfamiliar harsh lighting, high noise level, and unfamiliar people. Further, the absence of Mrs. Martino's daughter to provide support makes any intrusive touching and prodding from staff members a frightening experience for her. You are concerned that if any form of restraint is used, it will negatively affect Mrs. Martino. This situation is not safe for the patient or the staff. It is your responsibility to advocate for this patient.

Discussion Questions
1. Outline the feedback that you would give to the team members present to prevent the situation from escalating and adversely affecting Mrs. Martino.
2. When would you provide the feedback?
3. How would you communicate your feedback to the individual members of the team?
4. What response do you expect from the team members?
5. If your feedback is not respectfully received, how would you respond to support positive patient outcomes?

identify more positive nursing interventions to be implemented in similar situations in the future.

Self-Evaluation of CC5

Give timely, sensitive, instructive feedback to others about their performance on the team, responding respectfully as a team member to feedback from others.
1. Identify a potential incident that may occur in your own practice that may require you to give timely, sensitive, instructive feedback to others about their performance.
   a. Reflect on how you might prepare to give that feedback to your colleague in a way that is prompt and respectful.
   b. Anticipate the response that you might receive from your colleague about your feedback.
2. Reflect on past responses to feedback you have received from others related to your team performance.
   a. What was your response on hearing this feedback? What did you think? What did you do?
   b. Was it respectful? If it was not respectful, reflect on how you might have responded differently.

When you are able to give timely, sensitive, instructive feedback to others about their performance on the team and respond respectfully as a team member to feedback from others, you have demonstrated the CC5 Sub-competency.

CASE STUDY

Mrs. Martino's Confusion, Part 2

The scenario continues after the nurse exclaims, "I'm going to need some help here. Can one of you hold her arm for me so I can get this IV started? We're going to need to restrain this one."

The first nurse was concerned that if any form of restraint was used now, Mrs. Martino would probably become more frightened and agitated. She knew she had a responsibility to intervene immediately. She first acknowledged the second nurse's concern nonverbally, with a slight shake of her head, a smile, and a casual gesture intended to ask the nurse to stop her actions and "wait a minute." Next, she calmly and slowly moved closer to Mrs. Martino. She addressed her directly, saying softly but loud enough to be heard, "Hello Mrs. Martino, I'm your nurse. My name is Maria, I'm going to take care of you." Mrs. Martino focused on Maria's face and visibly calmed. Next, Maria looked at the second nurse and quietly said, "Let's try this again." Her colleague responded, "Okay." The nurse calmly introduced the nursing assistant to Mrs. Martino, asking the two of them to spend some quiet time together. She then dimmed the overhead light and quietly left the room with the other nurse to discuss the situation and plan for the intravenous (IV) line insertion.

Discussion Questions

1. What forms of communication did Maria use to deescalate the situation?
2. What feedback do you think Maria should give to her colleague once they leave the room?
3. What should be the second nurse's response to Maria's concern?

CC6: Use Respectful Language Appropriate for a Given Difficult Situation, Crucial Conversation, or Interprofessional Conflict

How we use language affects others. Sub-competency CC6 is specific in requiring that you use respectful language when involved in difficult situations, crucial conversations, and interprofessional conflicts. The intent of this Sub-competency is to create an atmosphere that supports communication in difficult situations by avoiding language that shuts down or impairs communication. Furthermore, CC6 requires team members to use communication that facilitates problem solving and supports positive patient and population outcomes. Healthcare professionals are expected to demonstrate effective communication by using language that respects the strengths, skills, talents, and individuality of all. This respect extends to all professionals, patients and families, nonprofessionals and volunteers, organizations, and communities. Refer to Chapter 10 to review content related to having a difficult conversation and to the basic components of respectful communication.

Respect is conveyed verbally and nonverbally. Regardless of patient or population health focus, all of our behaviors should confirm that we are on the same team and share the same goals. Trust is essential in all relationships. How we greet and address each other is crucial in setting the stage for a respectful relationship. Our interactions must demonstrate respect for each other's autonomy in decision making and the assertion of different opinions and points of view and a desire to avoid conflict or quickly resolve one that is apparent. Ensuring privacy, using active listening skills, providing necessary information honestly, being objective, and controlling facial expression and body language during challenging interactions are crucial.

The situation in Caselet 11.2 requires a crucial and difficult conversation for the healthcare professional and the patient. Camila Perez, the patient, is expressing uncertainty related to her surgery. You should explore this nonjudgmentally with a prompt such as: "You seem unsure about the surgeon who is doing your surgery." After listening carefully and empathetically to her response, you need to determine whether she is no longer sure about having the surgery. It is not your responsibility to "convince" a patient to have the surgery or to defend the reputation of the surgeon in question. It might be useful to ask the patient if she would like to see the surgeon to discuss the surgery and her questions. You could offer to be present for support. It is your responsibility to advocate for the patient and support her autonomy in making an informed decision. If it is clear that the patient is unsure, the surgeon who obtained the informed consent from the patient for the procedure should be consulted and informed respectfully about that uncertainty. This proposed communication between you and the surgeon is representative of what also may be seen as a difficult conversation and may result in the need for conflict resolution. Refer to Chapter 10 for additional guidelines related to the use of respectful language and how to approach a difficult conversation.

CASELET 11.2 Camila Perez

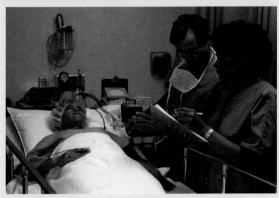

(Photo © Purestock/Thinkstock.)

Camila Perez is a 36-year-old single woman scheduled for a hysterectomy because of severe uterine fibroid tumors. Her operative consent form was signed, and she is being prepped for surgery. During the process, Ms. Perez seemed a little anxious, but you did not find that unusual. As you established rapport and attempted to make her more comfortable, Ms. Perez told you that she heard some rumors about her surgeon, specifically that she heard he has a bad surgical record in performing hysterectomies. She asks you if you heard anything like that about the surgeon. You did not hear anything specific about this surgeon's outcomes with hysterectomies.

Discussion Questions
1. How would you respond to this patient?
2. Knowing that the patient will be receiving her preoperative medication soon, what are your concerns?
3. Besides the patient, who else on the interprofessional team should you communicate with?

Self-Evaluation of CC6

Use respectful language appropriate for a given difficult situation, crucial conversation, or interprofessional conflict.

1. Read the caselet involving Camila Perez and the discussion that followed. Prepare yourself for contacting the surgeon.
2. When will you contact the surgeon? What mode of communication will you use?
3. Role play your conversation with the surgeon with one of your peers playing the role of the busy surgeon just hours before the scheduled surgery.
4. In the role play, demonstrate timely, sensitive, and respectful communication.

When you are able to use respectful language appropriate for a given difficult situation, crucial conversation, or interprofessional conflict, you have demonstrated an understanding of the CC6 Sub-competency.

CC7: Recognize How One's Own Uniqueness, Including Experience Level, Expertise, Culture, Power, and Hierarchy Within the Healthcare Team, Contributes to Effective Communication, Conflict Resolution, and Positive Interprofessional Working Relationships

Each of us is unique. It is not only our professional roles that provide us with unique perspectives on care; we each possess other unique perspectives that stem from our level of experience in like situations, our real or perceived power within the team, our individual religious and cultural beliefs, and other unique life experiences. It is important for each team member to recognize and value his or her own uniqueness because it is the uniqueness that each person brings to the team that provides a rich source of options for problem solving and care planning. To make the best use of this resource, a receptive atmosphere needs to exist within the team. All team members should know they are expected to clearly communicate their own unique perspectives in relation to specific care issues. Team members should listen carefully and not interrupt during this process as they carefully consider how the shared perspective might contribute to the collaboration. A respectful and open forum is essential to allow all aspects of an issue to be illuminated, discussed, and considered. Team collaboration provides a forum in which we share our uniqueness with other team members as we contribute to optimal care solutions and outcomes. The patient situation in Caselet 11.3 requires the team to demonstrate receptiveness to a unique contribution from a team member.

In Caselet 11.3, the rehabilitation team was pondering a patient care problem. Mr. Patel was doing well in physical therapy, yet he seemed resistive to the efforts of the occupational therapist and the nurse to assist him in making progress toward his own self-care and independence. The occupational therapist was not able to form a positive care relationship with Mr. Patel, and to complicate the problem, Mr. Patel's family was participating in his care in ways that fostered his dependence on them rather than his own independence, in direct opposition to the rehabilitation team's plan.

CASELET 11.3   Respect for Father

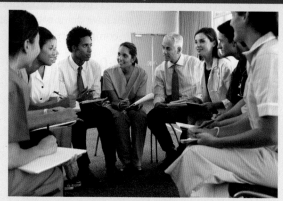

(Photo © bowdenimages/iStock/Thinkstock.)

Veer and Fátima Patel are a middle-aged professional couple who have been in the United States since 1983. In 2010 the couple and their extended family decided to permanently relocate Veer's father, Raj Patel, from his native India to the United States after the death of his wife (Veer's mother). Mr. Patel is now 82 years old and is a patient on a rehabilitation unit after a cerebrovascular accident, or stroke.

After his third day on the unit, the rehabilitation team meets to discuss Mr. Patel's uneven progress. The occupational therapist reports that Mr. Patel is not making much progress in self-feeding or dressing. She says she is puzzled because Mr. Patel seems resistant to everything she has tried; in fact she reported that he will barely look at her or speak to her. The physical therapist on the team reports

that Mr. Patel is showing expected progress in physical therapy. He also shares that they communicate and work well together. He asks the nurse how Mr. Patel is doing from a nursing perspective. The nurse on the team says that Mr. Patel is pleasant and usually cooperative with the unit routine but that she too has had some resistance when encouraging him to be more independent in caring for himself. The social worker asks if there has been any family involvement in his care; the nurse says, "Oh yes, more than enough. Now that I think about it, I wonder if his daughter-in-law isn't the problem. She really babies him; in fact, his whole family does." The nursing assistant, who has an Indian cultural background, says, "You know, Mr. Patel reminds me of my own grandfather who is a devout Hindu with strong spiritual and family beliefs. I think I know what the problem might be." The nurse says, "Great, what can you tell us that might help us work better with him and his family?" The team listens to the nursing assistant share and explain his perspective.

Discussion Questions

1. Why do you think that the team was not getting positive results when working with Mr. Patel?
2. What uniqueness did the nursing assistant bring to the team to help them understand the patient care problem?
3. The nursing assistant recognized his own "uniqueness" in this scenario. What positive elements of interprofessional team collaboration dynamics made it possible for this team member to contribute so effectively to the collaboration process?

This caselet suggested a lack of cultural understanding on the part of some team members rather than a lack of role expertise. In this example the team was dynamic, inclusive, and receptive to all team members' perspectives on the care of Mr. Patel. In this case the nursing assistant, who had the least formal education and the lowest "power" position in the team hierarchy, was the one with the cultural competence most needed by the team. His "uniqueness" rested in his knowledge of the patient's cultural background and his perspective was welcomed by the team.

The nursing assistant emphasized the importance of involving family members, along with Mr. Patel, in all aspects of his care planning. He explained that in the Indian culture the family unit is expected to be the first source of support. He further explained that direct eye contact with older family members is often considered

a sign of disrespect in the Indian culture; Mr. Patel is the family elder, and deference to him is expected. He explained that in communicating with Mr. Patel about his care planning and progress, the professionals should ask direct questions and provide concrete information because Indians expect professionals to be experts. He suggested that the team members use empathetic listening to help them be supportive of Mr. Patel and his family. The physical therapist said, "That's interesting because that's pretty much what has worked for me with him, now I know why." The occupational therapist said, "I see now that I have been communicating only with Mr. Patel and not with his family. I need to include his family in his care. Not communicating with all of them together was interfering with him getting the maximum benefit and must have been confusing for all of them. I see how he might have thought that I was pushing his family away from him at a time when he needs them so much!" The team's receptiveness to the contribution of the nursing assistant on the team benefited the patient and contributed to building the team's overall level of cultural competence.

Recognizing your own uniqueness and the contributions that you can make to improving outcomes of care is important. It is equally important that you are able to recognize the uniqueness of other team members. Being open to, and respectful of, the perspectives of all team members will provide you with valuable information for use throughout your career.

Self-Evaluation of CC7

Recognize how one's own uniqueness, including experience level, expertise, culture, power, and hierarchy within the healthcare team, contributes to effective communication, conflict resolution, and positive interprofessional working relationships.

1. What are your own areas of professional and personal "uniqueness"?
2. Can you identify any situations in which team-related communication resulting from any area of your "uniqueness" has contributed to improved patient outcomes, or to the resolution of a problem or a conflict?
3. Reflect on the value of your unique contribution to the outcome.

When you are able to recognize how your own uniqueness, including experience level, expertise, culture, power, and hierarchy within the healthcare team, contributes to effective communication, you have demonstrated an understanding of the CC7 Sub-competency.

CC8: Communicate the Importance of Teamwork in Patient-Centered and Population Health Programs and Policies

The existence of an identified patient or population-centered problem or need often spurs program and policy development in healthcare settings and in our communities. Bringing the representative voices of all stakeholders together to clearly articulate and understand the need should be an expected early step in planning to meet the need. Consider Caselet 11.4.

Clear, open communication and a comprehensive team made up of all stakeholders is essential in planning and implementing programs and policies. The example used here may appear simple at first, but it is complex. The problem, or issue, clearly involves a health

recommendation based on epidemiologic studies: that higher intake of added sugar is associated with cardiovascular disease risk factors (Yang et al., 2014). However, there are many other issues, including ethical considerations, such as individual freedom to choose what to drink, and financial concerns, such as loss of profit or income from the sale of sweetened drinks. Solving the problem will require all of the stakeholders to be represented; these may include representatives from many different hospital divisions, vendors who sell to or within the hospital, patients, volunteers, and employees. Most general patient and population problems can be classified as system problems because they affect many different aspects of an organization or community at many different levels. To develop effective policies and programs, the perspective of all stakeholders is essential. Difficult conversations will occur and issues will arise that require open and fair negotiation and compromise. A collaborative team effort is a powerful force in producing seamless and effective policy and program implementation and outcomes (Fig. 11.3).

Self-Evaluation of CC8

Communicate the importance of teamwork in patient-centered care and population health programs and policies.

1. Identify one patient- or population-centered problem that you are aware of.
2. Why is teamwork important in resolving the problem?
3. Suggest the composition of a collaborative team that could work to solve the problem through the development of a project or policy.
4. Discuss your rationale with a colleague.

When you are able to communicate the importance of teamwork in patient-centered care and population health programs and policies, you have demonstrated an understanding of the CC8 Sub-competency.

Demonstrating the Sub-competencies of Interpersonal Communication

Exemplar Case Study: Removing Sweet Soft Drinks From the Hospital Center demonstrates the application of the Sub-competencies of Interprofessional Communication in the provision of optimal interprofessional collaborative care. The presence of specific Sub-competencies is indicated throughout the exemplar case study.

The interactions described in the exemplar case study provide positive examples of using the Sub-competencies of Interprofessional Communication in team collaboration

CASELET 11.4   Banning Sweetened Drinks

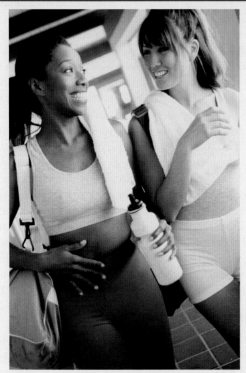

(Photo © Ingram Publishing/Thinkstock.)

A group of healthcare professionals regularly use the medical center's fitness facility after work. One afternoon, after their workout, they gathered at the juice bar. Looking at the menu, Rob said, "I can't believe that they still have sweetened drinks, energy drinks, and even soda here. It makes no sense to me. This is a 'fitness center,' and we know these sweetened drinks aren't part of anyone's fitness plan." Beth said, "You know I've been thinking a lot about that very same thing, but I was thinking about it throughout the medical center itself. Here I am, teaching patients about healthy diets and all of the negative health effects that added sugar can bring, and sugary drinks and snacks are for sale everywhere in the building. I think it's a problem when we tell patients and families to avoid all that stuff and then we sell it to them!" Jim says, "You're right, it is a problem." Meg says, "Hey, let's do something about it." They all look at Meg. Jim says, "Us? What do you have in mind?" Meg says, "Well, we can't do it ourselves, it is going to take a team effort to make this happen. Let's put together a team of the right people throughout the medical center to make this change happen!"

Discussion Questions

1. This group of health-conscious colleagues is thinking about how to have sugary drinks removed from the hospital environment.
   a. Identify those who would benefit from this plan and how they will benefit from it.
   b. Identify those who may oppose this plan and why they would oppose it.
2. Who should they invite to join them in collaborating about this project?

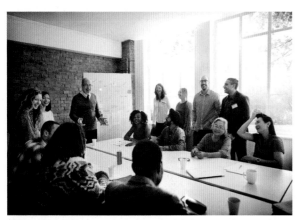

FIG. 11.3 Teamwork is essential in creating patient-centered care and population health programs and policies. (© Rawpixel Ltd/iStock/Thinkstock.)

toward the development of a healthcare system policy. The application of these Sub-competencies as a matter of routine provides us with a roadmap for clear, complete, open, and respectful team communication. There will be difficult conversations along the journey, but expecting conflicts and problems and being open to listening to the perspectives of others are essential to resolution. Mastering these Sub-competencies requires continuous practice and self-reflection for all healthcare providers. The key to success in achieving goal-directed patient and population outcomes is to maintain clear and respectful communication in all collaborations. Never lose sight of the value of your own uniqueness and that of your colleagues and patients because it is from these unique perspectives that team understanding is born.

◎ **EXEMPLAR CASE STUDY**

Removing Sweet Soft Drinks From the Hospital Center

A group of healthcare professionals employed at a comprehensive community medical center shared the values of health promotion and disease prevention. The mission of the medical center was consistent with these values. The group identified that selling sugar-added and high-fructose beverages on the medical center campus was not consistent with health promotion. They decided to spearhead an effort to remove these beverages from every coffee shop, cafeteria, snack cart, and vending machine on the medical center campus and replace them with healthier options. They knew that this ambitious project would require the cooperation and joint effort from many stakeholders within and outside of the medical center [CC8]. Their initial brainstorming session focused on how best to communicate their intention to potential project team members [CC1, CC3]. They needed to enlist the participation of all of those who would be affected by this potential change in policy. They decided to compile a database with the names and contact information of key individuals and approach them with a brief email to introduce the project. Next, they planned to contact these key people by email to arrange an initial meeting with them or their designee to see if they had any questions or concerns [CC1]. They planned to design and produce an electronic information packet and a simple flyer that would clearly provide the message and evidence related to the health issue [CC1, CC2]. Before the initial meeting, the information packet would be sent electronically to prospective team members. At their initial meetings with key individuals, they would offer additional information and education; seek out the attendees' unique perspectives related to the project, including any predicted obstacles to success; answer questions; and ask for their commitment of participation on the planning team [CC2, CC3, CC4, CC5, CC6, CC7]. To conclude the meeting, they would invite referrals to others who should be contacted to participate in the effort [CC4, CC7, CC8]. Informational flyers for distribution would be made available to those interested in distributing them [CC1, CC2].

As meetings progressed, support grew for the project. The project team now consisted of varied representation; for example, there were representatives from the divisions of administration, finance, medicine, dentistry, nursing and all clinical specialties, dietary services, laboratory and other diagnostic services, housekeeping, maintenance, and volunteer services. However, there were two main concerns. The first area of concern came from administration and finance; it concerned the long-time soft drink vendor who had established a positive working relationship with the institution. They were concerned about how this proposed change might negatively affect that working relationship and that company. The second area of concern came from employees who were accustomed to purchasing sugar-added drinks from the vending machines and the cafeteria during their lunch hour and breaks. They insisted that they had the right to make a choice related to the beverages they would drink [CC6].

In response, the team decided to invite representatives from the soft drink vendor to meet with them to explore how they might work together toward a positive solution for all. The invitation was extended by the hospital's liaison to that company, and a meeting with select team members followed [CC6, CC7, CC8]. The meeting was an informational and collaborative experience in which all participants shared their unique perspectives related to the proposed project. The team clearly explained the health risks associated with sugary soft drinks and juices; they also shared concerns related to the continued working relationship with the vendor and of employees and visitors who objected to the change in product availability [CC6]. Together they explored solutions. The vendor offered other options for the vending machines; for example, water, zero-calorie, and low-calorie options could replace the sugar-added products. These same products and a variety of others could be offered in the coffee shops and cafeterias. The vendor expressed his thanks for being included in the project. He acknowledged that although his sales may drop initially, he believed that working together they could provide healthy options and meet customer needs [CC4, CC7, CC8].

An invitation to an open forum was extended to all hospital employees, staff, and those who had practice privileges at the hospital center. Press releases were prepared by the medical center's public relations staff inviting members of the community to attend; posters throughout the medical center invited interested patients and visitors to join in as well [CC1, CC2, CC3, CC8]. The team worked with the partnering vendor to provide an assortment of non–sugar-added beverages and healthy snack options for those who attended. Informational packets were distributed. An open forum was used to provide information, hear concerns, and answer questions. The project team acknowledged

Continued

◎ **EXEMPLAR CASE STUDY**

Removing Sweet Soft Drinks From the Hospital Center—cont'd

the right of the employees and others to free choice and specifically the right to drink their choice of beverage while in the hospital setting. It was agreed that those who wanted to drink those products that will no longer be available could do so by bringing them in from home [CC5]. The audience acknowledged that it did not make sense for healthcare professionals to encourage patients to cut back on sweetened beverages while the hospital continued to sell those same drinks [CC4, CC6]. Some audience members commented positively about the drink options offered at the meeting. One man, in particular, said, "I never tried these flavored seltzers before. I think they could grow on me; no calories and healthy, too. Not bad" [CC5].

▮ KEY POINTS

- The ability to appropriately share information within the healthcare team, with patients and families, and with those in wide-reaching networks involving the patient is essential for interprofessional collaboration.
- You are communicating with everyone in the patient's proximity by your mere presence. Be constantly aware of what you are communicating both verbally and nonverbally to all members of the team, including colleagues, the patient, and others involved in the care.
- Interprofessional communication is a deliberate process that involves communicating clearly to all members of the team. Attend to the entire communication process; be aware of the listener's response to ensure that both your verbal and nonverbal communication is accurately understood.
- Avoid the use of unnecessary discipline-specific terminology and jargon, including the use of abbreviations, special words, or expressions used by your particular profession that may be difficult for others to understand.
- Use respectful language.
- Give timely, sensitive, and instructive feedback to others when you have a reason to do so.

- Be open to feedback that you might receive from others related to your own performance on the team. Receiving constructive feedback requires openness and a degree of humility. It requires that you pause and actively listen to what is being communicated to you by others. Use self-reflection as you consider and interpret the feedback you received and then respond respectfully.
- Use active listening. Give the speaker your full attention and make a determined effort to understand what is being communicated without being judgmental or argumentative. Interrupting, by interjecting your own thoughts and opinions, is not a part of active listening; demonstrate behaviors that communicate your interest, openness, and understanding by using verbal and nonverbal cues.
- Recognize your own uniqueness and be open to the uniqueness of the patient, community, and others involved in the team collaboration.
- Effective patient care, as well as policy and program development, requires clear and respectful team communication among all stakeholders.

REFERENCES

Interprofessional Education Collaborative Expert Panel (IPEC) (2011). *Core competencies for interprofessional collaborative practice: Report of an expert panel.* Washington, DC: Interprofessional Education Collaborative.

Interprofessional Education Collaborative Expert Panel (IPEC) (2016). *Core competencies for interprofessional collaborative practice: 2016 update.* Washington, DC: Interprofessional Education Collaborative.

University of Toronto (2008). *Advancing the interprofessional education curriculum.* Toronto. Canada: University of Toronto.

Yang, Q., Zhang, Z., Gregg, E., et al. (2014). Added sugar intake and cardiovascular diseases mortality among US adults. *JAMA Internal Medicine, 174*(4), 516–524.

12

Interprofessional Communication Case Studies

LEARNING OUTCOMES

After successfully working through the case studies in this chapter, you will be able to:

1. Apply the Interprofessional Communication Sub-competencies to problem-based case studies.
2. Operationalize the behaviors of Interprofessional Communication through case study application.

3. Demonstrate an understanding of the Sub-competencies of Interprofessional Communication through case study discussions.
4. Identify the importance of Interprofessional Collaboration as it applies to each case.

This chapter provides specially designed patient- and population-based case studies to provide practice opportunities related to the Core Competency of Interprofessional Communication (IPEC, 2011; 2016). Case studies are intended for use in group discussions or debates, as role playing exercises, or as individual learning exercises. The authors acknowledge that all four Core Competencies may apply in each case; however, learning in this chapter is purposefully focused on Interprofessional Communication Sub-competencies. Carefully crafted discussion questions will provide direction for learners and faculty facilitators.

CASE STUDY ACTIVITY GUIDELINES

For each case study, you will be directed to consider and apply specific Sub-competencies of Interprofessional Communication. These will be clearly indicated to you before you begin to read the case study. The Sub-competencies of Interprofessional Communication are provided for your reference in Box 12.1.

Case studies can be used as individual problem-based learning activities or incorporated as part of a variety of group learning activities. You can independently determine how each case study will be used after considering your specific learning needs and educational setting. Basic discussion questions and/or suggested learning activities

are provided after each case study. You are encouraged to modify these questions and activities, or to pose your own, to meet specific learning needs. Chapter 10 of this text provides foundational theory related to Interprofessional Communication and its Sub-competencies; Chapter 11 provides examples to help readers operationalize specific Sub-competencies; both chapters will be useful in considering the case studies that follow.

CASE STUDY: COMMUNICATING ACCURATE INFORMATION IN A CARE SITUATION

Specific Sub-competency to consider and apply: CC1.

You are a new nurse working on a cardiac step-down unit. Eva Schmidt is a 76-year-old patient who was admitted 4 days ago with a diagnosis of congestive heart failure. She was transferred to your step-down unit from the cardiac intensive care unit (CICU). This is your first day working with her and her second day on the unit. Mrs. Schmidt mentions to you how much better she is feeling since she is finally getting some "good food." She tells you the food on your unit is great compared with the "cardboard" tasting food in CICU. She describes the breakfast that she had this morning (scrambled eggs with ham and cheese) and last night's "delicious" dinner. You

---

BOX 12.1   Interprofessional Communication Core Competency and Related Sub-competencies (IPEC, 2016, p. 13)

Statement: General Core Competency of Interprofessional Communication
Communicate with patients, families, communities, and professionals in health and other fields in a responsive and responsible manner that supports a team approach to the maintenance of health and the treatment of disease.

The Specific Sub-competencies of Interprofessional Communication
CC1. Choose effective communication tools and techniques, including information systems and communication technologies, to facilitate discussions and interactions that enhance team function.
CC2. Communicate information with patients, families, community members, and health team members in a form that is understandable, avoiding discipline-specific terminology when possible.
CC3. Express one's knowledge and opinions to team members involved in patient care and population health improvement with confidence, clarity, and respect,

working to ensure common understanding of information, treatment, care decisions, and population health programs and policies.
CC4. Listen actively, and encourage ideas and opinions of other team members.
CC5. Give timely, sensitive, instructive feedback to others about their performance on the team, responding respectfully as a team member to feedback from others.
CC6. Use respectful language appropriate for a given difficult situation, crucial conversation, or conflict.
CC7. Recognize how one's uniqueness (experience level, expertise, culture, power, and hierarchy within the health team) contributes to effective communication, conflict resolution, and positive interprofessional working relationships (University of Toronto, 2008).
CC8. Communicate the importance of teamwork in patient-centered care and population health programs and policies.

---

notice that her weight is up 2.2 pounds from her weight on admission to your unit and that she has 2+ pitting edema in her feet and ankles. You check her diet order and it is for a "regular diet."

You are the nurse calling the physician to update the patient's status to avert future complications. You think that an oral diuretic (water pill) is indicated because Mrs. Schmidt's blood pressure is rising, her weight is up, pitting edema is present, and she has had no diet or fluid restrictions.

Learning Activity

1. Use SBAR, or any other handoff method you are familiar with, to communicate this information to the physician.

CASE STUDY: COMMUNICATION IN AN EMERGENCY

Specific Sub-competencies to consider and apply: CC1, CC2, CC6.

Mr. Walsh is a 68-year-old man who was admitted to the cardiac care unit (CCU) 2 days ago after a myocardial infarction (MI; "heart attack"). It was determined that

he had a 95% blockage in his left anterior descending coronary artery, and a stent was inserted. He showed steady improvement and was able to ambulate short distances without difficulty. He was transferred to the cardiac step-down unit. He has advance directives on file and is to be resuscitated in the event of a cardiac arrest. His wife and daughter are visiting.

Mr. Walsh's monitor begins to alarm as you enter the room. His daughter says, "He says he can't breathe." You (the respiratory therapist) quickly assess the abnormal cardiac rhythm on the monitor (ventricular tachycardia) and call the rapid response team. His wife and daughter are confused by the sequence of events and anxious. As you begin to assess him, he goes into cardiac and respiratory arrest. After finding no carotid pulse, you begin cardiopulmonary resuscitation just as the rapid response team arrives.

Discussion Questions

1. What information needs to be communicated to Mr. Walsh's wife and daughter, by whom, and in what form?
2. Should Mr. Walsh's wife and daughter be given the choice to stay in the room?

3. Explain your choice. How will you communicate this (your choice) to them?
4. Anticipate the feedback that you might get from Mr. Walsh's wife and daughter after your communication. Propose how you will respond to that.
5. What (and how) will you communicate to the rapid response team?

CASE STUDY: STIMULATING INTERPROFESSIONAL EDUCATION AND COLLABORATION DURING A CLINICAL ROTATION

Specific Sub-competencies to consider and apply: CC3, CC4, CC6, CC7, CC8.

Dr. Brush is the clinical instructor for a group of eight nursing students, assigned to a 4-week clinical rotation in a state hospital for patients with mental illness. This psychiatric setting serves as a clinical practicum site for many students, including dental, medical, music therapy, nursing, occupational therapy, physician's assistant, psychology, social work, and therapeutic recreation students. This setting will provide many opportunities for practicing communication skills (e.g., therapeutic communication, active listening, patient teaching, and interprofessional communication). Dr. Brush is excited about this clinical experience because he anticipates that students will have the opportunity to assess and care for persons with chronic mental illnesses in collaboration with the interprofessional treatment teams on each unit. He believes that this is the perfect opportunity for the students to engage in a true Interprofessional Education (IPE) learning experience in which they can demonstrate some of the Core Competencies of Interprofessional Collaborative Practice that they have been learning.

In planning for the students' clinical rotation, Dr. Brush communicates with the educational liaison on each of the clinical units to which students would be assigned. He finds that the staff enjoys having students and are used to them caring for one or two specific patients during their entire clinical rotation. However, the liaisons report that they have observed that the students are often "just sitting around" during their clinical shift when the patient(s) to which they are assigned do not require their constant attention. The liaisons explain that staff have very little direct "control" of the students' learning experiences.

Some staff have overheard students complaining that they find this clinical rotation to be boring. Many staff members say they would like to have more involvement and collaboration with students but do not know how to accomplish this, or if it is "their place" to do so. Students sometimes attend interprofessional treatment team meetings, but, depending on the unit, they have varied levels of contribution to the overall plan of care.

Dr. Brush explains to the liaison that his goal is to provide a positive and collaborative learning experience for the students focused on interprofessional communication. He wants the students to be excited about mental health nursing and see how the mental health concepts they will learn here can be applied in all healthcare settings. All of the unit liaisons agree that true interprofessional communication and team collaboration involving professional and nonprofessional staff, a variety of students, and the patients are possible and would improve the quality of patient care on the units. The liaisons agree to collaborate with Dr. Brush, interested staff members, and others providing care in the setting to encourage and create effective IPE experiences, not just for nursing students, but for all staff and students providing care in this setting.

Discussion Questions

1. Review the definition of a true IPE experience in Chapter 1. Identify at least three benefits of participation in IPE activities centered on Interprofessional Communication for the students and staff who provide care on the psychiatric units referred to in this case study.
2. Give one example of an IPE activity that might be easy to implement on one of these units. Include any professions with which you are familiar who may be in this type of setting.
3. Identify at least three possible barriers to the implementation of this IPE activity.
4. Propose a strategy to reduce each of the three identified barriers to IPE on the unit, and identify specifically how you will demonstrate Sub-competencies CC3, CC4, CC6, and CC7, as appropriate, in addressing these barriers.
5. Identify at least three intended and measurable outcomes (for staff, students, and/or patients) of the successful implementation of your IPE activity on a unit. Be sure to identify how you will "measure" the difference in behaviors of staff, patients, and/or

students from before your IPE activity to after it has been implemented. Keep in mind that terms such as "more" and "less" are not measurable unless you can quantify them.

CASE STUDY: LOOKING AT PATIENTS THROUGH DIFFERENT LENSES

Specific Sub-competencies to consider and apply: CC1, CC3, CC4, CC7.

Moya Potter is an 81-year-old woman who lives alone in her single-story home since the sudden death of her husband 2 years ago. She has an adult daughter living nearby and remains independent and self-sufficient; she still drives her car and maintains control of her financial affairs. Her daughter noticed that she was becoming forgetful about recent events and seemed confused at times. In addition, Mrs. Potter began complaining about headaches and worsening vision. The day that Mrs. Potter repeated the same story to her daughter four times, her daughter became alarmed and called Mrs. Potter's primary care physician.

Five days ago, Mrs. Potter was hospitalized related to her worsening vision, cognitive changes (e.g., forgetfulness, repetitiveness, and periods of confusion), and headache. During her hospitalization, she was diagnosed with metastatic brain cancer secondary to previously undiagnosed lung cancer. In addition to a small brain mass, Mrs. Potter showed evidence of having had several strokes that had resulted in changes to her visual field. It was believed that the strokes were related to the intermittent presence of a cardiac arrhythmia known as *atrial fibrillation;* an injectable anticoagulant was ordered by a cardiologist as a preventive measure. Mrs. Potter's prognosis was guarded at best. Cancer treatment options were discussed with Mrs. Potter and her daughter by the medical oncologist and the radiation oncologist; Mrs. Potter agreed to "try" radiation therapy, followed by chemotherapy.

In the opinion of her radiation oncologist, Mrs. Potter could be discharged to her home after her first radiation treatment, which was scheduled for the next day. The oncologist trusted her family to manage her transportation to the cancer center for outpatient treatments and follow-up. In the opinion of her primary care provider (an internist), with medications for management of her chronic conditions (atrial fibrillation and hypertension) and an appointment for a follow-up visit, she could

be discharged the next day if a family member could administer her injectable anticoagulant. In the opinion of the physical therapist who evaluated her, Mrs. Potter's functional status was ambulatory with a walker for safety and stability. No follow-up physical therapy was required.

Megan Miller, the nurse caring for Mrs. Potter, is concerned about discharging her too quickly. She approached the internist with her concerns: "Mrs. Potter lives alone and I'm not sure any arrangements have been made for how she will be cared for after discharge. Her daughter works full time and hasn't been in to visit very much. I don't know how involved her daughter can be in her care. Mrs. Potter is not able to care for herself and is unable to complete any of her activities of daily living independently since her vision is so severely compromised. I'm worried about us discharging her without a comprehensive plan in place."

Discussion Questions

1. This case study demonstrates how healthcare providers view an individual patient in their care from their own professional perspectives. Each provider has his or her own way of seeing and treating patients, looking through his or her specific "professional lens." This lens is colored by the specific profession, specialty, experience, and background; it often leads individuals to pay attention to specific patient issues that others may not notice. Their perspective influences how they approach problems. For example, the physician might assess a patient through a clinical lens, focusing on whether the patient meets the clinical criteria for discharge, whereas the nurse or social worker might see the patient through a personal or social lens, considering the patient's broader support system at home. Each way of seeing a particular issue is important; it is crucial that providers communicate and consider one another's perspectives when working together to meet specific care needs and planning effective, robust, and safe treatment approaches. Identify the individual perspective of each healthcare provider mentioned in this case study related to Mrs. Potter's discharge readiness.

2. Identify communication tools and methods that could have been used by the interprofessional team throughout Mrs. Potter's care experience to facilitate team discussions and interactions about her readiness for discharge.

3. Considering time constraints of individual team members, explain in which ways efficient communication could have been promoted within the team (i.e., in person, electronically, in a group meeting, in pairs, formally, informally).

4. How could you (as one professional on the team) use active listening to encourage the ideas and opinions of other team members to make better decisions during patient care?

CASE STUDY: INTERVENING DURING A DANGEROUS SITUATION

Specific Sub-competencies to consider and apply: CC5, CC6, CC7.

Julia Marsh, a certified nursing assistant (CNA) in a long-term care setting, enters a resident's room and sees that Mark, one of the nursing students on the unit, is struggling to help Mr. Lu move from the chair to the bathroom. Mr. Lu is a resident who has several oozing wounds on his arms and legs. The CNA observes that Mark is not using proper wound and skin infection control precautions, nor proper body mechanics, in transferring Mr. Lu. Julia's immediate concern is that either Mr. Lu or the student will be injured if she does not intervene immediately.

Discussion Questions

1. Describe how you would provide sensitive and instructive feedback to this student in a timely manner.
   a. Would you address both the lack of infection control and the poor body mechanics at the same time? Why or why not?
   b. Demonstrate respect for both the patient and the student.

2. Did you consider any issues of experience level, power, or hierarchy between the CNA and healthcare professional student in planning your approach? If so, explain any impact that had on your planned approach.

Role Play Activities

1. Role play the situation presented here, assigning the role of the patient, student, and CNA to three participants.

2. After the person playing the CNA provides feedback to the "student" related to the unsafe body mechanics, ask for feedback from those playing the student and the patient.

   a. Was the feedback instructive to both?
   b. Was the feedback sensitive and respectful to both?
   c. Was the feedback given at the right time?

3. Repeat activity 2, a to c, as appropriate related to the lack of skin infection control precautions.

4. Repeat this role play until you can all conclude that you have given "timely, sensitive, instructive feedback," using respectful language, to the "student" about his or her performance.

CASE STUDY: PROVIDING COMMUNITY ACCESS TO PRENATAL CARE FOR TEENS

Specific Sub-competencies to consider and apply: CC1, CC2, CC3, CC4, CC8.

You (choose your profession) are the head of the Maternal, Infant, and Reproductive Health program in a city with a high rate of adolescent pregnancy. Many teenagers do not receive prenatal care until late in their pregnancies. You are working with community-based organizations that serve teens to develop some strategies to increase access to comprehensive prenatal care.

Discussion Questions

1. Identify the community-based organizations that you would be working with to provide comprehensive prenatal care, if this program were in your city.

2. What is a common goal (in terms of a population health program for pregnant teenagers) that the group might work toward?

3. What barriers to open communication and coalition-building (working collaboratively) might exist between these groups (i.e., religious, social, political)?

4. How might these barriers be eliminated?

5. How would you present or frame your invitation to potential group members to respectfully ensure common understanding of the need to provide early access to prenatal care for pregnant teenagers?

Role Play Activity

1. Roleplay an interaction between yourself and a peer in which your peer is in the role of a representative of a faith-based agency who is opposed to Planned Parenthood. In that role, your peer is questioning how he or she can work collaboratively with representatives of Planned Parenthood on this project. Use Sub-competencies CC3, CC4, and CC8 in this role play exercise.

CASE STUDY: TEAMWORK IN A SCHOOL SETTING

Specific Sub-competencies to consider and apply: CC1, CC3, CC8.

Mya is a 5-year-old girl who is diagnosed with autism spectrum disorder (ASD). She attends a half-day general education preschool class in her community elementary school each day. Because of her disability, Mya has her own individualized education plan (IEP), an important legal document, that spells out her individual learning needs, the services the school will provide, and how her progress will be measured. Several people, including Mya's parents, her teacher, a special education teacher, and the school psychologist, were involved in creating this document. Although Mya's IEP stipulates that she is entitled to speech, occupational, and physical therapy services in school, Mya's parents decline. Her parents prefer to continue the private speech, occupational, and physical therapy services that she has participated in for the past 3 years. Mya's parents are very active participants in all of her therapies and decide they can communicate her strengths and areas of special need to her IEP team so that her therapeutic goals can be supported in her daily school activities. As part of her IEP, an aide accompanies Mya to school each day.

Mya's class consists of 21 children, ages 4 to 5 years, who are entering kindergarten in the fall. The classroom has three adults: Mya's teacher, one teacher's aide, and Mya's own aide. In the classroom, Mya demonstrates emerging verbal skills and can put together up to four-word sentences. She has good large motor skills; however, her fine motor skills are still emerging. For example, she has trouble using scissors and eating with a fork and spoon. Mya has some sensory issues with different textures and does not like getting things, like paint or glue, on her hands. One of Mya's greatest challenges is socialization. She usually engages in solo play and rarely interacts with the other children. Mya displays behaviors such as hand flapping and makes a "growling" type of sound when she is overstimulated.

The teacher has a positive relationship with Mya and makes the required adaptations. Mya is a visual learner, and the teacher has adapted the classroom to accommodate her learning style. For example, all the learning materials in the classroom are located on shelves that have been clearly labeled with a picture of the type of learning material that is located on that shelf. This adaptation helps Mya, as well as her classmates, to easily find class materials and be able to return them to the appropriate place in the room when their work is completed. The teacher also provides the class with a picture schedule of the sequence of events that will occur each day at school. Although this was originally done only to help Mya in making transitions, the teacher found that all the students benefited from having a picture schedule. It is now a class tool for all children.

Mya's aide assists her throughout the day and tries to be as "low key" as possible to allow Mya to "blend in" better with the other children. The aide rotates around the room and assists other children as well as Mya. Even though the teacher and the aide make a sincere effort to naturally include Mya in all class activities, the children interact with her cautiously. The teacher and aides wonder what more they can do, especially in helping Mya to communicate more clearly with the other children and in improving her fine motor skills.

Discussion Questions

1. Describe the importance of input from the speech–language pathologist (SLP), occupational therapist (OT), and physical therapist (PT) in developing Mya's IEP.

2. What is the present method of communicating information from Mya's SLP, OT, and PT to the IEP team?
   a. Is it effective? Why or why not?
   b. If you found it ineffective, identify at least two more effective and efficient ways to communicate her speech, occupational, and physical therapy needs to the IEP team.

3. Compare and contrast the quality of Mya's future IEP with her existing IEP, if the future IEP is developed under the following circumstances:
   a. The IEP team, as described in the case study, develops the future IEP with additional input from the SLP, OT, and PT, using the communication tools and techniques that you identified in 2, b.
   b. The IEP team, as described in the case study, develops the future IEP with the actual presence of the SLP, OT, and PT at the IEP meeting to collaborate.

REFERENCES

Interprofessional Education Collaborative Expert Panel (IPEC). (2011). *Core competencies for interprofessional collaborative practice: Report of an expert panel.* Washington, DC: Interprofessional Education Collaborative.

Interprofessional Education Collaborative Expert Panel (IPEC). (2016). *Core competencies for interprofessional collaborative practice: 2016 update.* Washington, DC: Interprofessional Education Collaborative.

University of Toronto (2008). *Advancing the interprofessional education curriculum.* Toronto. Canada: University of Toronto.

Foundations of Teams and Teamwork

LEARNING OUTCOMES

After studying this chapter, you will be able to:

1. Distinguish the characteristics of true teams from those of groups or pseudoteams.
2. Identify the relationship of effective teamwork to the provision of patient-centered care and optimization of healthcare outcomes.
3. Describe the characteristics of effective teams.
4. Identify factors that contribute to collaborative leadership practices for healthcare teams.
5. Describe strategies for performance appraisal for individuals and teams.
6. Apply process improvement strategies to individual and team performance.

This chapter presents the basic elements of groups and group dynamics to inform the process of team development and collaborative teamwork in health care. Effective teamwork is the foundation of Interprofessional Collaborative Practice. Classic views of team leadership are addressed in this chapter. Key concepts of effective decision making, conflict management, shared problem solving and shared accountability are introduced. The processes of quality improvement and outcome evaluation are explored through the lens of individual and team performance evaluation. Strategies to improve individual and team performance are presented.

WHY IS TEAMWORK IMPORTANT IN HEALTH CARE?

In the complex environment of health care, team members must rely on one another's expertise to provide optimal patient-centered care. In 1999 the Institute of Medicine (IOM) published a report titled "To Err Is Human: Building a Safer Health System" (Kohn et al., 1999). The IOM estimated that 98,000 preventable deaths occurred annually because of medical errors. Further studies reported the impact of these concerns, with 70% of medical errors attributed to poor teamwork (Studdert et al., 2002). Consequently, improved teamwork and communication have become priorities for the US government and accreditation agencies such as The Joint Commission for Hospital Accreditation Organization (JCHAO) and the Agency for Healthcare Research and Quality (AHRQ) (AHRQ, 2008; King et al., 2008; Plonien & Williams, 2015). Interprofessional Collaborative Practice is not only a national issue but also was identified as a priority of the World Health Organization (WHO, 2010). Frankel and colleagues noted that "we can assure our patients that their care is always provided by a team of experts, but we cannot assure our patients that their care is always provided by expert teams" (Frankel, Leonard, & Denham, 2006, p. 1690). Effective teamwork reduces errors and reduces mortality and morbidity, thus improving patient safety and care (Neily et al., 2010). Hospitals with high teamwork ratings reap the benefits of higher patient satisfaction, greater staff retention, and lower costs (O'Leary et al., 2012). This chapter explores factors that characterize effective teamwork in health care.

THE HEALTHCARE TEAM

What is a team? Grumbach and Bodenheimer (2004) defined a team as "a group with a specific task or tasks, the accomplishment of which requires the interdependent and collaborative efforts of its members" (p. 1247). Healthcare services are frequently delivered by individuals from different professions. Traditionally, groups of healthcare personnel are called *teams,* whether or not they collaborate in providing care. One key difference between a healthcare team and a group of providers delivering care, however, is intentional collaboration. A team works together, with shared responsibility for making decisions, planning, and delivering care (D'Amour et al., 2005; Grumbach & Bodenheimer, 2004). A sense of shared commitment and mutual accountability also characterize teams (Katzenbach & Smith, 1993). In contrast, a group of individuals from different professions providing care for a patient does not (Dufour & Lucy, 2010). In the latter circumstance, providers focus on individual contributions and accountability rather than combined performance of the group (Katzenbach & Smith, 1993).

Although the vast majority of health services staff reported that they work within a team, only 40% reported the presence of essential characteristics that define a true team (West & Lyubovnikova, 2013). Three essential team characteristics are (1) having clear, shared objectives; (2) working closely and interdependently; and (3) reflecting, which means the team meets regularly and reviews its effectiveness. West and Lyubovnikova (2013) used the term *pseudo teams* to describe groups of individuals working together but lacking these essential characteristics.

Related terms describing the work of healthcare providers are *multidisciplinary* or *multiprofessional teams, interdisciplinary teams,* and *interprofessional teams.* Although these terms were used interchangeably in the past, there is increasing agreement about their distinctions (Thistlethwaite, 2012). Thistlethwaite (2012) described the distinction: "Multi, with its connotations of many, leads to a definition of multiprofessional as: two or more professionals working side by side, without any particular cooperation or collaboration" (p. 18). This means that the multidisciplinary "team" consists of multiple professionals working independently, or in parallel (D'Amour et al., 2005). Multidisciplinary teams often lack the level of communication and collaboration needed for delivery of coordinated patient care. In essence, they are a group of providers, each offering individual contributions to patient care.

In contrast, an interdisciplinary team involves collaboration among team members toward achieving a common goal and integration of the knowledge and expertise of each professional within a shared decision-making process (D'Amour et al., 2005). A foundation of mutual trust and respect supports collaborative relationships in which each member understands and values the contributions and perspective of other professionals. These characteristics closely align with today's definition of Interprofessional Collaborative Practice: "when multiple health workers from different professional backgrounds work together with patients, families, carers, and communities to deliver the highest quality of care" (WHO, 2010).

Thistlethwaite (2012) echoed this distinction between interprofessional and multiprofessional teamwork: "As inter means between, among and mutually, the interprofessional approach to patient care may be defined as involving practitioners from different professional backgrounds delivering services and coordinating care programs to achieve different and often disparate service client needs. Ideally goals are set collaboratively (including the patient) with decision-making through consensus. The result should be an individualized patient care plan, which may be delivered by one or more professionals" (p. 18).

The Interprofessional Education Collaborative (IPEC) 2011 Report and 2016 Update provided operational definitions for interprofessional teamwork and interprofessional team-based care. *Interprofessional teamwork* is defined as "the levels of cooperation, coordination and collaboration characterizing the relationships between professions in delivering patient-centered care" (2016, p. 8). *Interprofessional team-based care* is defined as "care delivered by intentionally created, usually small work groups in health care who are recognized by others as well as by themselves as having a collective identity and shared responsibility for a patient or group of patients (e.g., rapid response team, palliative care team, primary care team, and operating room team)" (2016, p. 8). These definitions emphasize collaborative interprofessional teamwork for providing patient-centered care.

🌐 GLOBAL PERSPECTIVES

The Canadian Family Health Team initiative is part of a paradigm shift that extended the concept of primary care to that of primary health care. Primary health care includes services along the entire healthcare continuum, from health promotion to curative and/or rehabilitative care (WHO, 2002). The Canadian Family Health Team initiative specifically addressed the need to establish interprofessional healthcare teams to improve the delivery of primary health care to meet the needs of local communities (Meuser et al., 2006; Ministry of Health and Long Term Care [MOHLTC], 2006). Inherent in this initiative was transforming the provision of services by groups of individual practitioners to collaborative team practice.

HEALTHCARE TEAM DEVELOPMENT

Creating and maintaining an effective team is challenging, dynamic, and ongoing. All members must be engaged in the process and committed to the overall success of the team in providing optimal patient outcomes. Healthcare leaders and administrators must foster this viewpoint and actively cultivate it as part of the organizational culture and structure. For example, administrators who model collaborative behavior set that expectation for teams (Gratton & Erickson, 2007). Supporting a sense of community fosters sharing of information among team members. Providing employee development activities on topics such as communication, relationship building, and conflict resolution fosters interpersonal skills needed for collaboration. Dedicating time for team members to build trusting relationships helps create an atmosphere of respect for all members' contributions.

Creating clearly defined, mutual goals provides direction for teams (Cooper-Duffy & Eaker, 2017; Gratton & Erickson, 2007). The processes with which to achieve patient-centered, team-based goals typically include developing a plan of care that integrates the expertise of individual members. Team members meet to discuss progress on the plan of care and implement the steps needed to achieve shared goals. An important part of team development is establishing processes to determine whether goals have been achieved and evaluate team functioning (Cooper-Duffy & Eaker, 2017).

Although teams or pseudoteams are common in the delivery of healthcare services, effective teamwork is "a goal that requires training and cultivation" (Clancy & Tornberg, 2007, p. 214). Simply bringing healthcare providers from different disciplines together within a team does not guarantee they will be able to integrate their services while providing care. There is often duplication of care and conflicting care if the responsibilities of members overlap and are not understood by all team members. Clearly defined team member roles and responsibilities improve collaboration (Cooper-Duffy & Eaker, 2017; Gratton & Erickson, 2007). All providers must be able to explain their own roles and responsibilities as well as those of other team members as a precursor to clarify how the team will work together in specific patient-care situations. A shared understanding of each member's contribution is particularly important in light of overlapping skill sets among professions in various work settings.

One challenge for interprofessional teams is the development of ways to share professional responsibilities against the backdrop of professional boundaries or territories. Cultivating the perspective that patient care is a team endeavor and not an individual responsibility is important because it influences the willingness to work collaboratively with others (MacNaughton et al., 2013). Collaborative healthcare teams demonstrate enhanced coordination and continuity of care. It is particularly important for patients and families to perceive that "providers know what has happened before, that different providers agree on a management plan, and that a provider who knows them will care for them in the future" (Haggerty et al., 2003, p. 1221). Providers need to know that their contributions to the plan of care are valued and supported by other team members. Developing a coordinated plan of care necessitates shifting role responsibilities within the team to best meet individual patient-care needs, rather than perpetuating a "siloed" approach with multiple disciplines working independently. Specifically, adopting "the view that a patient is 'ours' instead of 'mine' seems to encourage more interchangeability of responsibilities (where applicable) and also more interactions and knowledge exchanges to inform patient care" (MacNaughton et al., 2013). This mirrors language adopted in the original IPEC Report (2011):

Working in teams involves sharing one's expertise and relinquishing some professional autonomy to work closely with others, including patients and communities, to achieve better outcomes. Shared accountability, shared problem-solving, and shared decisions are characteristics of collaborative teamwork and working effectively in teams. (p. 24)

BOX 13.1 **Interprofessional Education Collaborative Report 2011**

Learning to be interprofessional means learning to be a good team player. Teamwork behaviors apply in any setting where health professionals interact on behalf of shared goals for care with patients or communities. Teamwork behaviors involve cooperating in the patient-centered delivery of care; coordinating one's care with other health professionals so that gaps, redundancies, and errors are avoided; and collaborating with others through shared problem-solving and shared decision-making, especially in circumstances of uncertainty (IPEC, 2011, p. 24).

This means that in addition to developing a professional identity as part of one's training, healthcare providers also need to develop an interprofessional identity. The link between adopting an interprofessional identity and teamwork is described in Box 13.1.

Development of interprofessional healthcare teams is an essential element of Interprofessional Collaborative Practice as defined by the World Health Organization and adopted by IPEC (2011, 2016): "When multiple health workers from different professional backgrounds work together with patients, families, [carers], and communities to deliver the highest quality of care" (IPEC, 2016, p. 8; WHO, 2010). The Core Competencies of Interprofessional Collaboration illustrate the "Integrated enactment of knowledge, skills, values and attitudes that define working together across the professions, with other health care workers, and with patients, along with families and communities, as appropriate to improve health outcomes in specific care contexts" (IPEC, 2016, p. 8). Salas et al. (2008) advocated for explicit team training to improve overall effectiveness. Their model includes elements to develop team leadership, mutual performance monitoring, backup behavior, adaptability, and team orientation.

It is important to note that the Core Competencies explicitly include patients, families, and communities as members of the team.

One example of an evidence-based training program to develop and optimize team performance in health care is *Team Strategies and Tools to Enhance Performance and Patient Safety* (TeamSTEPPS®) (AHRQ, 2010; AHRQ, 2013a). TeamSTEPPS® was developed by AHRQ to improve safety and quality in health care (King et al., 2008). The curriculum is based on more than 25 years of research

and evidence on team performance and can be adapted to any healthcare setting (Plonien & Williams, 2015). The training program includes tools to enhance communication within teams and improve patient outcomes (King et al., 2008). Training is focused on improving three types of teamwork outcomes: knowledge, attitudes, and performance, as depicted in Fig. 13.1. Knowledge refers to a shared understanding with team members working toward the same goal. Attitude encompasses mutual trust and a team orientation, meaning working as a team rather than as individuals. For example, team members consider "our patient" rather than "my patient" in providing team-based care (Plonien & Williams, 2015). Performance outcomes include improved efficiency, adaptability, safety, and productivity. The inner circle of the figure highlights teamwork skills of mutual support, situation monitoring, communication, and leadership (see Fig. 13.1). Each of these skills is part of the TeamSTEPPS® training curriculum (Curriculum Materials, AHRQ, 2013b). Integration of these skills leads to effective, team-based patient care. More information can be found in the Additional Resources section at the end of the chapter.

Roles of Team Members and Group Dynamics

The topic of professional roles and responsibilities is presented at length in Chapter 7 and operationalized in Chapter 8. Stereotypes about perceived roles, or other member characteristics, can be a barrier to collaborative practice. This section emphasizes the relationship between teamwork and interactions among group members.

One influence on group dynamics is the homogeneity versus heterogeneity of group membership. Homogenous groups share similar values, views, and beliefs. For example, a group of female healthcare providers of similar age and cultural background is likely to share similar perspectives. On the other hand, a group comprising men and women of different ages and cultural backgrounds is likely to have more diverse perspectives, values, and beliefs. Such differences must be acknowledged, appreciated, and navigated to provide effective team-based care. Different perspectives also lead to a wider range of solutions in providing patient-centered care.

Consider public stereotypes about generational characteristics as an example of group heterogeneity that may influence group dynamics. Today's healthcare workforce includes individuals from three generations: Baby Boomers, Generation X, and Generation Y, also known

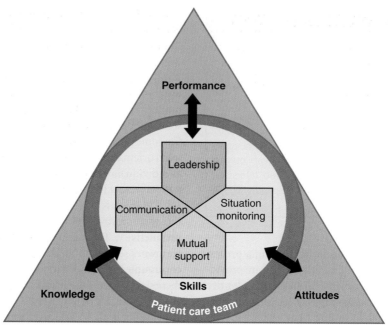

FIG. 13.1 TeamSTEPPS triangle model. (Reprinted with permission of the U.S. Agency for Healthcare Research and Quality." The suggested reference citation for TeamSTEPPS® 2.0 is: Team Strategies & Tools to Enhance Performance & Patient Safety (TeamSTEPPS®) 2.0. Agency for Healthcare Research and Quality; Rockville, MD. December 2012. https://www.ahrq.gov/teamstepps/index.html.)

as millennials. Public stereotypes about generational characteristics may lead to misunderstandings and conflict among team members, between managers and employees, or between patients and providers (Clark, 2017). For example, Baby Boomers tend to prefer face-to-face communication and be less comfortable with technology, whereas members of the more tech-savvy Generations X and Y may prefer electronic communication. Also, differing views about working overtime versus guarding a work-life balance, or the reliance on life experience versus reliance on technology, are potential sources of misunderstanding and conflict among team members. These are some of the many factors that may influence team interactions. One key to effective team interactions is respectful recognition of differences to reach mutual understanding (Clark, 2017). In all situations of differences between members, it is important to treat each member of a team as an individual and learn his or her strengths rather than relying on public stereotypes.

Team members also benefit from awareness of group dynamics and the roles people play within group interactions. For example, assigning silent group members the

> **ACTIVE LEARNING**
>
> Look up characteristics of Baby Boomers, Generation X, and Generation Y.
> 1. Do the characteristics listed describe your perspectives and values?
> 2. How do your characteristics differ from the stereotype?
> 3. Can you think of an example from your experience where generational differences influenced an interaction?
> 4. How could these differences influence the dynamics of interactions among healthcare team members, patients, and families?

role of taking minutes increases those members' participation. Another strategy is for a leader to sit next to a member who is reluctant to speak up during meetings. This simple step increases the likelihood that he or she will do so. Other members may take on the role of facilitator and encourage communication both during and between meetings. Being aware of group dynamics, and taking steps to capitalize upon them, contributes to effective team functioning.

LEADERSHIP OF HEALTHCARE TEAMS

Any team member can take on the role of leader depending on the context of the specific patient-care situation. A collaborative leadership style is particularly important in health care. Effective leaders in team-based care value all team members' potential contributions in meeting the needs of patients and communities (IPEC, 2011). Leadership is one of the primary teamwork skills influencing improved team performance (Hjortdahl et al., 2009). Specifically, leadership is defined as the "ability to coordinate the activities of team members by ensuring team actions are understood, changes in information are shared, and that team members have the necessary resources" (AHRQ, 2010, p. 5). The following section explores characteristics of leadership and management of healthcare teams.

Leadership Theory

Leadership refers to the ability to influence, motivate, and enable others to contribute. A leader should "inspire, facilitate and direct rather than to dictate the way in which work is undertaken" (Ellis & Abbott, 2013, p. 96). Effective team leaders fulfill several important roles as they "organize the team, articulate clear goals, make decisions through collective input of members; empower members to speak up and challenge, when appropriate; actively promote and facilitate good teamwork; are skillful at conflict resolution" (TeamSTEPPS®, AHRQ, 2010, p. 9).

An individual must adapt his or her leadership style to the needs of the team and clinical task. Ezziane (2012a) described the differences in leadership styles among clinical leaders: "*Authoritarian leaders* like to be in charge, expect people to perform as they are told, and do not like to be questioned" (p. 265). This style of leadership provides little opportunity for group decisions and may be appropriate in select clinical situations such as managing a cardiac arrest. In contrast, a *shared leadership style* is often preferred for clinical leaders (Ezziane, 2012a). Team members are engaged in decision making with shared responsibility by all members. Effective leaders offer guidance rather than dictating how things will be done. They promote input from team members and rely on follower participation to accomplish teamwork tasks. A collaborative, participative, team-centered leadership style is essential in promoting IPCP. *Transformational leadership* (Ellis & Abbott, 2013) includes the ability to motivate and inspire others by appealing to individual values. Transformational leaders express vision for how the organization operates, providing direction for teams about establishing priorities and goals.

Leadership is more challenging to describe than management, which is often linked to a specific job description and associated responsibilities (Page, 2015). Managers typically have clearly delineated roles within an organization and the authority to carry out specific responsibilities. In contrast, leaders may not have such clearly defined authority, instead relying on teaching or persuasion, rather than controlling, to carry out activities. Leadership roles may shift for different projects in an organization (Ellis & Abbott, 2013; Page, 2015). Sometimes the healthcare team leader will also be a manager, at other times a manager may need to be consulted by the team to get things done. Both management skills and leadership abilities are important elements in health care for smooth, efficient operations and delivery of optimal patient-centered care.

HEALTHCARE TEAM BEHAVIORS

Effective leadership contributes to team performance, but equally important is the concept of "followership" (Ezziane, 2012b). Team members who hold a positive attitude toward one another and who avoid "antiteam" behaviors are critical to successful teamwork. The following characteristics of healthcare professionals align well with qualities of effective followership. First, they share a common commitment to the patient and the shared purpose of providing optimal care. Second, health professionals are able to self-manage their specific responsibilities to patients and their sensitive information. Third, most professionals continue to build their competence by improving their knowledge and skills needed for the health service context. Finally, healthcare training includes clearly articulated standards and expectations for honesty and ethical behavior. The characteristics needed for good followership clearly align with development of well-functioning healthcare teams (Ezziane, 2012b).

The complexity of healthcare systems requires providers to shift between the roles of leader and follower according the specific context of patient-care needs. This expectation is articulated in the Core Competency of Teams and Teamwork, where members "apply relationship-building values and the principles of team dynamics to perform effectively in different team roles to plan, deliver and evaluate patient/population-centered care and population health programs and policies that are safe, timely, efficient, effective, and equitable" (IPEC, 2016, p. 10). Essential teamwork behaviors include "coordinating one's care with other health professionals so that gaps, redundancies, and errors are avoided; and collaborating with others through shared problem-solving and shared decision-making" (IPEC, 2011, p. 24).

In the busy healthcare environment, providers are sometimes reluctant to ask for assistance because they want to avoid imposing on others, or are fearful that others may question their competence if they need assistance. Concerns such as these contribute to a perspective of solo responsibility rather than shared responsibility for patient care. Similarly, a provider who lacks a clear understanding of the roles and responsibilities of other team members is less likely to collaborate with others. The concept of cross-monitoring on the healthcare team is one strategy to promote team behaviors. Cross-monitoring entails watching out for one another, rather than placing blame for performance gaps, redundancies, or mistakes. Despite the uncertainties and complexities of the healthcare environment, with rapid changes in knowledge and practice, decisions have to be made and actions have to be taken. An atmosphere of mutual trust and respect promotes cooperation, with a focus on achieving cooperative versus individual goals. Likewise, all team members look out for one another and address errors openly rather than placing blame on others. The key is being willing to admit and learn from mistakes, and to learn from one another through shared problem solving (Edmondson, 2012). Chapter 5 discusses the importance of mutual respect among healthcare professionals.

Organizational, Interpersonal, and Team Interactions

Communication is an essential component of effective teamwork. The Joint Commission Report (2006) indicated that communication failures were the underlying cause of close to 70% of sentinel events. A sentinel event is an unanticipated event resulting in serious injury or death to a patient (The Joint Commission, 2006, 2013). Some communication failures can be attributed to fear related to personal interactions and social risk, which may hamper collaboration. Individuals may be reluctant to speak up because of fear of embarrassment, rejection, or punishment (Edmondson, 2012). Likewise, team members may not want to "rock the boat" by expressing differences of

opinion. A person who perceives risk in speaking up may remain silent, but the failure to speak up can have significant consequences in health care and affect the well-being of patients. Communication is discussed extensively in Chapters 10 and 11.

Leaders must encourage, empower, and support team members' willingness to speak up when they have concerns about care, especially to protect quality and patient safety. (AHRQ, 2010; O'Sullivan, Moneypenny, & McKimm, 2015). Simulation training on mannequins provides training opportunities for healthcare professionals to work through patient case scenarios without risk to actual patients. St. Pierre et al. (2012) examined residents' and nursing staff's willingness to challenge physician errors during simulation training. The attending physician was only challenged in 28% of situations because of significant reluctance to speak up during simulation scenarios. In a similar study, medical students were reluctant to speak up when senior colleagues made potentially life-threatening errors during simulation (Moneypenny et al., 2013). See the Research Highlight for a more detailed description of this study. Taken together, these studies emphasize the importance of shifting from leadership based on hierarchies to collaborative leadership (O'Sullivan, Moneypenny, & McKimm, 2015).

RESEARCH HIGHLIGHT

Researchers studied medical students' willingness to challenge a senior colleague who made serious, potentially life-threatening errors in care during simulation training (Moneypenny et al., 2013). When medical students failed to challenge the medical errors, the leader prompted students by questioning, "That's right, isn't it?" Medical students did not challenge errors of the senior colleague in 16 of 36 opportunities during the study. During debriefing sessions after the simulation, several reasons underlying failure to speak up were identified: assumed hierarchy, fear of being wrong, fear of embarrassment, and deference to more experience of the senior colleague. Errors were not addressed by study participants because of their reluctance to challenge the leader, even when participants recognized that errors were made by the senior colleague. The authors recommended including erroneous decisions as part of simulation training to provide medical students with opportunities to practice speaking up (Moneypenny et al., 2013). They also recommended training senior physicians to adopt more receptive attitudes toward discussion of care decisions.

Hierarchy of positions influences team interactions. Those with lower status feel more risk in speaking up. For example, a laboratory technician may be reluctant to question a nurse who is perceived to hold a position of greater status. This hierarchy may decrease the likelihood of some members seeking help, or lead to feeling less able to bring up problems, or feeling that others do not value their contributions. Leaders must recognize the potential influence of hierarchy on interactions and actively provide opportunities for those lower in the hierarchy to offer ideas or ask questions. Edmondson (2012) notes "when people in power speak authoritatively and speak first, it often results in greater self-censorship by others, even if this was not the original intention" (p. 635). As a result, it is the leader's responsibility to actively seek and welcome differences of perspective. When individuals on the team embrace the following behaviors, speaking up is encouraged: communicating respect, acknowledging skills and expertise of all members, and admitting when you do not know something. Leaders can encourage reporting mistakes by team members when they acknowledge their own vulnerability and when they frame failures as learning opportunities (Edmondson, 2012).

Setting Goals and Meeting Objectives in the Context of a Team

One of the key elements of a healthcare team involves clear, shared objectives (West & Lyubovnikova, 2013). This means mutual goal setting so that all team members are working toward the same purpose. The patient and family are essential members of the team and should be active participants in goal setting. The second part of this process is ensuring that mechanisms are in place to assess whether the patient, family, or team goals are being met; this includes measuring outcomes and identifying processes related to patient-centered care. For example, achievement of goals such as "return to home" can be evaluated through direct measures of discharge destination. In these circumstances, the focus is on coordinating care with others to avoid gaps, redundancies, or errors (IPEC, 2011).

Shared Problem Solving and Decision Making

Two essential components of effective healthcare teams are collaboration and shared decision making processes. This means engaging and integrating the knowledge and

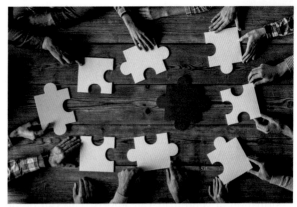

FIG. 13.2 All pieces of the puzzle are needed to create the whole picture. (© ALotOfPeople/iStock/Thinkstock.)

experience of other professionals as valuable contributors to patient-centered or population-focused problem solving. The importance of considering multiple perspectives can be understood through the analogy of a puzzle. Each piece is important but only provides a part of the big picture. It takes putting all the pieces together to create the entire seamless picture (Fig. 13.2)

Shared problem solving begins by clearly defining the problem(s), and generating multiple ideas for potential solutions. The team considers the merits of potential options and then comes to a decision about the plan of action (Cooper-Duffy & Eaker, 2017).

Consensus Building and Motivation

Reaching consensus means coming to an agreement about a decision. Establishing consensus is an important step in planning care. Teams start with a range of ideas and concerns, working to refine the plan until it is acceptable to all members. Being able to have productive conversations and creatively resolve differences supports collaboration (Gratton & Erickson, 2007). Having the opportunity to articulate different perspectives as part of the decision-making process also fosters a greater sense of "buy in" for the team's purpose, goals, and processes. In turn, this shared commitment translates into greater motivation to follow through with team decisions. When multiple perspectives strengthen team knowledge and understanding, effective teams are able to reach consensus to guide team planning and provision of care. Keeping the focus on providing optimal patient-centered care and valuing the integrated collaborative approach enhances team members' support of group decisions.

Shared Accountability

We demonstrate the importance of developing consensus-based goals and plans to achieve team goals related to provision of care. To "close the loop," teams need to foster a sense of shared accountability to one another, to patients and families, and to their communities. This means that all team members are responsible for working interdependently to achieve team goals. In the absence of a strong sense of shared accountability, providers may not share information or coordinate care efforts. This can result in errors or gaps in care and compromise patient safety and wellbeing.

One example of making the concept of shared accountability explicit is the practice of situation monitoring built into the TeamSTEPPS model. Situation monitoring means actively scanning situations and maintaining awareness in order to "support functioning of the team" (AHRQ, 2010, p. 5). This is closely related to the key principle of mutual support, which is the "ability to anticipate and support other team members' needs through accurate knowledge about their responsibilities and workload" (AHRQ, 2010, p. 5). Implementing these strategies creates an atmosphere of mutual trust where team members offer and seek assistance from others.

Managing Conflict

Interprofessional teams with diverse abilities and areas of expertise provide a more comprehensive plan of care. Inevitably, there will be different perspectives about optimal care for specific patients. Such differences have the potential to lead to conflict among team members. Differences in professional and personal values and perspectives may be a source of potential conflict and difference of approaches to problem solving. For example, medical schools focus more on a scientific approach than humanistic, whereas nursing schools adopt a more holistic, humanistic perspective (McNeil et al., 2013). Yet another potential source of disagreement is differing views about team leadership. Regardless of the source of differences, "staying focused on patient-centered goals and dealing with the conflict openly and constructively through effective interprofessional communication and shared problem-solving strengthen the ability to work together and create a more effective team" (IPEC 2011, p. 24). Team members need to find ways to resolve conflict, yet

maintain shared commitment to team goals and mutual respect for differences of perspective.

Conflict, negative emotions, and withholding of information can negatively affect teamwork. A key barrier to effective collaboration is interprofessional conflict associated with threats to professional identity. Specifically, identity threats may result from differential treatment of disciplines, different values between professions, expectations for assimilation, or insults or humiliating actions (Mitchell, Parker, & Giles, 2012). Differential treatment among healthcare professionals is often discussed with examples of dominance of the medical profession. Several authors note the traditional hierarchy of medicine holding a dominant position in the workplace over other professions in areas such as communication, recognition of specialist expertise, economic advantages, and authority over others (Long et al., 2006; Nugus et al., 2010; Reeves, 2011; Reeves et al., 2009). Long et al. (2006) found that medical professionals unintentionally interacted in dominant roles during team meetings, medical procedures, and case conferences, whereas interactions were more evenly distributed during informal discussions on the floor.

The organizational culture of the healthcare setting may perpetuate hierarchies as well. Physicians are traditionally seen as the key decision makers for patient care in the acute setting, overseeing other healthcare professionals, whereas collaborative decision making is more likely in community settings (Nugus et al., 2010). All team members need to be aware of the potential influences of hierarchical relationships on their interactions. Active listening with an underlying mutual respect for others are key elements of collaborative and collegial team interactions.

The World Health Organization (2011) offers specific strategies to empower team members in their interactions despite hierarchy differences. One strategy to manage differences of opinion in patient-care situations is the "two challenge rule," which means team members must (1) voice concerns and (2) restate them. Another three-step communication strategy is abbreviated CUS (I am *Concerned,* I am *Uncomfortable,* this is a *Safety* issue) (AHRQ, 2013a, p. 30). Use of specific strategies like these during interactions among healthcare professionals notifies all team members to pause and attend to the concerns being raised. Additional communication strategies are covered in more depth in Chapters 10 and 11.

Resource Management

One of the most challenging resources to manage in healthcare environments is time. Coordination of optimal care encompasses competing demands for healthcare professionals and for patient availability. Consider the example of an inpatient rehabilitation facility. All patients must receive at least 3 hours of therapy each day from two or more disciplines. When a patient requires a radiograph or other imaging procedure, staff must communicate and coordinate efforts to reschedule therapy times to ensure patients receive their required therapy hours. This can be further complicated by limited staffing of one or more disciplines. For example, if there is only one speech therapist to see all clients with a diagnosis of cerebrovascular accident, then the physical and occupational therapists will have to work around the speech language pathologist's availability to schedule their sessions and achieve the team goal for 3 hours of therapy per day. Ongoing interprofessional collaboration ensures all aspects of the patient's plan of care are addressed.

Another example is staffing shortages. The census of the hospital can be unpredictable. The number of beds in the hospital or a given unit is a rough guide, but the number of patients admitted can fluctuate over time. On an orthopedic surgical unit, elective surgeries can be scheduled with predictable staffing needs. However, an influx of trauma patients through the emergency department can lead to a shortage of staff to provide patient care. Once again interprofessional collaboration assists in providing coverage of patient-care needs.

TEAM EFFECTIVENESS

A central element of Interprofessional Collaborative Practice is working effectively to plan, deliver, and evaluate optimal patient- or population-centered care (IPEC, 2016). The following sections differentiate characteristics of effective and dysfunctional teams. Strategies to appraise team performance and apply process improvement strategies to healthcare teams are also presented.

Characteristics of Effective Teams

Three essential practices of effective healthcare teams are developing shared objectives, working interdependently to achieve those objectives, and meeting regularly to review team effectiveness (Dawson, Yan, & West, 2007; West & Lyubovinkova, 2012). Of particular importance

is having clear team goals with shared commitment to the goals (Reeves et al., 2010). Members of effective teams respect one another's time and expertise and trust each member to do his or her part in achieving mutual goals (Cooper-Duffy & Eaker, 2017). To work closely together, there must be good communication and active engagement among team leaders and team members as necessary elements for collaborative problem solving (Cooper-Duffy & Eaker, 2017; Reeves et al., 2010; Thistlethwaite, 2012) to effectively plan, deliver, and evaluate care. Effective teams embrace collective and individual accountability for achieving their goals and implement explicit plans to evaluate outcomes. High-performing teams collect data, encourage critical appraisal and peer review of their work, and are transparent about their abilities and processes (Ezziane, 2012b; Gawande, 2008).

Characteristics of Dysfunctional Teams

There are a number of challenges to developing and demonstrating the characteristics of an effective team. Lencioni (2002) identified five key characteristics of dysfunctional teams: absence of trust, fear of conflict, lack of commitment, avoidance of accountability, and inattention to results (Fig. 13.3). At the foundation is an absence of trust that team members will fulfill their roles. For example, if one team member doubts the competency of others, this can lead to a perspective that "the only way things get done is if I do them myself." This siloed

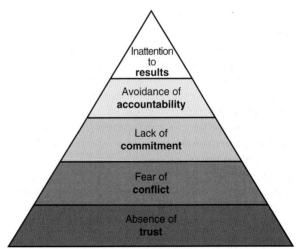

FIG. 13.3 Five dysfunctions of teams. (From Lencioni, P. [2002]. *The five dysfunctions of a team.* San Francisco, CA: Jossey-Bass.)

approach can lead to redundancies or gaps in patient care. A lack of trust may stem from prior experiences (Lencioni, 2002) or stereotypes about other healthcare professions.

The second dysfunction, fear of conflict, leads to avoidance behaviors. This can mean not raising valid concerns about patient care because of fears that you are "stepping on the toes" of another team member, which might anger the other individual. A culture where varied perspectives are encouraged and valued will help reduce this. Although uncomfortable, speaking up and learning to constructively manage conflict are essential skills for healthcare professionals.

Third, lack of commitment to group decisions or administrative directives means that team members may continue to act of their own accord and simply refuse to participate in new initiatives or follow established guidelines. A reluctance to change or lack of agreement with the need to do things differently may contribute to a lack of commitment to team goals. A team member may have an underlying belief of "I know best." Even when based on good intentions, individual or siloed actions can be detrimental to effective team functioning. Lack of commitment to team goals may stem from underlying lack of trust (Lencioni, 2002) or lack of team leadership.

The fourth dysfunction, avoidance of accountability, may lead to the blame game. Individuals hold the perspective that "It's not my job" to make sure "x" happens. Placing blame is more likely from a silo perspective of responsibility versus a team perspective of patient-centered care, where everyone is accountable for optimal patient outcomes. In health care, avoidance of accountability means that patient care suffers. This is in direct contrast to the concept of situation monitoring (AHRQ, 2010), discussed earlier in the chapter. Implementing specific strategies to counter avoidance of responsibility can enhance team performance and outcomes. For an example, see the Research Highlight.

Finally, inattention to results can happen if each person has tunnel vision of his or her silo perspective, instead of appreciating responsibilities for the big picture outcome of providing optimal patient-centered care. This dysfunction is closely linked to avoidance of accountability. Healthcare providers may report being "too busy" to evaluate the results or the process in achieving patient outcomes. Adopting this perspective can lead to gaps or redundancies in patient care.

RESEARCH HIGHLIGHT

A study of 4863 cases in the operating room (OR) examined performance after team training using Team-STEPPS tools of briefings and debriefings. After training, the OR team (surgeons, anesthesia professionals, and perioperative personnel) implemented preoperative briefings in the OR. To encourage input by all team members, surgeons asked for concerns from everyone. This promoted communication and teamwork before and throughout the procedure, rather than reinforcing the strict hierarchy of the surgeon "in charge." Postoperative debriefings were conducted to review team performance, identify any missteps or problems, and thank team members for positive contributions.

Six months after implementation, there was a 95% compliance rate for the new procedures. Participants surveyed reported that the program improved patient safety and collegiality, with better resolution of emerging issues. Evidence from medical records revealed fewer delayed start times (32%–19%), fewer delays for equipment (24%–6.8%), and fewer issues requiring follow-up (44%–0%) (Wolf, Way, & Steward, 2010).

Impact on Optimal Patient Outcomes

One of the criticisms of discipline-specific care delivered with a "siloed" approach has been episodic and fragmented delivery of services with resulting gaps in care for ongoing patient needs. The Triple Aim describes an approach to optimizing health system performance by (1) improving the patient experience of care (including quality and satisfaction), (2) improving the health of populations, and (3) reducing the per capita cost of health care (IHI, 2017). These concepts were applied at one organization. Significant gaps in care were observed in the management of children with chronic conditions, with patients receiving only half of their recommended care (Mangione-Smith et al., 2007). Cincinnati Children's Hospital Medical Center implemented the Condition Outcomes Improvement Initiative (COI) to improve clinical outcomes for children with chronic conditions through enhanced coordination of care by the healthcare team, population management, improvements of the delivery system, and application of evidence-based care (Lail et al., 2017). For specific details, see the Research Highlight.

Collectively, COI improved outcomes for 13,601 children over the 3-year initiative. Eighteen chronic condition teams participated in the initiative; eleven achieved the goal of 20% improvement in their selected clinical outcome over the 3-year initiative (Lail et al., 2017). Two additional teams showed smaller improvements. Successful COI teams shared several characteristics. Team leaders were motivated to change and committed to standardization and shared accountability. The teams had prior quality improvement (QI) training or experience, a physician champion, and prior experience working together. The successful teams showed commitment to application of evidence-based care through consistent implementation of identified processes and accountability for data collection. Successful teams used provider- or team-specific feedback and actively sought family perspectives through team meetings, focus groups, and development of patient education materials. Broad representation of providers and parent or family involvement fostered selection of meaningful goals and outcome measures and improved clinic processes and communication strategies.

COI teams that were unable to demonstrate or sustain improvement had inconsistent implementation of changes in care delivery processes and inconsistent data collection. Changes in leadership or staffing challenged some teams. They also identified implementation barriers of time for QI work, staff turnover, and competing clinical priorities. In summary, the outcomes of this initiative highlight the essential role of effective teamwork in transforming care delivery to provide optimal patient-centered and population-centered care.

Performance Appraisal (Individual and Team)

Most healthcare professions require some form of performance appraisal to ensure that an individual is able to carry out his or her designated roles and responsibilities. In addition to discipline-specific abilities, healthcare providers are expected to be effective team members. For this reason, performance appraisals also need to include assessment of, and feedback regarding, an individual's ability to function as a team member. This assessment may include skills and behaviors such as willingness to speak up, ability to constructively manage conflict, engaging in shared planning and decision making, and shared accountability for patient care. Individual performance and each individual's interactions within the team directly influence healthcare team performance.

Providing explicit feedback on team performance, in addition to patient outcomes, reinforces team goals,

---

RESEARCH HIGHLIGHT

The Condition Outcomes Improvement Initiative's (COI) goals were "the delivery and measurement of the right care to each patient, data feedback to clinical teams, and planned, deliberate population management strategies for groups of children/youth with a specific chronic conditions, while identifying and addressing the family's self-management needs" (Lail et al., 2017, pp. 108–109). Optimal management of children with chronic and complex conditions required explicit training and support for teams providing care for children with conditions such as asthma, epilepsy, juvenile idiopathic arthritis, sickle cell disease, and torticollis.

Specific elements of COI that addressed teamwork were practice redesign and deliberate planning and coordination of care that bridged the outpatient clinic and inpatient and acute care settings. Leaders worked with teams to clarify roles and responsibilities to optimize care and streamlined processes by reducing duplication of services while identifying the most appropriate team member for specific care. Improvement required dedicated time with team leaders, who were committed to accountability and standardization of processes and data collection. COI teams included physicians, nurses, care managers, family members, mental health providers, and social workers. Families participated on clinical teams, in team meetings, on conference calls, and in focus groups and completed electronic surveys.

COI also embraced the importance of improving population health through development of clinical registries and "planned, deliberate population management strategies for groups of children / youths with a specific chronic condition, while identifying and addressing the family's self-management needs" (Lail et al., 2017, pp.108–109). They analyzed baseline data to identify processes to reduce variation and enhance consistency of care, using evidence-based interventions. The quality improvement efforts led to establishing previsit planning as part of enhanced care coordination. As a result, teams were able to identify and prioritize care needs before, during, and after office visits, including laboratory work, imaging studies, and referrals (both prior and for follow-up care).

---

expectations, and performance. In one example, the clinicians and staff of a large healthcare organization received training specifically dedicated to team-oriented care. This orientation emphasized the organization's commitment to developing effective interprofessional teams for delivering patient care. After implementation, each team within the healthcare system received regular feedback on team functioning and staff satisfaction, in addition to patient care outcomes (Grumbach & Bodenheimer, 2004). Establishing expectations and explicit mechanisms for feedback on performance as part of the planning and implementation process helped build shared accountability for outcomes without damaging trust among team members. Teams were informed ahead of time regarding who would provide feedback and the type of performance measures.

Process Improvement Strategies

The expectation for engaging in process improvement to promote effective team-based care is explicitly addressed in the Teams and Teamwork Sub-competencies (IPEC, 2011, 2016). However, few clinical care providers receive formal training in quality-improvement strategies, or the management of healthcare organizations, as part of their professional training. Several approaches have been used to improve quality and performance in healthcare organizations, including Six Sigma, Lean/Toyota Production System, or Studer's Hardwiring Excellence (Koning et al., 2006; Vest & Gamm, 2009). A systematic review of implementing various quality-improvement strategies to address common clinical issues revealed improved processes and outcomes in areas such as clinic appointment access, hand hygiene compliance, incidence of urinary tract infections, patient falls, and patient satisfaction (Vest & Gamm, 2009). Quality-improvement activities yielded changes in both practices and organizational culture, which in turn led to better health care.

Training healthcare team members in quality-improvement strategies equips them with the tools to actively engage in continuous improvement of patient care and interprofessional team performance. Workshops and coaching for healthcare organizations can move participants from discipline-specific perspectives within individual silos, to a sense of shared ownership for process improvement (Studer, 2003). Engaging front-line providers in quality-assurance activities through collaborative problem solving to generate creative solutions, rather than recommending "top down" solutions, yields greater "buy in" when strategies to enhance overall patient care experiences are implemented. Fostering a collaborative problem-solving approach to quality improvement improves satisfaction of patients, employees, and physicians (Studer, 2003) while creating a shared

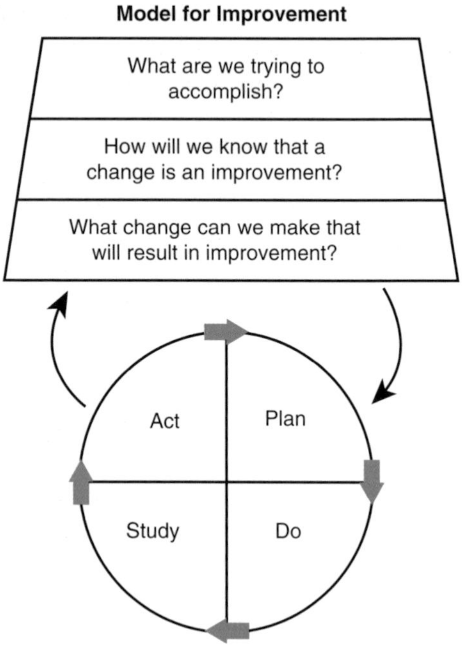

FIG. **13.4** Model for improvement: Plan-Do-Study-Act cycle for quality improvement. (Developed by Associates in Process Improvement. [2009]. In G. L. Langley, R. Moen, K. M. Nolan, T. W. Nolan, C. L. Norman, & L. P. Provost. *The improvement guide: a practical approach to enhancing organizational performance* [2nd ed.]. San Francisco, CA: Jossey-Bass.)

commitment to a culture of excellence in healthcare organizations.

Improvement in provision of services requires planning, action, and evaluation. Another process improvement strategy is the Plan-Do-Study-Act (PDSA) cycle to identify and analyze a problem, followed by planning actions for improvement (Institute for Healthcare Improvement, 2009) (Fig. 13.4). In essence, this cycle adapted the scientific method for action-oriented learning. The PDSA cycle describes a deliberate process for testing change in the work setting by planning it, trying out the change, observing the results, and then evaluating and acting on what was learned. Teams collect enough data to describe and understand an existing process, and then identify aspects of that process to begin to address. The cyclical process of testing change on a small scale, and subsequently refining changes, continues through repeated PDSA cycles. Teams can then decide to implement change in a more widespread manner. PDSA cycles offer a structured improvement process for multidisciplinary teams to identify and solve complex problems that can be applied to health care (Simons et al., 2014). More information can be found in the Additional Resources section at the end of the chapter.

There are several examples of applying this process improvement strategy in health care. Simons et al. (2014) used a structured problem-solving process based on a Plan-Do-Check-Act (PDCA) cycle (an earlier version of the PDSA cycle, Deming, 2000) to improve patient safety in operating rooms. They determined that one factor in the development of surgical site infections was traffic flow and door movement in the operating room (OR). First, they tracked the high number of OR door movements to develop a clear description of the problem. The team identified three actions to reduce OR door movement. The team also determined a feasible target outcome. During the implementation phase, they reduced the number of door movements, including a 78% reduction during orthopedic surgeries (Simons et al., 2014). The authors concluded that the PDCA process was a feasible and relevant mechanism for quality improvement.

ADDITIONAL RESOURCES

The following resources are provided to assist you in identifying tools and techniques to facilitate effective teamwork as the foundation for interprofessional collaboration.

TeamSTEPPS®

This resource is an evidence-based teamwork system developed by Department of Defense's Patient Safety Program in collaboration with the Agency for Healthcare Research and Quality. The TeamSTEPPS system is designed to improve communication and teamwork skills among healthcare professionals and provides ready-to-use materials and a training curriculum that can be used to integrate teamwork principles into all areas of the healthcare system. The training curriculum materials also include an updated pocket guide (AHRQ, 2013b) and an application that can be ordered online (TeamSTEPPS® Pocket Guide App).

For more information, access https://www.ahrq.gov/teamstepps/about-teamstepps/index.html. Curriculum materials available at https://www.ahrq.gov/teamstepps/curriculum-materials.html

TeamSTEPPS Pocket Guide 2.0 Strategies and Tools to Enhance Performance and Patient Safety. AHRQ Pub. No. 14-0001-2. (2013a). Available at https://www.ahrq.gov/sites/default/files/wysiwyg/professionals/education/curriculum-tools/teamstepps/instructor/essentials/pocketguide.pdf

TeamSTEPPS® Pocket Guide App provides a quick-reference tool for the TeamSTEPPS® communication framework. Information about obtaining this app is available at https://www.ahrq.gov/teamstepps/instructor/essentials/pocketguideapp.html

Distinguishing Teams From Groups*

The following table is a useful guide to distinguish characteristics of working groups from teams.

Not All Groups Are Teams: How to Tell the Difference

Working Group	Team
Strong, clearly focused leader	Shared leadership roles
Individual accountability	Individual and mutual accountability
The group's purpose is the same as the broader organizational mission	Specific team purpose that the team itself delivers
Individual work-products	Collective work-products
Runs efficient meetings	Encourages open-ended discussion and active problem-solving meetings
Measures its effectiveness indirectly by its influence on others (e.g., financial performance of the business)	Measures performance directly by assessing collective work-products
Discusses, decides, and delegates	Discusses, decides, and does real work together

Canadian Interprofessional Health Collaborative (CHIC)

Three of the Domains from the Canadian Interprofessional Health Collaborative (CHIC) have relevance for the Sub-competencies of Teams and Teamwork. The CHIC Domain and Competency Statements are provided below. Readers are encouraged to explore this resource further for additional information.

Domain: Team Functioning (CIHC, 2010, p. 14).

Competency Statement: Learners/practitioners understand the principles of teamwork dynamics and group/

Continued

ADDITIONAL RESOURCES—cont'd

team processes to enable effective interprofessional collaboration.

Domain: Collaborative Leadership (CIHC, 2010, p. 15).

Competency Statement: Learners/practitioners understand and can apply leadership principles that support a collaborative practice model.

Domain: Interprofessional Conflict Resolution (CIHC, 2010, p. 17).

Competency Statement: Learners/practitioners actively engage self and others, including the client/patient/family, in positively and constructively addressing disagreements as they arise.

The Teamwork Assessment Scale

This tool was developed to train and to assess undergraduate medical students' ability to work in teams. The tool can be accessed free in the website of the National Center for Interprofessional Education and Practice.

Kiesewetter, J., & Fischer, M. R. (2015). The teamwork assessment scale: A novel instrument to assess quality of undergraduate medical students' teamwork using the example of simulation-based ward-rounds. *GMS Zeitschrift für Medizinische Ausbildung*, 32(2), 1-9. https://nexusipe.org/advancing/assessment-evaluation/teamwork-assessment-scale-tas

Four Habits of High Performance Teams

Using a person-centered perspective, this course explores four habits of high performance teams and teamwork.

This online course is provided free by the Center for Advancing Interprofessional Practice, Education and Research from Arizona State University.

Saewert, K. J. (2017, May). Four habits of high performance teams & teamwork from a person-centered perspective (Y. Price, Designer.) [Interactive video module]. Center for Advancing Interprofessional Practice, Education & Research, Arizona State University, Phoenix. https://ipe.asu.edu/curriculum/elearning-module-four-habits-high-performance-teams-teamwork-person-centered-perspective

Healthcare Quality Improvement Processes

Readers interested in the Institute for Healthcare Improvement Model for Improvement (2009) are encouraged to explore this website further. These resources provide practical strategies for improving individual and team performance. A wide variety of resources, tools, white papers, and audios/videos are provided. Individuals can learn the fundamentals of quality improvement (QI) through online courses that are free with registration. Resources include Plan-Do-Study-Act (PDSA) Worksheets and Project planning forms. Registered users can access and download the Quality Improvement Essentials Toolkit.

*From Katzenbach J. R., & Smith D. K. (1993). The discipline of teams. *Harvard Business Review*, 71(2),111-120. https://hbr.org/1993/03/the-discipline-of-teams-2

KEY POINTS

- Effective teamwork is essential when healthcare professionals interact to provide care to achieve optimal patient outcomes.
- Essential team characteristics include (1) clear, shared objectives; (2) working closely and interdependently; and (3) shared accountability and reflection on team processes and outcomes.
- A key difference between a team and a group of providers delivering care is intentional collaboration.
- Coordination of patient care through effective interprofessional teamwork reduces gaps in care, redundancies, and errors.

- Shared problem solving includes building consensus to integrate multiple perspectives among team members and constructively managing differences of perspectives.
- Effective leadership influences team performance.
- A collaborative, shared leadership style is often preferred for clinical teams.
- Ongoing assessment and improvement of individual performance and team performance improves quality and coordination of care.

REFERENCES

AHRQ. (2008). *Advances in patient safety: New directions and alternative approaches.* Rockville, MD: Agency for Healthcare Research and Quality.

AHRQ. (2010). *TeamSTEPPS Pocket Guide: Strategies and Tools to Enhance Performance and Patient Safety.* AHRQ Pub. No. 14-0001-1. Retrieved from www.ahrq.gov/teamsteppspocketguide.pdf.

AHRQ. (2013a). *TeamSTEPPS Pocket Guide 2.0 Strategies and Tools to Enhance Performance and Patient Safety.* AHRQ Pub. No. 14-0001-2. Retrieved from www.ahrq.gov/teamsteppspocketguide.pdf.

AHRQ. (2013b). *Curriculum Materials.* Agency for Healthcare Research and Quality. Rockville, MD Content reviewed November 2017. Retrieved from https://www.ahrq.gov/teamstepps/curriculum-materials.html.

Canadian Interprofessional Health Collaborative (CIHC). (2010). *A National interprofessional competency framework.* Vancouver, Canada. Retrieved from https://www.cihc.ca/files/CIHC_IPCompetencies_Feb1210.pdf.

Clancy, C. M., & Tornberg, D. N. (2007). TeamSTEPPS: Assuring optimal teamwork in clinical settings. *American Journal of Medical Quality*, 22(3), 214–2017.

Clark, K. R. (2017). Managing multiple generations in the workplace. *Radiologic Technology*, 88(4), 379–396.

Cooper-Duffy, K., & Eaker, K. (2017). Effective team practices: Interprofessional contributions to communication issues with a parent's perspective. *American Journal of Speech-language Pathology*, 26, 181–192.

D'Amour, D., Ferrada-Videla, M., Sam Martin Rodriguez, L., et al. (2005). The conceptual basis for interprofessional collaboration: Core concepts and theoretical frameworks. *Journal of Interprofessional Care*, 5(S1), 116–131.

Dawson, J. F., Yan, X., & West, M. A. (2007). *Positive and negative effects of team working in healthcare: Real and pseudo-teams and their impact on safety.* Birmingham: Aston University.

Deming, W. E. (2000). *The new economics for industry, government, and education.* Cambridge, MA: MIT Press.

Dufour, S. P., & Lucy, S. D. (2010). Situating primary health care within the International Classification of Functioning, Disability and Health: Enabling the Canadian Family Health Team Initiative. *Journal of Interprofessional Care*, 24(6), 666–677.

Edmondson, A. C. (2012). *Teaming: How organizations learn, innovate, and compete in the knowledge economy.* Ebook. San Francisco, CA: Jossey-Bass.

Ellis, P., & Abbott, J. (2013). Leadership and management skills in health care. *British Journal of Cardiac Nursing*, 8(2), 96–99.

Ezziane, Z. (2012a). The Importance of clinical leadership in twenty-first century health care. *International Journal of Health Promotion and Education*, 50(5), 261–269.

Ezziane, Z. (2012b). Building effective clinical teams in healthcare. *Journal of Health Organization and Management*, 26(4), 428–436.

Frankel, A. S., Leonard, M. W., & Denham, C. R. (2006). Fair and just culture, team behavior, and leadership engagement: The tools to achieve high reliability. *Health Services Research*, 41, 1690–1709.

Gawande, A. (2008). *Better: A surgeon's notes on performance.* New York, NY: Picador.

Gratton, L., & Erickson, T. J. (2007). Eight ways to build collaborative teams. *Harvard Business Reviews*, 11, 1–19.

Grumbach, K., & Bodenheimer, T. (2004). Can health care teams improve primary care practice? *Journal of the American Medical Association*, 291, 1246–1251.

Haggerty, J. L., Reid, R. J., Freeman, G. K., et al. (2003). Continuity of care; a multidisciplinary review. *British Medical Journal*, 327, 1219–1221.

Hjortdahl, M., Ringen, A., Naess, A. C., et al. (2009). Leadership is the essential non-technical skill in the trauma team—results of a qualitative study. *Scandinavian Journal of Trauma, Resuscitation Emergency Medicine*, 17, 48.

Institute for Healthcare Improvement. (2009). *Model for Improvement.* Retrieved from http://www.ihi.org/resources/Pages/HowtoImprove/ScienceofImprovementHowtoImprove.aspx.

Institute for Healthcare Improvement (IHI). (2017). *Initiatives: The Triple Aim Initiative.* Retrieved from http://www.ihi.org/Engage/Initiatives/TripleAim/Pages/default.aspx.

Interprofessional Education Collaborative. (2016). *Core competencies for interprofessional collaborative practice: 2016 update.* Washington, D.C.

Interprofessional Education Collaborative Expert Panel (IPEC). (2011). *Core competencies for interprofessional collaborative practice.* Retrieved from http://www.aacn.nche.edu/education-resources/IPECReport.pdf.

Katzenbach, J. R., & Smith, D. K. (1993). The discipline of teams. *Harvard Business Review*, 71(2), 111–120.

King, H. B., Battles, J., Baker, D. P., et al. (2008). TeamSTEPPS: Team strategies and tools to enhance performance and patient safety. In K. Henriksen, J. Battles, M. A. Keyes, et al. (Eds.), *Advances in patient safety: New directions and alternative approaches.* Rockville, MD: Agency for Healthcare Research and Quality. Retrieved from http://www.ahrq.gov/downloads/pub/advances2/vol3/advances-king_1.pdf.

Kohn, L., Corrigan, J., Donaldson, M., et al. (1999). *To err is human: Building a safer health system*. Washington DC: National Academies Press.

Koning, H. D., Verver, J. P. S., van den Heuvel, J., et al. (2006). Lean six sigma in healthcare. *Journal for Healthcare Quality, 28*(2), 4–11.

Lail, J., Schoettker, P. J., White, D. L., et al. (2017). Applying the Chronic Care Model to improve care and outcomes at a pediatric medical center. *Joint Commission Journal on Quality and Patient Safety, 43*, 101–112.

Lencioni, P. (2002). *The five dysfunctions of a team*. San Francisco, CA: Jossey-Bass, A Wiley Company.

Long, D., Forsyth, R., Iedema, R., et al. (2006). The (im) possibilities of clinical democracy. *Health Sociology Review, 15*(5), 506–519.

MacNaughton, K., Chreim, S., & Bourgeault, I. (2013). Role construction and boundaries in interprofessional primary health care teams: A qualitative study. *BioMed Central Health Services Research, 13*, 486. Retrieved from http://www.biomedcentral.com/1472-6963/13/486.

Mangione-Smith, R., et al. (2007). The quality of ambulatory care delivered to children in the United States. *New England Journal of Medicine, 357*, 1515–1523.

Ministry of Health and Long Term Care (MOHLTC). (2006). *How family health teams work*. Toronto, Ontario: Ministry of Health and Long Term Care.

Mitchell, R., Parker, V., & Giles, M. (2012). Open-mindedness in diverse team performance: Investigating a three-way interaction. *International Journal of Human Resource Management, 23*(17), 3652–3672.

McNeil, K. A., Mitchell, R. J., & Parker, V. (2013). Interprofessional practice and professional identity threat. *Health Sociology Review, 22*(3), 291–307.

Meuser, J., Bean, T., Goldman, J., et al. (2006). Family health teams: A new Canadian interprofessional initiative. *Journal of Interprofessional Care, 20*(4), 436–438.

Moneypenny, M. J., Guha, A., Mercer, S. J., et al. (2013). Don't follow your leader: Challenging erroneous decisions. *British Journal Hospital Medicine, 74*(12), 687–690.

Neily, J., Mills, P. D., Young-Xu, Y., et al. (2010). Association between implementation of a medical team training program and surgical mortality. *Journal of the American Medical Association, 304*, 1693–1700.

Nugus, P., Greenfield, D., Travaglia, J., et al. (2010). How and where clinicians exercise power: Interprofessional relations in health care. *Social Science & Medicine, 71*(5), 898–909.

O'Leary, K. J., Sehgal, N. L., Terrell, G., et al. (2012). Interdisciplinary teamwork in hospitals: A review and practical recommendations for improvement. *Journal of Hospital Medicine, 7*(1), 48–54.

O'Sullivan, H., Moneypenny, M. J., & McKimm, J. (2015). Leading and Working in Teams. *British Journal of Hospital Medicine, 76*(5), 264–269.

Page, C. (2015). Managers and leaders in contemporary healthcare organizations. In *Management in physical therapy practices* (pp. 21–38). Philadelphia, PA: F. A. Davis Company.

Plonien, C., & Williams, M. (2015). Stepping up teamwork via TeamSTEPPS. *AORN Journal, 101*(4), 465–470.

Reeves, S. (2011). Using the sociological imagination to explore the nature of interprofessional interactions and relations. In S. Kitto, J. Chesters, J. Thistelthwaite, et al. (Eds.), *Sociology of interprofessional health care practice: Critical reflections and concrete solutions* (pp. 9–22). New York, NY: Nova Science.

Reeves, S., Lewin, S., Espin, S., et al. (2010). *Interprofessional teamwork for health and social care*. London: Blackwells.

Reeves, S., Rice, K., Conn, L., et al. (2009). Interprofessional interaction, negotiation and no-negotiation on general internal medicine wards. *Journal of Interprofessional Care, 23*(6), 633–645.

Salas, E., Diaz Granados, D., Weaver, S. J., et al. (2008). Does team training work? Principles for health care. *Academic Emergency Medicine, 15*(11), 1002–1009.

Simons, F. E., Aij, K. H., Widdershoven, G. A. M., et al. (2014). Patient safety in the operating room theatre: How A3 thinking can help reduce door movement. *International Journal for Quality in Health Care, 26*(4), 366–371.

St. Pierre, M., Scholler, A., Strembski, D., et al. (2012). Do residents and nurses communicate safety relevant concerns? Simulation study on the Influence of the Authority Gradient. *Anaesthetist, 61*, 857–866.

Studdert, D. M., Brennan, T. A., & Thomas, E. J. (2002). What have we learned from the Harvard Medical Practice Study? In M. M. Rosenthal & K. M. Sutcliffe (Eds.), *Medical error: What do we know? What do we do?* (pp. 3–33). San Francisco, CA: Jossey-Bass.

Studer, Q. (2003). *Hardwiring excellence: Purpose, worthwhile work, making a difference*. Gulf Breeze, FL: Firestarter Publishing.

TeamSTEPPS® Pocket Guide App. Information about obtaining this App is available at: https://www.ahrq.gov/teamstepps/instructor/essentials/pocketguideapp.html.

The Joint Commission. (2006). *Root causes for sentinel events*. Retrieved from www.jointcommission.org/sentinel_event.aspx.

The Joint Commission. (2013). *Comprehensive accreditation manual for hospitals*. Retrieved from www.jointcommission.org/sentinel_event.aspx.

Thistlethwaite, J. E. (2012). Teamwork and collaborative practice in modern health care. In *Values-based interprofessional collaborative practice: Working together in health care*. Cambridge UK.: Cambridge University Press.

Vest, J. R., & Gamm, L. D. (2009). A critical review of the research literature on Six Sigma, Lean and Studer Group's Hardwiring Excellence in the United States: The need to demonstrate and communicate the effectiveness of transformation strategies in healthcare. *Implementation Science, 4*, 35.

West, M. A., & Lyubovnikova, J. (2012). Real teams or pseudo teams? The changing landscape needs a better map. *Industrial and Organizational Psychology, 5*(1), 25–28.

West, M. A., & Lyubovnikova, J. (2013). Illusions of team working in health care. *Journal of Health Organization and Management, 27*(1), 134–142.

Wolf, F. A., Way, L. W., & Steward, L. (2010). The efficiency of medical team training: Improved team performance and decreased operating room delays: A detailed analysis of 4863 cases. *Annals of Surgery, 252*(3), 477–483.

World Health Organization. (2002). *Health for all: Origins and mandate*. Geneva: WHO.

World Health Organization. (2010). *Framework for action on interprofessional education and collaborative practice*. Geneva: WHO.

World Health Organization. (2011) *WHO patient safety curriculum guide*. www.who.int/patientsafety/education/curriculum/en/.

14

The Competency of Teams and Teamwork

LEARNING OUTCOMES

After studying this chapter, you will be able to:

1. Describe the process of team development and the roles and practices of effective teams.
2. Develop consensus on the ethical principles to guide all aspects of teamwork.
3. Engage health and other professionals in shared patient-centered and population focused problem-solving.
4. Integrate the knowledge and experience of health and other professions to inform health and care decisions, while respecting patient and community values and priorities/preferences for care.
5. Apply leadership practices that support collaborative practice and team effectiveness.
6. Engage yourself and others to constructively manage disagreements about values, roles, goals,

and actions that arise among health and other professionals and with patients, families and community members.

7. Share accountability with other professions, patients, and communities for outcomes relevant to prevention and health care.
8. Reflect on your own performance as an individual, and as a team member, for performance improvement.
9. Use process improvement strategies to increase the effectiveness of interprofessional teamwork and team-based services, programs, and policies.
10. Use available evidence to inform effective teamwork and team-based practices.
11. Perform effectively on teams and in different team roles in a variety of settings.

The Core Competency of Teams and Teamwork, as defined by the Interprofessional Education Collaborative Expert Panel (IPEC, 2011, 2016), is explained and operationalized in this chapter. Teamwork behaviors are essential in all settings in which healthcare professionals interact to care for individual patients or communities (IPEC, 2011). In considering the Core Competency of Teams and Teamwork, it is important to clearly identify characteristics of effective healthcare teams and strategies to coordinate care "so that gaps, redundancies, and errors are avoided" (IPEC, 2011, p. 24). Interprofessional team-based care requires the enactment of shared identity and responsibility in providing services for patients, families, and communities (IPEC, 2016). This means respecting and engaging other professionals and learning to constructively manage different perspectives to arrive at shared decisions about patient care.

After the presentation of the Teams and Teamwork (TT) Core Competency Statement and specific

Sub-competencies, case studies, and caselets are used as appropriate to set the stage and illustrate each specific behavior. Not every possible profession or team member is involved in the provided patient-care scenarios. Additional case studies are provided in Chapter 15. You are encouraged to apply each specific Sub-competency to examples in your own clinical practice and experience to determine any missed opportunities for Interprofessional Collaborative Practice that you may discover. Learning to use the Sub-competencies is an ongoing process and continues throughout one's professional career.

THE TEAMS AND TEAMWORK CORE COMPETENCY STATEMENT

Apply relationship-building values and the principles of team dynamics to perform effectively in different team roles to plan, deliver, and evaluate patient/population-centered care and population health programs and policies that are safe, timely, efficient, effective, and equitable (IPEC, 2016, p. 14).

THE SUB-COMPETENCIES OF TEAMS AND TEAMWORK

Recognizing the need for cooperation, coordination, and collaboration with other healthcare professionals begins the process of interprofessional teamwork that is essential to achieve optimal patient-care outcomes (IPEC, 2011). Preparing future healthcare professionals to function effectively as members of an interprofessional collaborative team better equips them to address the prevention of population health problems (Evans, Cashman, Page, & Garr, 2011).

Healthcare services are often provided to one person or community by individuals from multiple professions. As presented in previous chapters, one of the key differences between a team and a group of providers delivering care is collaboration. A team works together with shared responsibility for making decisions, planning, and delivering care (D'Amour et al., 2005; Grumbach & Bodenheimer, 2004). In contrast, a group of providers from different professions providing care for an individual patient, but who do not actively collaborate with one another, do not constitute a team (Dufour & Lucy, 2010). Engaging other professionals in patient-centered problem solving requires achieving consensus on the optimal course of action. This means developing a sense of team identity in addition to a profession-specific identity. To be an effective collaborative team member, you need to demonstrate the specific behaviors, or Sub-competencies, associated with Teams and Teamwork. The specific Sub-competencies of Teams and Teamwork are listed in Box 14.1.

TT1: Describe the Process of Team Development and the Roles and Practices of Effective Teams

The focus of this Sub-competency is for you to be able to describe how healthcare teams develop and identify the behaviors and practices that characterize effective teamwork. As discussed in Chapter 13, collaborative practice entails more than a group of individuals simply working alongside one another. Effective healthcare teams must include three essential elements: shared objectives,

---

> **BOX 14.1 Specific Sub-competencies of Teams and Teamwork (IPEC, 2016, p.14)**
>
> TT1. Describe the process of team development and the roles and practices of effective teams.
>
> TT2. Develop consensus on the ethical principles to guide all aspects of teamwork.
>
> TT3. Engage health and other professionals in shared patient-centered and population-focused problem-solving.
>
> TT4. Integrate the knowledge and experience of health and other professions to inform health and care decisions, while respecting patient and community values and priorities/preferences for care.
>
> TT5. Apply leadership practices that support collaborative practice and team effectiveness.
>
> TT6. Engage self and others to constructively manage disagreements about values, roles, goals, and actions that arise among health and other professionals and with patients, families and community members.
>
> TT7. Share accountability with other professions, patients, and communities for outcomes relevant to prevention and health care.
>
> TT8. Reflect on individual and team performance for individual, as well as team, performance improvement.
>
> TT9. Use process improvement strategies to increase the effectiveness of interprofessional teamwork and team-based services, programs, and policies.
>
> TT10. Use available evidence to inform effective teamwork and team-based practices.
>
> TT11. Perform effectively on teams and in different team roles in a variety of settings.

---

working interdependently, and meeting regularly to review team effectiveness (West & Lyubovinkova, 2012, 2013). Consider the unfolding Case Study: The Case of Nancy King, Part 1.

The new employee orientation presenters specifically addressed essential elements of effective healthcare teams. In Case Study: The Case of Nancy King, Part 1, King did not fully understand or embrace the importance of team development or the practices of effective teams. Like many professionals, she was focused primarily on discipline-specific care for her patients and assumed that by doing her own "job" well, teamwork would "just happen." She was used to being a part of a group of healthcare providers, not a healthcare team. Because she had no experience working collaboratively in a healthcare team, the suggested process of dedicated time for team

CASE STUDY

The Case of Nancy King, Part 1

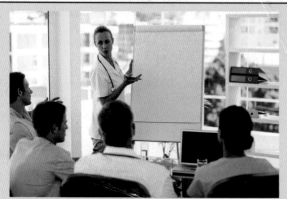

(Photo © Wavebreakmedia/iStock/Thinkstock.)

Nancy King is a newly hired nurse at a subacute rehabilitation center. Before working with patients, she participated in an orientation for new employees. During the training session, she noticed that an entire afternoon was devoted to presentations on team building and teamwork. Eager to start working with patients on the unit, she wondered if all this special training was needed, thinking "Don't teams just happen when you are assigned a caseload? Is there really more to it than working with other colleagues? Can't I just figure it out once I get to my unit like I did at my last job?" The presenter described how teams are established, and three essential elements of healthcare teams: collaboration, shared accountability, and communication strategies to resolve conflicts. She explained the differences between effective teams and dysfunctional teams. Nancy King smiled to herself thinking about some of the "dysfunctional" teams she had worked with in the past. Nancy wondered if there had been staffing problems in the past that led to including these topics in orientation. She reassured herself that all she needed to worry about was doing a good job working with her patients. The presenter talked about regularly scheduled team meetings for planning patient care, and "debriefing" sessions to evaluate and improve team performance. Nancy thought, "I can't imagine having time for all those meetings! I have patients to care for!"

Discussion Questions

1. What assumptions does Nancy King make about providing patient care?
2. What barriers does she anticipate to providing team-based patient care?
3. Do you think these views and concerns are common in health care?

planning, problem solving, and debriefing meetings seemed unrealistic and unnecessary. In particular, the idea of meetings to review team effectiveness seemed unnecessary and burdensome given the busy pace of patient care on the unit that she was expecting. She wondered about this heavy emphasis on "the team," not realizing that the collaborative team-based care given to the patient would far surpass fragmented siloed care in quality and patient outcomes. She completed the required new employee orientation but was not really sure how all of this information about forming and functioning as part of a team applied to her. You will revisit this unfolding case study in the discussion of Sub-competencies TT4, TT5, TT8, and TT9.

Self-Evaluation of TT1

Describe the process of team development and the roles and practices of effective teams.

1. List the three essential characteristics of an effective team. Refer to Chapter 13 as needed for review.

2. Explain how effective teams are developed. Refer to Chapter 13 as needed for review.
3. Identify an example from your own experience of an effective team (any type of team).
4. List three practices that define your example as an effective team.
5. As a contrast, list three characteristics that would describe an ineffective team.

✳ ACTIVE LEARNING

To learn how to describe the characteristics and practices of effective teams, try the following:

1. Develop a 2-minute "elevator pitch" that describes the differences between a group of providers and an interprofessional collaborative healthcare team.
2. Ask for feedback from a peer.
3. Refer to Chapter 13 to see if you highlighted the key differences between a group and a team of healthcare providers.

When you are able to describe how teams develop and the roles and practices of effective teams, you have demonstrated an understanding of the TT1 Sub-competency.

TT2: Develop Consensus on the Ethical Principles to Guide All Aspects of Teamwork

Members of an interprofessional healthcare team may hold different personal values and perspectives about certain aspects of patient care. Individual heathcare team member values may also differ from those of the patients and families on the team. Team members should recognize and respect one another's individual differences while coming to consensus on how to approach new or recurring patient-care situations that they encounter. Demonstrating mutual respect for one another is a key element in reaching team consensus on ethical issues.

Consider the following example of a patient who has a terminal condition and a team that has to make a difficult decision about the plan of care. Mr. Smith is a 57-year-old man diagnosed with amyotrophic lateral sclerosis (ALS), commonly referred to as *Lou Gehrig's disease.* This degenerative disease involves progressive loss of motor function, including the muscles of respiration (breathing) and swallowing. Mr. Smith and his family must make important decisions such as whether to initiate the use of a mechanical ventilator to sustain life. Navigating individual patient, family, caregiver, and healthcare provider perspectives with respect to these decisions is a challenging and ongoing part of the process as the disease and its manifestations progress. In this scenario, the healthcare professionals need to develop consensus on the ethical principles that will guide all aspects of patient care and teamwork within their team. The overriding principle that they all agree upon is respect for patient autonomy and self-determination—that is, the patient's right to be in control and make informed choices. Even when the patient's decision differs from perspectives of these individual healthcare providers, the team members agree to respect the right of patients to make informed decisions about their care. This means that team members' individual preferences and values regarding quality of life should not influence the patient's care. These concepts are exemplified in Caselet 14.1.

Some may consider entering a nursing home where the patient has constant medical care to supervise and manage respiration through mechanical ventilation the best option. Others may consider the emotional well-being of the patient to be the paramount consideration and feel that keeping him at home with his loved ones is the best medical decision. Some team members may consider end-of-life decisions to be a matter of "God's will," whereas healthcare providers should offer all possible interventions to extend life as long as possible.

In Caselet 14.1, perspectives about the "best medical decision" may have differed among team members, yet as a result of working together through a number of difficult patient care decisions, this team maintained the consensus that the autonomy of the patient will be honored. In respecting the patient's right to make informed choices about care, the team presented alternative treatment options for Mr. Smith and his family to consider in making their decision.

Self-Evaluation of TT2

Develop consensus on the ethical principles to guide all aspects of teamwork.

1. Imagine that you are one of the team members who disagrees with the recommendation to begin mechanical ventilation and plan for discharge to a nursing home. How would you approach your colleagues?
2. Reflect on team member values and perspectives that differ.
3. Describe the process you will use to arrive at consensus with the shared values of the team.

When you have successfully identified how to develop consensus on an ethical principle that your team might use to guide an aspect of care, you have demonstrated an understanding of the TT2 Sub-competency.

TT3: Engage Health and Other Professionals in Shared Patient-Centered and Population-Focused Problem-Solving

The key word in Sub-competency TT3 is "engage." This means actively involving others in making care decisions. Reconsider Caselet 14.1. Mr. Smith and his family were seriously considering their options when questions began to emerge related to their religious beliefs. The family members wondered if the use of mechanical ventilation might interfere with "God's will," and they wondered if it was selfish of them to want to use such interventions to extend his life as long as possible. They shared their concern with the nurse on the team, who recognized the need to engage other professionals in assisting the patient and family in making their decision. The

CASELET 14.1   Mr. Smith

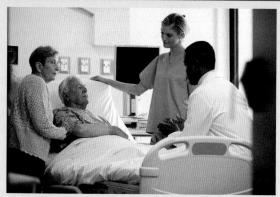

(Photo © monkeybusinessimages/iStock/Thinkstock.)

Mr. Smith is a 57-year-old man with amyotrophic lateral sclerosis (ALS), commonly referred to as *Lou Gehrig's disease*. He and his family have been dealing with the effects of this disease for 6 years. Over the years they have modified their activities and their home to accommodate his progressive loss of muscle strength. At this point he requires total assistance for all activities of daily living (e.g., positioning in bed, feeding and grooming, etc.). Over the past year, his breathing and swallowing ability significantly declined. He was recently admitted to the hospital for a respiratory infection.

His declining respiratory function has reached the point where the need for mechanical ventilation will likely continue after the infection resolves. The respiratory unit team meets with the family to discuss the options related to his breathing. The first option presented is to consider whether to begin the use of mechanical ventilation on a long-term basis. The respiratory therapist explains that use of a ventilator will likely extend his life, but it will not change the fact that he will eventually succumb to this disease. If Mr. Smith chooses mechanical ventilation, he and the family need to consider whether this will be done in their home or in a skilled nursing facility. Home mechanical ventilation would require 24-hour care with nurses and respiratory therapists in the home. Mechanical ventilation in a nursing home would provide round-the-clock care by skilled professionals. The other option is to take a hospice approach to care, making Mr. Smith as comfortable as possible, but not using mechanical ventilation to prevent respiratory arrest. After presenting these options for care, the team recommends that Mr. Smith enter a nursing home upon discharge with mechanical ventilation and round-the-clock care by skilled professionals. Mr. Smith and his family expressed their strong desire to remain at home rather than have him spend the remainder of his life in a nursing home. Mr. Smith also voiced concerns about "being a burden" to his family and recognizes the toll the last several years have taken on him and his loved ones. Mr. Smith informs the team that he needs some time to consider his options.

Discussion Questions

1. What are some of the ethical concerns presented in this case?
2. What are your personal views about this patient case? What would you recommend if this were your family member?

nurse suggested that Mr. Smith and his family meet with their pastor to consider how to navigate decisions about end-of-life care in the context of their faith. The family agreed and the nurse arranged for the pastor to visit. The pastor met together with the family and the team to explore Mr. Smith's treatment options. Engaging the pastor to participate in patient-centered decision making illustrated respect for patient autonomy and self-determination. The process of engaged collaboration used the collective expertise, perspectives, and resources available to enable the patient to make an informed decision about his own care. After much thought and prayer, Mr. Smith and his family declined mechanical ventilation and chose to be discharged home with the support of hospice to make Mr. Smith as comfortable as possible.

Self-Evaluation of TT3

Engage health and other professionals in shared patient-centered and population-focused problem solving.

1. Identify other professionals, based on their role and expertise, who could be engaged to provide the specific aspects of Mr. Smith's care as part of the team to promote optimal patient-centered care.
2. Choose one of the healthcare or other professionals whom you identified. Describe the process that you would use to engage these professionals in Mr. Smith's care.

When you are able to identify other professionals who could be engaged in providing care in patient scenarios and you can describe the process to engage them in care of the patient, you have demonstrated awareness of the TT3 Sub-competency.

TT4: Integrate the Knowledge and Experience of Health and Other Professions to Inform Health and Care Decisions, While Respecting Patient and Community Values and Priorities/Preferences for Care

The TT4 Sub-competency addresses the importance of integrating the knowledge and experience of other professionals to inform decisions while honoring the values of those we serve. The specific healthcare situation determines who needs to be involved in making care decisions that respect patient and family priorities and preferences for care. Case Study: The Case of Nancy King, Part 2, describes what may be considered "routine" patient care, yet there are opportunities where the application of the Sub-competencies associated with Teams and Teamwork could transform "routine" care into a true example of Interprofessional Collaborative Practice to improve patient outcomes.

When attending the new employee orientation, Nancy did not fully appreciate the recommended strategies for collaborative teamwork. Now she recognizes that she might need to use what she learned there to provide better patient care by enhancing teamwork and shared problem solving on the unit where she works. As the nurse for each of these patients, she is deeply concerned about what can be done to ensure patient safety on her unit but is frustrated that her input is not being sought in addressing the problem. She clearly recognizes the need to integrate the knowledge and expertise of all members of the healthcare team, to look beyond the specific circumstances of each individual patient's fall and find solutions to this recurrent unit problem. To achieve an interprofessional team approach to fall prevention, Nancy suggested establishing a collaborative fall prevention program. This suggestion would actively engage the knowledge and expertise of all team members in shared problem solving and delivery of care. To completely demonstrate the TT4 Sub-competency, the team will need to be aware of individual patient perceptions of, and especially their objections to, fall prevention strategies now in place. Patient input must be sought so that the team can pose solutions and strategies that are consistent with the patients' values and preferences for their own care.

Another important role for the fall prevention team is to identify interprofessional team (IP) members who will work closely together in a coordinated way. Each

CASE STUDY

The Case of Nancy King, Part 2

Nurse Nancy King is now working the night shift in the subacute rehabilitation center. During the past month, three patients have fallen on her unit. The circumstances of each fall differed. The most recent incident involved a patient who refused previous staff recommendations to wear a diaper and got out of bed in the middle of the night to go to the bathroom without ringing the call bell for assistance. The patient fell and broke her wrist as she tried to break her fall. After each fall, an incident report was completed according to subacute unit established procedures. In each situation, appropriate precautions were implemented, including patient education on the use of nursing call bells in bed and the bathroom, and keeping the bed height low.

Each incident was discussed at weekly utilization review meetings attended by the rehabilitation supervisor, a nursing supervisor, and the safety administrator of the subacute unit. However, attendance of direct care providers was not part of the utilization review meetings. Instead, the decisions from the meetings were communicated to staff the following week for implementation. Nancy King, the nurse for each of the patients who fell over the course of the month, had no direct input. She realized that there might be an opportunity to improve patient care, promote safety, and prevent future falls by shifting to team-based care. She approached the nursing supervisor and suggested creating a "fall prevention team" for the subacute rehabilitation unit.

Discussion Questions
1. Who would you identify to be members of the fall prevention team?
2. What are the "missed opportunities" for interprofessional care in this example of routine care?

team member has a role in ensuring patient safety. The following individuals have expertise related to reducing falls risk: nurse, certified nurse assistant (CNA), physical therapist (PT), occupational therapist (OT), physician, physician assistant (PA), nurse practitioner (NP), pharmacist, and safety administrator. The nurse conducts a baseline assessment of fall risk factors on admission and educates the patient and family about risk factors, the use of the call bell, and requesting assistance for specific activities. The CNAs report any new fall risks to nurses, assist with toileting as needed, and make sure that assistive devices are within reach. The physician, PA, or the NP reviews the patient status, prescribes medications, and consults with rehabilitation therapies as needed. The pharmacist reviews the medication list for patients identified at risk for falls, and notifies the team of medications (including drug interactions) that may increase fall risk, making recommendations for changes as needed. The PT assesses the patient's functional mobility, recommends assistive devices and level of assistance needed, and educates the patient and family. The PT also provides therapeutic exercise to improve strength and balance. The OT educates the patient and family on self-care and activities of daily living to ensure safety and may provide adaptive devices. As circumstances warrant, additional staff are involved from environmental services and housekeeping to maintain the environment to reduce fall risks, such as keeping hallways free of clutter, placing signs to indicate wet floors, and so on. Although each individual has a role to play, the fall prevention team will foster interprofessional collaboration to establish an integrated plan of care.

To effectively integrate the knowledge and expertise of healthcare professionals, the fall prevention team implements two new strategies: "fall huddles" and "debriefing sessions." The "fall huddle" is a brief meeting for on-the-spot problem solving by the healthcare team members who are directly involved in providing care to the patient who experiences a fall, as well as a facility safety administrator. Together they discuss the specific circumstances surrounding the fall and develop team-based prevention strategies to maximize patient safety. The results of the "fall huddle" are discussed with the patient and family, who indicate their understanding and preferences for care. The team also recognizes the importance of reflecting upon and evaluating their efforts, and sets quarterly "debriefing" meetings to monitor the team process and outcomes.

Self-Evaluation of TT4

Integrate the knowledge and experience of health and other professions to inform health and care decisions, while respecting patient and community values and priorities/preferences for care
1. Identify all of the team members involved in Case Study: The Case of Nancy King.
2. Describe how the knowledge and experience of each identified team member contributes to decisions about patient care.

3. Discuss how patient values and preferences might influence the decisions of the IP fall prevention team.
4. Provide specific suggestions related to how team members can demonstrate their respect of patient values, priorities, and preferences for care in making decisions related to Case Study: The Case of Nancy King.

When you are able to describe integrating the contributions of at least three professional team members with patient values and preferences for care to inform health and care decisions, you are demonstrating an understanding of the TT4 Sub-competency.

TT5: Apply Leadership Practices That Support Collaborative Practice and Team Effectiveness

The IP fall prevention team described in Case Study: The Case of Nancy King, Part 2, is moving forward with their initiatives. Their meetings have gone fairly well, although not all team members have been able to attend the "huddles" on short notice. Although all staff support the concept, some have more "buy-in" to the process than others. Read Case Study: The Case of Nancy King, Part 3, to consider how interactions between the team leader and team members, and assumptions about hierarchy, influence the exchange.

Most members assumed that the physician was responsible for leading the team. In further discussion, team members realize that they have been "deferring" to the physician during meetings, and have been reluctant to offer alternative perspectives and solutions because of subtle perceptions of differences in status and power among team members. The majority of team members see their role as contributing expertise in support of the physician's role as leader. They have not fully embraced the perspective that each of them are empowered partners in this team collaboration process. Shared leadership is essential to team effectiveness (O'Sullivan, Moneypenny, & McKimm, 2015).

As the team reviews the previous year's reports, several different scenarios emerge. In situations in which falls were attributed to toileting needs, the nurses and CNAs have the primary role in addressing prevention. Other times, the pharmacist was the key player in resolving medication interactions that precipitated dizziness or hypotension-related falls. When patients were admitted to subacute rehabilitation for impaired mobility related

CASE STUDY

The Case of Nancy King, Part 3

Dr. Hite starts the Fall team meeting by sharing her frustration about this new responsibility being added to her caseload, saying, "I'm too busy with patient care throughout the facility to organize fall meetings." The team members nod but do not respond. Dr. Hite continues, saying, "Meghan, the OT has a team conference and cannot be here but we may as well get started. I know we are all busy with patients, so let me summarize the details for Mrs. Young's fall." Dr. Hite reviews the patient's medical record, summarizes the circumstances and outcomes of Mrs. Young's fall, and then says: "Does that about sum it up? Going forward we should implement the following steps …"

Dr. Hite continues looking at the medical record without pausing to see if any of the team members have additional information to share. Nancy King thinks of something but is hesitant to speak up, rationalizing that it's probably not important anyway.

Discussion Questions

1. How could Dr. Hite encourage greater participation by other members during the meeting?
2. How should the group handle the perspective of the absent team member?
3. What assumptions do the individuals in this case study appear to hold about the leadership role?
4. How could members shift to a collaborative perspective with shared accountability?

---

to weakness and balance deficits, the PT was the primary person addressing fall prevention. The team members acknowledge support for a team approach, recognizing that their siloed efforts at implementation have faltered at times.

After discussion, the team recognizes that the common "player" in previous patient falls was the safety administrator of the subacute unit. Her prior experience in evaluating safety concerns across the hospital and her collaborative leadership style make her well suited for leading the IP fall prevention team. They will continue working collaboratively but with more effective leadership. She actively works to encourage all team members to speak up and ask questions and raise concerns during huddles and debriefing meetings. She pauses periodically in the discussion and solicits input from team members who have not yet spoken. As team leader, the safety administrator

encourages team efforts and fosters a sense of shared responsibility in which team members hold each other accountable for team goals and plans.

It is important to note that this team decision to make a change in leadership of the fall prevention team was not the only viable option. In this scenario, each of the team members held certain assumptions about the role of the physician as "being in charge" and saw themselves in "supporting roles." The physician was more familiar with the role of "giving orders" that were implemented by others. Similarly, the other team members were used to their role in carrying out physicians' orders. Uncovering these assumptions about hierarchy was the basis for all team members to work toward changing their behaviors, to foster true collaboration and shared accountability for effective team performance. In addition, the leader could actively cultivate her role by empowering team members to communicate and collaborate to achieve successful outcomes, thus shifting away from hierarchical relationships and encouraging full participation by all team members (Edmondson, 2012). In particular, leaders need to affirm the importance of input from team members to foster a sense of shared ownership and a shared sense of purpose. This may include soliciting input and assistance from others, actively listening to suggestions, encouraging reciprocal communication, and explicitly recognizing the contributions of team members. All participants are viewed as valued partners with the expertise needed to address shared team goals. Team members need to believe they can make meaningful contributions to fully "buy in" and make the effort. Team members also recognize that changing familiar interaction patterns is never easy, but together they can succeed.

✴ ACTIVE LEARNING

Think of prior experiences where you were part of a team (working on a group project, playing on a sports team, etc.) where there was effective leadership.
1. What contributed to the effectiveness?
2. How did this differ from an experience where there was less-effective leadership?

Self-Evaluation of TT5

Apply leadership practices that support collaborative practice and team effectiveness.
1. Describe leadership behaviors and skills that foster collaboration. Refer to Chapter 13 as needed.

2. Describe leadership behaviors and skills that discourage collaboration. Refer to Chapter 13 as needed.
3. Explain how these behaviors and interactions potentially influence patient care.
4. Identify an opportunity to begin practicing leadership skills and behaviors that foster collaboration.

When you are able to apply leadership practices that support collaborative practice and team effectiveness, you have demonstrated an understanding of the TT5 Sub-competency.

TT6: Engage Self and Others to Constructively Manage Disagreements About Values, Roles, Goals, and Actions That Arise Among Health and Other Professionals and With Patients, Families, and Community Members

There may be situations where team members disagree about values, goals, or actions to be taken. Likewise, there are times when healthcare professionals disagree with patients and families about the course of action. For example, patients may have health conditions that require dietary restrictions such as low-salt or low-fat diets for individuals with high blood pressure or cardiac conditions. Patients and families may not adhere to recommended dietary restrictions, instead preferring familiar meals and comfort foods. When a patient is a resident in a setting such as an assisted living facility, the need to manage these disagreements may become prominent. To illustrate this concept, read Case Study: The Case of John Williams, Part 1.

In Case Study: The Case of John Williams, Part 1, it was clear to the nursing staff that they were providing the appropriate diet to support Mr. Williams's overall health. Similarly, it was clear to the dietary staff that they were cooking and providing nourishing meals to promote Mr. Williams's well-being. However, the family wanted John to be happy, and if that meant eating the restricted food that he enjoyed rather than his recommended diet, they were going to honor that. After all, John was 83 years old, and they doubted he would enjoy a healthier diet at this stage of life. Everyone valued doing what was best for Mr. Williams, although they all differed in their perspectives about what that was. In this case the interprofessional team caring for John needs to engage him and his family, as well as members of the assisted living community, in managing the disagreements that have arisen related to

CASE STUDY

The Case of John Williams, Part 1

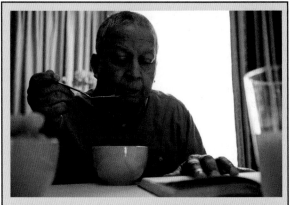

(Photo © Wavebreakmedia/iStock/Thinkstock.)

John Williams is an 83-year-old man with a history of dementia related to Alzheimer's disease for several years. He resides in an assisted living facility. Mr. Williams, who has a past history of cardiac disease, is supposed to be on a low-salt, low-fat cardiac diet. Recently he has been taking salt packets and butter from other residents' trays at mealtimes. When nursing staff confront him about his food choices, he replies, "The food here is terrible…it needs more salt! I don't want those stinking vegetables, I want a cheeseburger and fries!" The dietary staff attempts to appease John by periodically preparing his requested favorite dishes. John complains to family members about the food, and they bring in his favorite salty snacks and fast food on a regular basis.

Discussion Questions
1. How would you respond to this patient?
2. Identify positive and negative aspects of the approaches to managing disagreements described in this caselet.
3. Who would you include as members of the team to address these concerns?

Mr. Williams's dietary restrictions. Consider Case Study: The Case of John Williams, Part 2.

Self-Evaluation of TT6

Engage self and others to constructively manage disagreements about values, roles, goals, and actions that arise among health and other professionals and with patients, families, and community members.

1. Consider the scenario described in the first part of Case Study: The Case of John Williams. Which perspective would you most likely support?

CASE STUDY

The Case of John Williams, Part 2

The nursing staff called in Susan Kenny, a registered dietician, to meet with Mr. Williams, his family, and the dietary staff at the assisted living facility. She began by asking Mr. Williams and his family about his food preferences. When Mr. Williams listed pizza, cheeseburgers, fries, bacon, and other high-fat, salty options, the nursing staff objected that his choices were not allowed on the cardiac diet. A member of the dietary staff described how challenging it was to cook and serve residents food permitted on modified diets, and hear their complaints that "the food here is terrible!" Susan Kenny educated the patient and family about the importance of his cardiac diet. She then worked with them and the dietary staff to modify his favorite foods and suggested acceptable alternatives such as substituting low-fat, low-salt cheeses on the pizza and adding alternative seasonings for flavor instead of salt. By engaging the patient, family, and assisted living facility staff in the discussion, the team was able to find compromises and alternative solutions to manage the disagreements about Mr. Williams's diet.

Discussion Questions

1. How did Susan Kenny's nonjudgmental approach influence these interactions?
2. What strategies were used to constructively manage disagreements in this scenario? Can you suggest additional approaches?

2. Find peers who can role play the team members involved in the differences of perspective on what is the best course of action for Mr. Williams.

3. In the role play, demonstrate constructive discussion about differences of perspective among nursing, the dietary staff, family members, and Mr. Williams.

When all team members in your role play can respectfully verbalize their differing perspectives, consider alternatives, and come to mutual agreement of the course of action, you have demonstrated an understanding of the TT6 Sub-competency.

TT7: Share Accountability With Other Professions, Patients, and Communities for Outcomes Relevant to Prevention and Healthcare

Effective teams cultivate a shared responsibility and shared accountability for healthcare outcomes and prevention.

 GLOBAL PERSPECTIVE

Teams and Teamwork

The Canadian Interprofessional Health Collaborative (CHIC) National Interprofessional Competency Framework (2010) includes Team Functioning, Collaborative Leadership, and Interprofessional Conflict Resolution as three of their six competency domains. Their competency statement and descriptors are similar to those in this chapter. In addition, they also include the importance of interprofessional communication to address conflicting viewpoints and reach reasonable compromises.

A common example in a hospital setting is the importance of handwashing to prevent the spread of infection from patient to patient. It is important to remember that hospital staff are not the only ones who transmit microorganisms and spread infection: patients, families, and others who interact with patients also share this accountability. All people in the hospital setting should wash their hands before and after any direct contact with a patient or his or her environment. Though a simple idea, it only takes one person to forget to observe this simple practice to transmit infection. Caselet 14.2 illustrates this point.

Busy healthcare providers may overlook routine procedures in their haste to see all of their patients. All hospital personnel are instructed in the importance of handwashing as the most effective mechanism to prevent the spread of infection. Knowing the established procedure and consistently carrying it out are two different things. In addition, staff members may be reluctant to "speak up" and point out a lapse to another care provider. Differences in status or perceived power between the surgical resident and the CNA, in this example, may have contributed to her reluctance to speak up. Imagine instead that shared accountability was the culture of the workplace. The CNA could have offered to get examination gloves for the resident or felt empowered to direct the resident to the soap dispenser at the bedside as a gentle reminder. The patient should also be instructed, as a member of the team, not to allow anyone to touch her without first washing hands or using hand sanitizer and wearing examination gloves. Take a moment to consider the activities in the Active Learning box.

Several interprofessional communication strategies to address difficult situations using respectful language were

CASELET 14.2 Mary Brown

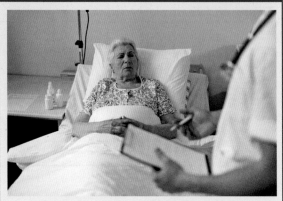

(Photo © shironosov/iStock/Thinkstock.)

Mary is recovering in the hospital from a total knee replacement. Immediately postoperatively she has a urinary catheter in place and bandages covering the incision on her knee. Throughout the course of the day the following individuals interact with Mrs. Brown: nurses, the certified nursing assistants (CNAs), the surgeon, the surgical resident, the physical therapist, the social worker, dietary staff, her family members, other visitors, and housekeeping personnel. The morning after surgery, Louise, the CNA, is giving Mary Brown her bed bath, and the surgical resident stops into the room. Louise observes the surgical resident approach the patient without first washing his hands or using hand sanitizer. He asks Mrs. Brown several questions and then asks to see her incision. He sees that the box of examination gloves at the patient's bedside table is empty. The resident is running late for surgical rounds so he proceeds to examine the knee incision and manually assists the patient in bending and straightening her knee to determine how much movement she has and whether there is swelling in the knee. Louise is uncomfortable speaking up and assumes the surgical resident must have washed his hands before entering the room. The next day, Mrs. Brown begins to run a fever.

Discussion Questions

1. How would you respond if you were the CNA in this scenario?
2. How could you provide feedback to the resident in this scenario? What response would you expect?
3. Who is accountable for preventing the spread of infection?

✷ ACTIVE LEARNING

Identify a situation from your past experience where you were reluctant to speak up and point out a mistake by another person.

1. Why were you reluctant?
2. What would have made you more willing to do so?
3. Role play the scenario described in Caselet 14.2: Mary Brown with a peer, acting out at least three different interactions. Suggest specific language the CNA could use to demonstrate shared accountability for preventing the spread of infection.

presented in Chapters 10 and 11. One example that might assist Louise, the CNA, in speaking up is to use the approach described by the acronym CUS (Concern, Uncomfortable, Safety). Specifically, Louise could have said, "I am Concerned about you not washing your hands before seeing the patient. I am Uncomfortable with you not using gloves to examine her. Handwashing and the use of gloves is a Safety issue" (AHRQ, 2013, p. 30). Refer to Chapter 10 for a more in-depth discussion of inter-professional communication strategies.

Self-Evaluation of TT7

Share accountability with other professions, patients, and communities for outcomes relevant to prevention and health care.

1. Describe an example from your experience where all team members shared accountability for an outcome.
2. Identify strategies individuals and team members could implement to ensure shared accountability in achieving the identified outcome.
3. How could those skills and behaviors apply to health-care teams?

When you are able to identify and implement strategies for sharing accountability with other team members, you have demonstrated an understanding of the TT7 Sub-competency.

TT8: Reflect on Individual and Team Performance for Individual, as Well as Team, Performance Improvement

Once again, we will revisit Case Study: The Case of Nancy King, Part 4. Six months after initiation of the fall preven-tion team, the team holds a debriefing meeting to review outcomes and to reflect on the performance of individuals,

CASE STUDY

The Case of Nancy King, Part 4

The team begins the debriefing meeting by noting their success with the immediate "fall huddle," including direct care providers and sharing recommendations with patients and families. They also note improved patient compliance with safety procedures after this interaction. They are pleased to see trends toward improvement from their efforts. Team members also report improved communication among individuals involved in patient care and increased collaboration when patients are considered to be at risk for falls.

The team also identifies areas for improvement. They identify a problem in that select members were unable to attend fall huddles on short notice. Megan, the occupational therapist (OT), feels uncomfortable with the discussion about her inability to attend several of the meetings. She comments "I am not quite sure why we spent so much time discussing team performance. The number of falls on the unit decreased, isn't that enough?" Nancy King responded, "I used to have that viewpoint but now I understand how the investment in assessing team performance means even better outcomes for all patients. It helps us work toward our shared goal of creating proactive strategies for prevention rather than simply reacting to each event in isolation." Megan reflects on her limited engagement and begins to recognize the benefits of providing integrated team-based care. After exploring this issue, the team identified alternative notification procedures to increase attendance by all parties.

Discussion Questions

1. Why is it important to reflect on individual performance as well as team performance?
2. What barriers to effective team performance do you see in this scenario?
3. Why do you think these barriers exist? What strategies would you suggest to address them?

as well as the entire team. The team will revise their plan as needed.

Although it is not possible to prevent all falls, this scenario represents a patient-centered approach by an interprofessional team aimed toward quality improvement. To further illustrate the importance of an integrated approach to care, subsequent debriefing meetings resulted in several changes. As part of a regular process of reflecting on team performance, the fall prevention team decided to create a clinical pathway that triggers proactive intervention by the team. The electronic health record includes a falls risk assessment screening tool. Patients identified as "at risk" receive a brightly colored arm band and have a sign posted over their bed, identifying the need for fall precautions. The fall prevention team collaborates with institutional technology department personnel to incorporate additional team recommendations into the electronic record. For example, screening documentation that identifies patients at high risk for falls automatically triggers computerized order sets for mobility protocols and pharmacist consultation.

Self-Evaluation of TT8

Reflect on individual and team performance for individual, as well as team, performance improvement.

1. Think about your previous experiences as a member of a team. Reflect on your individual performance and opportunities for improvement.
2. Reflect on the overall performance of the team and identify strategies to enhance team performance.
3. How would your individual performance and your performance as a team member enhance the overall outcome for the team?

When you can reflect on your individual performance, your contributions toward team performance, and overall team performance, you have demonstrated awareness of the process to achieve the TT8 Sub-competency.

TT9: Use Process Improvement Strategies to Increase the Effectiveness of Interprofessional Teamwork and Team-Based Services, Programs, and Policies

In addition to reflecting on individual and team performance, effective teams should explicitly implement a quality improvement or process improvement approach to increase the effectiveness of teamwork, team-based services, programs, and policies. For example, administrative support would further enhance a culture of patient safety and fall prevention. This could take place by revising institution policies and procedures related to screening and intervention for patients identified as being at risk of falling. An additional step might be instituting fall risk assessment competency testing for all staff members.

In Case Study: The Case Study of Nancy King, Part 4, the fall prevention team reviewed all incidences of falls and noted a number of falls related to patients attempting to get to the toilet. In an effort to reduce this causative factor, the subacute rehabilitation unit staff implemented a proactive toileting schedule whereby staff provided toileting assistance every hour for patients on the unit, rather than waiting for a call bell to request assistance. This schedule was more efficient than the previous "reactive" approach. Similar examples reported in the literature have resulted in significant reductions in the rate of falls (Shever et al., 2011).

Self-Evaluation of TT9

Use process improvement strategies to increase the effectiveness of interprofessional teamwork and team-based services, programs, and policies.
1. Think about how implementing any of Sub-competencies TT1 to TT8 has improved your effectiveness in working on team-based projects.

When you are able to identify and implement processes to improve effective teamwork, you have demonstrated awareness of the TT9 Sub-competency.

✴ ACTIVE LEARNING

Refer to Box 14.1.
1. Review each Sub-competency statement and place a check mark next to the ones you have mastered.
2. For those you have not mastered, reflect on how you might practice the skills needed to gain mastery.
3. Enlist appropriate support to reach your goals.

TT10: Use Available Evidence to Inform Effective Teamwork and Team-Based Practices

Effective teamwork requires training and cultivation (Clancy & Tornberg, 2007). As discussed in Chapter 13, some evidence-based resources for training healthcare professionals to enhance teamwork include Team Strategies and Tools to Enhance Performance and Patient Safety (TeamSTEPPS). Frankel and colleagues (2006) further emphasized the need for such training, noting that care delivered by a group of experts in their respective professions is not the same as care provided by an expert team.

TeamSTEPPS can be adapted to meet the specific needs of healthcare teams.

Lack of formal training or dedicated time for team development in healthcare settings may result in busy professionals seeing limited value in such activities. However, practicing professionals can benefit from practical, clinically relevant team development activities that provide opportunities for application and feedback (Bajnok, Puddester, MacDonald, Archibald, & Kuhl, 2012). In Ontario, the Teams of Interprofessional Staff (TIPS) Project provided a series of team development Interprofessional Education (IPE) workshops for practicing professionals from varied disciplines and settings. Structured learning sessions were interspersed with time to apply concepts in daily practice. Participants reported improved communication, enhanced understanding of team members' roles and responsibilities, and improved collaboration. They also articulated the importance of administrative support for resources and processes to foster effective teamwork (Bajnok et al., 2012).

The need for and benefits of intentional team development in the workplace are readily apparent in developing team protocols for the operating room (OR), where effective teamwork is essential for optimal patient outcomes. Wolf et al. (2012) reported improved performance after team training in several parameters, including reduced OR procedure delays, improved hand off, and improved adherence to prophylactic antibiotic guidelines. Tibbs and Moss (2014) combined TeamSTEPPS training with implementation of a surgical protocol leading to decreased turnover time between procedures and improved perceptions of teamwork. In particular, the surgical teams studied improved in staff members speaking up and correcting one another's mistakes and reevaluating goals when situations changed. Such improvements in teamwork and communication are vitally important to patient safety. These are powerful examples of shared accountability and decision making.

Self-Evaluation of TT10

Use available evidence to inform effective teamwork and team-based practices.
1. Use the literature to find articles related to effective teamwork.
2. Scan the article titles to select an article specific to healthcare teams.

3. Identify the level of evidence to support the recommendations of the study.

When you have demonstrated the ability to find and apply evidence to specific healthcare situations, you have demonstrated an understanding of the TT10 Sub-competency.

TT11: Perform Effectively on Teams and in Different Team Roles in a Variety of Settings

It is important for each individual to function effectively as a team member, and different situations may require different expertise. In particular, the specific details of performing a given role may vary based on the setting where the care is provided. For example, the physician is traditionally considered to be the "leader" of the healthcare team in the hospital setting; however, this may not be the case in another setting. Likewise, with the shift to Interprofessional Collaborative Practice, the team leader could be any one of a number of professionals. Consider the example of a patient receiving healthcare services in his or her own home. Physicians typically do not make house calls, so another provider, such as the home health nurse, may take the leadership role in this setting to manage and oversee the patient care. Similarly, in behavioral health, the team leader may be the psychiatrist in some settings, whereas in others an advanced practice nurse or social worker may perform this role. The Global Perspectives box illustrates considerations for effective performance on a global team.

Similarly, the dynamics of an effective team vary based on the specific needs of the patient case at a given time. Consider Caselet 14.1, in which the progression of a degenerative condition (ALS) affects Mr. Smith's primary care needs at different stages. If his primary needs are for physical mobility, the physical therapist may take the primary role in managing the patient's plan of care. If the primary focus of treatment is managing medications or catheters, then nursing may have the primary role. As the disease progresses, difficulties with swallowing and oral communication may be the primary concern and the speech–language pathologist or speech therapist may take the primary role. During the late stages when breathing becomes significantly impaired, the respiratory therapist may have the primary role. As in Caselet 14.1, the patient, the family, and team of professionals will need to work collaboratively to address the changing care requirements. As always, the team works together to provide a shared, patient-centered plan of care. Effective

GLOBAL PERSPECTIVE

Working in Multicultural Interprofessional Teams

Mastering the Core Competencies is important in the global health environment, which requires the ability to work effectively in multicultural interprofessional teams. Guerin (2014) pointed out that the silo approach to healthcare services is evolving into an interprofessional practice model that includes both preventive and reactive healthcare services. The following quote highlights the importance of effective teamwork in the global health environment. Global health "represents a dynamic field with diverse practitioners that rely upon partnerships and collaborations. Even with the best information, and resources, a project may never reach its full potential due to the people involved" (p. 39). Integration of social-emotional learning into global health education helps to manage conflicts, bridge gaps between professions, and improve team interactions. Social-emotional learning includes specific instruction in self-awareness, self-management, social awareness, relationship skills, and responsible decision making. Guerin suggests subtle changes in IPEC Competency language to fully integrate these social-emotional elements.

team members adapt to assume different roles based on the patient's care needs at the time.

Self-Evaluation of TT11

Perform effectively on teams and in different team roles in a variety of settings.

1. Choose two members of a healthcare team. Identify their role in a specific setting.
2. Choose three different settings where care may be provided (e.g., hospital, nursing home, outpatient, community, etc.). Explore differences in team roles for each of those settings.

When you are able to identify effective team performance in different roles and settings, you have demonstrated an understanding of the TT11 Sub-competency.

Demonstrating the Competency of Teams and Teamwork

Exemplar Case Study: The Competency of Teams and Teamwork demonstrates the application of the concepts in the provision of optimal interprofessional collaborative

◎ EXEMPLAR CASE STUDY

The Competency of Teams and Teamwork

Nancy King is a newly employed nurse at a subacute rehabilitation facility. While attending the Orientation for New Employees she learns about the facility's emphasis on teamwork, the process of team development, and effective team practices [TT1]. Nancy remembers examples from her previous job where individuals from different disciplines worked side by side, each with their own discipline-specific lens for providing patient care; she was surprised when she realized that that was not "teamwork." There was no real shared ownership, accountability, or teamwork in planning or providing care. She realizes now that her nursing skills alone cannot ensure the best patient outcomes and is eager to learn more about teamwork skills that she can use to enhance her own interprofessional collaboration skills.

After a few months in her new position, Nancy King recognizes an opportunity to create heightened interprofessional teamwork in addressing the problem of patient falls on her unit. Multiple disciplines are included in forming a fall prevention team to address the shared goals of learning more about past incidents and working toward preventing falls. The team is founded on key principles of mutual respect and the recognition of the unique expertise that each member/discipline brings to the table. They build in shared accountability and a problem-solving approach to enhance team strategies to achieve their shared goal of improved patient safety during their stay. The fall prevention team members develop consensus on underlying ethical principles to guide their team work [TT2, TT3]. In addition, they include patients and families in developing and implementing fall prevention strategies, respecting patient preferences while addressing safety concerns for toileting

[TT4]. The fall prevention team also consults literature in their planning stages to inform team-based practice. The evidence confirms underlying causes of falls are often multifactorial in nature, further supporting their desire to move from providing discipline-specific routine care and implement a collaborative, interprofessional team-based approach [TT10].

As they implement the new team, they share accountability and build in debriefing meetings to evaluate the outcomes of their effort and assess team performance. The team recognizes that initial plans for team leadership were not the most effective strategy and shift gears. The newly designated team leader actively encourages open discussion and sharing of ideas by all [TT5, TT6, TT7].

The decline in fall incidences on the unit is one successful outcome. Team members realize that process evaluation also offers valuable insights to further optimize patient-centered care. The fall prevention team reflects on individual and team performance, engaging in process improvement to increase the effectiveness of services, programs, and policies [TT8, TT9]. They decide to engage the information technology department to build a clinical pathway into the electronic health record to trigger proactive implementation of fall prevention strategies for high-risk patients to enhance effectiveness of care. When a patient identified as high risk for falls experiences a fall at home 2 days after discharge, the team extends their interprofessional collaboration and communication to include home care agency providers, recognizing that team leadership and teamwork will need to be adapted to effectively provide service in the home [TT11].

care. The presence of specific Sub-competencies has been indicated throughout the case study.

The interactions described here provide examples of using effective teamwork and integrating the expertise of all team members, including the patient and family, to enhance the quality of patient-centered care. The planning and provision of collaborative interprofessional care includes shared accountability by all team members, constructively managing disagreements as they arise. In addition, teams reflect upon individual and team performance to improve effectiveness of interprofessional teamwork. This Exemplar Case Study focusing on Nancy

King provides just one example of the type of high-quality patient-centered care that results from the operationalization and incorporation of the Competency of Teams and Teamwork. Every patient care scenario you encounter will be unique, with specific details varying based on factors such as the patient's own care needs, the setting, the organizational structure, the professionals involved, and the resources for care. Regardless of case-specific factors, moving beyond the traditional fragmented delivery of services by individual providers to interprofessional collaborative teamwork will enhance and improve patient-care outcomes.

KEY POINTS

- There is a need for healthcare professionals to shift from a discipline-specific perspective to an interprofessional, collaborative, patient-centered approach to care in all settings.
- Patients, families, communities, and other professionals must actively engage in shared problem solving and decision making.
- Shared accountability empowers all team members to advocate for patients and populations to foster prevention and optimal healthcare outcomes. Reluctance to speak up because of perceived differences in knowledge, responsibility, or status can negatively affect patients and must be overcome.
- Effective teamwork is essential to optimal patient care. Achieving this requires explicit efforts to reflect upon and improve team performance, in addition to individual contributions to patient care.
- All interprofessional team members must embrace attitudes, behaviors, and skills that contribute to effective team functioning and collaborative leadership.

REFERENCES

AHRQ. (2013). *TeamSTEPPS Pocket Guide 2.0 strategies and tools to enhance performance and patient safety*. AHRQ Pub. No. 14-0001-2. (2013). Retrieved from www.ahrq.gov/teamstepspocketguide.pdf.

Bajnok, I., Puddester, D., MacDonald, C. J., et al. (2012). Building positive relationships in healthcare: Evaluation of the teams of interprofessional staff interprofessional education program. *Contemporary Nurse*, 42(1), 76–89.

Canadian Interprofessional Health Collaborative (CHIC). (2010). *A national interprofessional competency framework*. Vancouver, Canada. Retrieved from http://www.cohc.ca/files/CIHC_IPCompetencies_Feb1210r.pdf.

Clancy, C. M., & Tornberg, D. N. (2007). TeamSTEPPS: Assuring optimal teamwork in clinical settings. *American Journal of Medical Quality*, 22(3), 214–2017.

D'Amour, D., Ferrada-Videla, M., San Martin Rodriguez, L., et al. (2005). The conceptual basis for interprofessional collaboration: Core concepts and theoretical frameworks. *Journal of Interprofessional Care*, 5(S1), 116–131.

Dufour, S. P., & Lucy, S. D. (2010). Situating primary health care within the International Classification of Functioning, Disability and Health: Enabling the Canadian Family Health Team Initiative. *Journal of Interprofessional Care*, 24(6), 666–677.

Edmondson, A. C. (2012). *Teaming: How organizations learn, innovate, and compete in the knowledge economy*. San Francisco, CA: Jossey-Bass.

Evans, C. H., Cashman, S. B., Page, D. A., et al. (2011). Model approaches for advancing interprofessional prevention education. *American Journal of Preventive Medicine*, 40, 245–260.

Frankel, A. S., Leonard, M. W., & Denham, C. R. (2006). Fair and just culture, team behavior, and leadership engagement: The tools to achieve high reliability. *Health Service Research*, 41, 1690–1709.

Grumbach, K., & Bodenheimer, T. (2004). Can health care teams improve primary care practice? *Journal of the American Medical Association (JAMA)*, 291, 1246–1251.

Guerin, T. (2014, Winter). Relationships matter: The role for social-emotional learning in an interprofessional global health education. *Journal of Law, Medicine & Ethics, Interprofessional Health Education Suppl*, 39–44.

Interprofessional Education Collaborative. (2016). *Core competencies for interprofessional collaborative practice: 2016 update*. Washington, D.C.

Interprofessional Education Collaborative Expert Panel (IPEC). (2011). *Core competencies for interprofessional collaborative practice*. Retrieved from http://www.aacn.nche.edu/education-resources/IPECReport.pdf.

O'Sullivan, H., Moneypenny, M. J., & McKimm, J. (2015). Leading and working in teams. *British Journal of Hospital Medicine*, 76(5), 264–269.

Shever, L., Titler, M., Lehan Mackin, M., et al. (2011). Fall prevention practices in adult medical-surgical units described by nurse managers. *Western Journal of Nursing Research*, 33, 385–397.

Tibbs, S. M., & Moss, J. (2014). Promoting teamwork and surgical optimization: Combining TeamSTEPPS with a specialty team protocol. *AORN Journal*, 100(5), 477–488.

West, M. A., & Lyubovnikova, J. (2012). Real teams or pseudo teams? The changing landscape needs a better map. *Industrial and Organizational Psychology*, 5(1), 25–28.

West, M. A., & Lyubovnikova, J. (2013). Illusions of team working in health care. *Journal of Health Organization and Management*, 27(1), 132–142.

Wolf, F. A., Way, L. W., & Stewart, L. (2012). The efficacy of medical team training: Improved team performance and decreased operating room delays, a detailed analysis of 4863 cases. *Annals of Surgery*, 252(3), 477–483.

15

Teams and Teamwork Case Studies

LEARNING OUTCOMES

After successfully working through the case studies in this chapter, you will be able to:

1. Demonstrate the ability to apply the Teams and Teamwork Sub-competencies to problem-based case studies in this chapter.
2. Operationalize the behaviors of Teams and Teamwork through case study application.

3. Evaluate how the Sub-competencies of Teams and Teamwork in Interprofessional Collaboration are demonstrated in the case study discussions.
4. Identify the importance of Interprofessional Collaboration as it applies to each case.

This chapter presents patient- and population-based case studies designed to highlight the application of teamwork concepts to practice. Case studies are intended for use in group discussions or debates, as role-playing exercises, or as individual learning exercises. The authors acknowledge that all four Core Competencies may apply in each case; however, learning in this chapter is purposefully focused on Teams and Teamwork (TT) Sub-competencies. Carefully crafted guiding questions provide direction for learners and faculty facilitators.

CASE STUDY GUIDELINES

For each practice case study, you are asked to consider and apply specific Sub-competencies of Teams and Teamwork. These will be clearly indicated to you before you begin to read the case study. The Sub-competencies of Teams and Teamwork are provided for your reference in Box 15.1.

Case studies can be used as individual problem-based learning activities or incorporated as part of a variety of group learning activities. You can independently determine how each case study will be used after considering your specific learning needs and educational setting. Discussion questions and/or suggested learning activities are provided after each case study. You are encouraged to modify these questions and activities or pose your own to meet specific

learning needs. Chapter 13 of this text provides foundational theory related to Teams and Teamwork; Chapter 14 provides examples to help readers operationalize specific Sub-competencies. Both chapters will be useful in considering the case studies that follow.

CASE STUDY: TEAM OR "PSEUDOTEAM"

Specific Sub-competencies to consider and apply: TT1, TT3; also consider resources from Chapter 13 describing the characteristics of "true teams" versus "pseudoteams."

Individuals with intellectual and developmental disabilities (IDD) often encounter challenges in maintaining a healthy lifestyle. Get FIT is a community-based program that was developed to promote access to physical activity, as well as education about healthy lifestyle choices, for individuals with IDD living in the community. You have the opportunity to volunteer at the Get FIT program at your local university and observe the following.

Clients with IDD arrive at the campus community center with their group home care providers. The clients gather around a table and socialize with one another and the individuals providing the program. The group home care providers sit in chairs toward the back of the room. The session begins with nursing students discussing the importance of healthy food choices. The discussion centers on sugary beverages, diet beverages, and water. Several

BOX 15.1 **Teams and Teamwork Core Competency and Related Sub–competencies (IPEC, 2016, p.14)**

Statement: General Core Competency of Teams and Teamwork

Apply relationship-building values and the principles of team dynamics to perform effectively in different team roles to plan, deliver, and evaluate patient/population-centered care and population health programs and policies that are safe, timely, efficient, effective, and equitable.

TT1. Describe the process of team development and the roles and practices of effective teams.

TT2. Develop consensus on the ethical principles to guide all aspects of teamwork.

TT3. Engage health and other professionals in shared patient-centered and population-focused problem-solving.

TT4. Integrate the knowledge and experience of health and other professions to inform health and care decisions, while respecting patient and community values and priorities/ preferences for care.

TT5. Apply leadership practices that support collaborative practice and team effectiveness.

TT6. Engage self and others to constructively manage disagreements about values, roles, goals, and actions that arise among health and other professionals and with patients, families and community members.

TT7. Share accountability with other professions, patients, and communities for outcomes relevant to prevention and health care.

TT8. Reflect on individual and team performance for individual, as well as team, performance improvement.

TT9. Use process improvement strategies to increase the effectiveness of interprofessional teamwork and team-based services, programs, and policies.

TT10. Use available evidence to inform effective teamwork and team-based practices.

TT11. Perform effectively on teams and in different team roles in a variety of settings.

to encourage everyone to "get moving." Students interact with their assigned clients throughout the session. Everyone seems to enjoy the physical activity and the social interactions. At the end of the session, student volunteers guide clients to their respective care providers to return to their home.

Discussion Questions

1. Based on your understanding of the case study presentation, were the individuals providing the Get FIT program functioning as a true team or pseudoteam? Provide specific examples as a rationale for your perspective.

2. Identify at least two potential benefits of interprofessional collaboration for the clients participating in this program.

3. Suggest additional team members who can engage in this client- and population-centered program. How would you rework the scenario to illustrate engaging other professionals in shared patient- and population-focused problem solving?

4. Offer at least three suggestions for team development and effective teamwork practices in this setting. Refer to Chapters 13 and 14.

CASE STUDY: PROVIDING TEAM-BASED CARE IN A SCHOOL SETTING

Specific Sub-competencies to consider and apply: TT1, TT4, TT5, TT11.

Sarah Edwards is an 8-year-old girl who was born prematurely in a complicated birth to a mother who was addicted to drugs. She lives with her grandmother, who is her legal guardian. Sarah has multiple physical, emotional, and cognitive challenges. She has limited verbal ability to express her needs and is prone to behavioral outbursts. She attends special education classes in her community school. The interprofessional team includes her special education teacher, instructional paraprofessionals, the school nurse, the case manager/social worker, a behaviorist, a speech therapist, an occupational therapist, and a school psychologist.

Sarah's physical, emotional, and psychological well-being is the focus for all team members. The team works together effectively to address behaviors and implement strategies to improve the fluctuating challenges in the classroom and at home. There are no turf battles; rather the team cohesively discusses and makes

clients actively interact with the nursing students and each other for half an hour. At that point, the physical activity portion of the session begins. Students from occupational therapy and physical therapy disciplines lead a gentle stretching and strengthening program for the group. Each client is assisted by a student volunteer who records the specific activities the client completes. This is followed by a group activity that is set to music recommendations, easily shifting the leadership role depending on the situation. Working in teams involves sharing expertise and relinquishing some professional autonomy to work closely with others to share the care and improve the client's outcomes. The entire team is valuable and provides essential resources in their area of knowledge. For example, adjustments in Sarah's medication may require the nurse or case manager to intervene. The behaviorist may change the behavioral management program, whereas the remaining team members implement the plan and provide feedback on its effectiveness. If the team determines that Sarah's increasing outbursts stem from frustration with a limited ability to express her needs, the speech therapist takes the lead and works closely with the teacher, paraprofessionals, and family to identify the most appropriate communication strategies. The team integrates individual expertise of all members in shared planning to develop, implement, and reinforce team-based care.

By working closely together, the team members are aware of one another's plans and can transition activities more smoothly. For example, one day the speech therapist was running late because of a team meeting for another student. The occupational therapist realized this, and rather than ending the therapy session on time and leaving Sarah to wait for the speech therapist, the occupational therapist continued to work on team goals by incorporating goals both the occupational therapist and speech-language pathologist were addressing. The occupational therapist made use of the extra time to address communication and recognition of objects along with the motor skills practice of reaching and grasping objects. This creative use of time helped Sarah smoothly transition to her speech therapy session.

At a team meeting, the team discusses a concern raised by Sarah's grandmother about recent behavioral problems at home that seem to stem from her school day. Sarah's grandmother reports that for the past few weeks, Sarah has been agitated and prone to outbursts when she arrives home from school. Team members share their experiences related to circumstances throughout the day that seem to trigger outbursts in Sarah and what strategies help in calming her. The special education teacher notes that unexpected schedule changes and disrupted routines are especially challenging for Sarah. The behaviorist and the paraprofessionals reports that fatigue, hunger, and toileting needs commonly lead to emotional outbursts. The occupational therapist shares observations from her sessions working on sensory integration that loud noises trigger strong emotional responses from Sarah and disrupt her ability to participate in activities. The speech-language pathologist notes that Sarah seems relaxed and calm when reading in a quiet environment. The team works together, troubleshooting to determine how to reduce potential triggers. The team recommends changing Sarah's schedule during the last period of the school day from a group physical activity held in the combined classroom with multiple students to quiet reading time to help Sarah adjust to the end of the school day transition to home.

Discussion Questions

This case study illustrates how each member of the healthcare team, from the teacher to the paraprofessionals to the speech therapist, was able to integrate the knowledge and experience of others to make decisions about Sarah's plan of care.

1. Why is interprofessional collaboration important in this case study?
2. Identify at least two of the practices that support effective teams that are illustrated in this case study.
3. Refer to Chapters 13 and 14. Who do you believe is the team leader in developing Sarah's plan of care? Explain your reasoning.
4. Give an example of a situation described in the case study in which leadership appropriately shifts from one team member to another member.
5. Who should be included in problem solving and planning related to Sarah's care? Can you suggest other healthcare professionals and other professionals who should be part of the team?
6. Describe how team members' roles in the school setting differ from other settings.

CASE STUDY: COMMUNITY HEALTH CONCERNS

Background

Provision of healthcare services typically focuses on individual patients, but broader consideration of population health needs is also warranted. The TT3 Subcompetency addresses population-centered problem solving, whereas TT7 addresses healthcare outcomes related to prevention. Public health initiatives such as Healthy People 2020 focus on population health beyond individual patients. For example, the obesity epidemic continues to rise in the United States. Although this has implications for the health of individuals, it is clearly a problem for the population as well. The chronic health conditions of diabetes and cardiovascular disease are associated with obesity. In some urban areas, limited access to healthy food choices and safe venues for physical activity magnify the problem. Interprofessional collaboration provides an opportunity to integrate the expertise or experience of multiple professions to address population health concerns. With complex problems, engaging other professionals outside of health care in shared problem solving is particularly important. Consider this case study, which highlights these challenges and offers an example of developing potential solutions.

Case Study

Specific Sub-competencies to consider and apply: TT3, TT7.

Maya Marquez is a 63-year-old woman living in a low-income senior citizen high rise in an impoverished inner city. She has diabetes, high blood pressure, and is obese. Her doctors tell her to exercise and make healthy food choices. Ms. Marquez does not feel safe walking the 5 blocks to the corner market. The corner store has a limited selection of fresh fruits and vegetables. Instead, the options included mostly prepackaged and processed foods with high sodium content and sugary beverages. She does not drive. The senior service transportation van provided through her high rise is limited to doctor's appointments and the neighborhood market.

University students majoring in public health provide monthly screening and education services at the senior citizen high rise as part of their fieldwork. During a presentation to the residents about preventing and reducing obesity, Ms. Marquez shares her concerns about not having reasonable access to healthy food and exercise. Lively discussion by the residents and students generates the idea of converting an adjacent abandoned lot into a community garden. Ms. Marquez engages other professionals, including the city's urban planning officer, the high-rise community board members, and faculty and students from the following university programs: public health, dieticians, and nursing. They get approval for the community garden proposal and seek donations from area hospitals, banks, the university, and a local hardware store.

The community members partner with the university's Day of Service and local church members to clean up and remove debris from the abandoned lot. They break ground and build the fences, walkways, and irrigation system. Once ready, local donations include soil, fertilizer, mulch, and gardening tools. Interested residents sign up for a designated plot to plant, tend, and harvest. Their efforts are so successful that they convert an unused storage shed into a farmers' market stand to sell their produce. The outcome of their efforts is increased access to fresh and healthy food for the all the community residents.

Emboldened by their success, the residents (with support of community partners) convert one of the first-floor common areas into a small fitness center with a treadmill, two stationary bicycles, and some free weights. Public health students recommend that they partner with the university exercise science program students to offer fitness screening and develop an exercise program for residents who obtain medical clearance to participate in a physical activity program. One of the residents is a retired yoga instructor and offers to provide weekly classes for the residents.

Discussion Questions

1. Why was it important to have interprofessional collaboration for this initiative? How might the outcome have differed if the efforts only included one partner (discipline)?
2. Identify the leadership approach that Ms. Marquez used in developing the community garden. Contrast this leadership style with others she could have used. (Refer to the discussion of team leadership in Chapter 13.)

CASE STUDY: WHEELCHAIR SEATING CLINIC

Specific Sub-competencies to consider and apply: TT4, TT5, TT11.

The outpatient department of a rehabilitation center offers a monthly wheelchair seating clinic to evaluate seating needs for patients and community members. Team members meet with patients and caregivers to determine optimal seating recommendations based on individual needs. The team includes a physician, the equipment vendor, a social worker, and a physical therapist.

Tom Hargrave is 26 years old, and 1 year past a motorcycle accident in which he sustained multiple injuries, including a severe head injury. He requires a custom wheelchair for mobility. The physician provides a brief medical history and opens the discussion asking for recommendations from the team. In discussing potential recommendations, the vendor suggests a particular wheelchair with modular inserts for postural alignment. The physical therapist and the family report the need for removable arm and leg rests. As the conversation continues, the physician notices that the social worker has not spoken and specifically asks for his input regarding insurance coverage for medical equipment. Before finalizing the prescription, the physician asks the team if there is anything else they should consider. After a pause, the caregiver mentions the new communication device that Tom has been working with in speech therapy. The team modifies earlier suggestions so that the wheelchair includes a lap tray to accommodate the communication system as well.

Discussion Questions

1. Why was it important to have interprofessional collaboration for this situation? What would likely happen if patient-care decisions were made "in a silo"?
2. Suggest other members of the team that should be involved in decision making for the wheelchair seating clinic. Provide a rationale for your answer.
3. Identify leadership practices demonstrated by the physician in this case that supported collaboration and team effectiveness. Suggest additional strategies or behaviors to enhance the interactions. Refer to Chapters 13 and 14.
4. Refer to Chapter 13 to explore how perceptions of hierarchy and empowerment could have influenced the team meetings described in this case.

CASE STUDY: DISCHARGE DILEMMA: MANAGING DISAGREEMENTS

Specific Sub-competencies to consider and apply: TT3, TT6, TT10.

Jack Flynn is a 60-year-old construction worker who had a total knee replacement 2 days ago. At this point, decisions about discharge from the hospital are being made. The surgeon recommends discharge to home with an exercise program provided by an application available on the computer or phone, without any other services until after the 6-week postoperative visit. The occupational therapist (OT) recommends discharge to home with immediate follow up by a home care nurse and OT via home therapy services. The physical therapist recommends

discharge with a short stay in a subacute rehabilitation facility. The nurse acknowledges that the patient and family can carry out incision care at home but would prefer one to two visits by a home care nurse to follow up with any questions or potential complications. Mr. Flynn and his family are worried about his ability to negotiate stairs when entering the home and regaining full motion in the knee considering the pain and swelling. Mr. Flynn says he does not like computer technology and prefers face-to-face care.

Discussion Questions

1. How can the team engage in shared patient-centered problem solving related to Mr. Flynn's discharge?
2. Provide at least three examples of decision-making strategies to plan for discharge and recovery. Refer to Chapters 13 and 14.
3. How can available evidence be used to guide effective team decision making in this case study?

CASE STUDY: CROSS-MONITORING FOR SMOOTH RECOVERY

Specific Sub-competencies to consider and apply: TT3, TT7.

Mrs. Ashburn is a patient on the cardiac care unit of the hospital recovering from triple bypass heart surgery. Her past medical history includes rheumatoid arthritis affecting both knees and ankles that requires the use of a wheeled walker for ambulation. Her cardiologist has consulted physical therapy to begin her cardiac rehabilitation walking program. At day 2 after surgery she is still wearing a heart monitor, which sends a signal to the electrocardiography (ECG) technician station. Nurses oversee her pain medication, her vital signs, and care of her incisions. The respiratory therapist instructed Mrs. Ashburn on use of the spirometer to encourage deep breathing and reduce the risk of developing pneumonia. Each healthcare team member has an important role in promoting successful recovery from surgery. The physical therapist checks in with the nurse caring for Mrs. Ashburn to see how she has been doing for the past 24 hours. The physical therapist also checks in with the ECG-monitor technicians to discuss the current readings from Mrs. Ashburn's heart monitor and to alert them that she will be taking the patient for a walk in the hallway. The physical therapist checks her heart rate, blood pressure, and oxygen saturation before walking with her in the hallway. Midway through the walk in the hallway with the physical therapist, the ECG technician notes an abnormal heart rhythm and calls the nurse to communicate this information. The nurse brings a wheelchair to the hallway and suggests they take a rest break. The physical therapist and nurse closely monitor her heart rate, blood pressure, and oxygen saturation. Mrs. Ashburn says that she feels a little tired but otherwise alright. After a few minutes of rest, the ECG technician notifies them that her heart rhythm has returned to normal. The nurse and PT walk Mrs. Ashburn back to her room.

Discussion Questions

1. Why was it important to have an interprofessional team cross-monitoring and communicating about the patient's status during activity? What could have happened if patient care decisions were made "in a silo"?

2. Imagine that the nurse had handled the situation differently, placing blame for the episode of abnormal heart rhythm rather than addressing it with the team. What would have been the impact on the patient? What would have been the impact on the physical therapist?

3. Identify at least three examples in this case study in which team members effectively engaged others in the plan of care. Can you suggest additional strategies that they could use?

CASE STUDY: INTERPROFESSIONAL TEAM ROUNDS IN ACUTE CARE

Specific Sub-competencies to consider and apply: TT8, TT9.

Lincoln County Hospital decided to implement interprofessional team rounds each morning to discuss each patient's condition and the events in the past 24 hours and to collaboratively develop a plan of care. The purpose of this new process was to minimize unnecessary services, reduce delays and gaps in care, and enhance collaborative patient-centered care. Previously, there were two formal processes for communicating patient information: the electronic medical record and the change-of-shift handoff by nursing held in a small conference room next to the nurses station.

The new interprofessional team rounds were implemented at the bedside with the nurse, the attending physician, and the patient and included any family members who were present. After a few weeks with the new process, staff noted enhanced communication and follow through on the plan of care. Preliminary feedback from patients and families was positive, and they valued regular updates on the plan of care. Staff realized there was further opportunity to include other members of the team in the interprofessional rounds.

Discussion Questions

1. Discuss any anticipated barriers to implementing daily interdisciplinary rounds in the hospital. For each of the anticipated barriers suggest specific, realistic strategies to address the concerns.

2. What are the potential benefits to implementing this new process?

3. Who should be included in the daily interprofessional rounds? Consider different patient examples and list any members you consider appropriate.

4. Suggest at least three strategies to monitor individual and team performance with implementation of this new process.

REFERENCES

Interprofessional Education Collaborative Expert Panel (IPEC). (2016). *Core competencies for interprofessional collaborative practice: 2016 update.* Washington, DC: Interprofessional Education Collaborative.

Interprofessional Collaborative Case Studies

LEARNING OUTCOMES

After successfully working through the case studies in this chapter, you will be able to:

1. Demonstrate the ability to apply multiple Core Competencies to a single healthcare situation.
2. Operationalize the behaviors described in the specific Sub-competencies of all four Core Competencies.

3. Demonstrate all four Core Competencies for Interprofessional Collaborative Practice (IPCP) through case study discussions.
4. Identify the importance of Interprofessional Collaboration as it applies to each case.

This chapter provides patient- and population-based case studies designed to promote practice related to the specific Sub-competencies associated with all four Core Competencies for Interprofessional Collaborative Practice (IPEC, 2011; 2016): Values/Ethics, Roles/Responsibilities, Interprofessional Communication, and Teams and Teamwork. For easy reference, the general statement for each Core Competency and their associated specific Sub-competencies are presented in Box 16.1. Readers are encouraged to apply the Core Competencies and Sub-competencies that best fit each case, considering all four Core Competencies, rather than applying the specific Sub-competencies of just one Core Competency as was done in the previous case study chapters. Readers are encouraged to adapt the case studies as appropriate; for example, the reader may add or switch a character in a case study to explore the specific Competencies and related Sub-competencies in a profession not highlighted in the case study. This may be particularly useful if your profession is not part of the case study, but you see a relevant role for your profession in the situation being described

in the case study. Similarly, although each case study is accompanied by basic discussion questions, readers and educators are encouraged to generate additional questions that may better meet the needs of the learner.

CASE STUDY ACTIVITY GUIDELINES

For each practice case study, you will have the opportunity to consider and apply specific Competencies of Interprofessional Collaborative Practice and their associated Sub-competencies (see Box 16.1). Case studies can be used as individual problem-based learning activities or incorporated as part of a variety of group learning activities. You can independently determine how each case study will be used after considering your specific learning needs and educational setting. Basic discussion questions or suggested learning activities are provided after each case study. You are encouraged to modify these questions and activities, or to pose your own, to meet your specific learning needs. Chapters 4, 7, 10, and 13 of this text provide foundational theory related to each Core

Competency. Chapters 5, 8, 11, and 14 provide examples to help readers operationalize specific Sub-competencies. Readers are encouraged to refer to those chapters when working through the case studies in this chapter.

The following general guiding questions apply to all the case studies in this chapter and can be used in addition to the specific discussion questions that accompany each case study. These general guiding questions are designed to help you better identify and target the appropriate Sub-competency.

1. For each of the four Core Competencies, decide which Competencies or specific Sub-competencies are best exemplified in the case study; keep in mind that some may be implied by the situation. For example, for these

---

BOX 16.1 Core Competencies of Interprofessional Collaborative Practice With Specific Sub-competencies (IPEC, 2016, pp. 11–14)

Statement: General Core Competency of Values/Ethics

Work with individuals of other professions to maintain a climate of mutual respect and shared values.

The Specific Sub-competencies of Values/Ethics

VE1. Place the interests of patients and populations at the center of interprofessional health care delivery and population health programs and policies, with the goal of promoting health and health equity across the lifespan.

VE2. Respect the dignity and privacy of patients while maintaining confidentiality in the delivery of team-based care.

VE3. Embrace the cultural diversity and individual differences that characterize patients, populations, and the health team.

VE4. Respect the unique cultures, values, roles/responsibilities, and expertise of other health professions and the impact these factors can have on health outcomes.

VE5. Work in cooperation with those who receive care, those who provide care, and others who contribute to or support the delivery of prevention and health services and programs.

VE6. Develop a trusting relationship with patients, families, and other team members (CIHC, 2010).

VE7. Demonstrate high standards of ethical conduct and quality of care in contributions to team-based care.

VE8. Manage ethical dilemmas specific to interprofessional patient/population centered care situations.

VE9. Act with honesty and integrity in relationships with patients, families, communities and other team members.

VE10. Maintain competence in one's own profession appropriate to scope of practice.

Statement: General Core Competency of Roles/Responsibilities

Use the knowledge of one's own role and those of other professions to appropriately assess and address the health care needs of patients and to promote and advance the health of populations.

The Specific Sub-competencies of Roles/Responsibilities

RR1. Communicate one's roles and responsibilities clearly to patients, families, community members, and other professionals.

RR2. Recognize one's limitations in skills, knowledge, and abilities.

RR3. Engage diverse professionals who complement one's own professional expertise, as well as associated resources, to develop strategies to meet specific health and healthcare needs of patients and populations.

RR4. Explain the roles and responsibilities of other care providers and how the team works together to provide care, promote health, and prevent disease.

RR5. Use the full scope of knowledge, skills, and abilities of professionals from health and other fields and healthcare workers to provide care that is safe, timely, efficient, effective, and equitable.

RR6. Communicate with team members to clarify each member's responsibility in executing components of a treatment plan or public health intervention.

RR7. Forge interdependent relationships with other professions within and outside of the health system to improve care and advance learning.

RR8. Engage in continuous professional and interprofessional development to enhance team performance and collaboration.

RR9. Use unique and complementary abilities of all members of the team to optimize health and patient care.

RR10. Describe how professionals in health and other fields can collaborate and integrate clinical care and public health interventions to optimize population health.

Continued

BOX 16.1   Core Competencies of Interprofessional Collaborative Practice With Specific Sub-competencies (IPEC, 2016, pp. 11–14)—cont'd

Statement: General Core Competency of Interprofessional Communication

Communicate with patients, families, communities, and professionals in health and other fields in a responsive and responsible manner that supports a team approach to the maintenance of health and the treatment of disease.

The Specific Sub-competencies of Interprofessional Communication

CC1. Choose effective communication tools and techniques, including information systems and communication technologies, to facilitate discussions and interactions that enhance team function.

CC2. Communicate information with patients, families, community members, and health team members in a form that is understandable, avoiding discipline-specific terminology when possible.

CC3. Express one's knowledge and opinions to team members involved in patient care and population health improvement with confidence, clarity, and respect, working to ensure common understanding of information, treatment, care decisions, and population health programs and policies.

CC4. Listen actively, and encourage ideas and opinions of other team members.

CC5. Give timely, sensitive, instructive feedback to others about their performance on the team, responding respectfully as a team member to feedback from others.

CC6. Use respectful language appropriate for a given difficult situation, crucial conversation, or conflict.

CC7. Recognize how one's uniqueness (experience level, expertise, culture, power, and hierarchy within the health team) contributes to effective communication, conflict resolution, and positive interprofessional working relationships (University of Toronto, 2008).

CC8. Communicate the importance of teamwork in patient-centered care and population health programs and policies.

Statement: General Core Competency of Teams and Teamwork

Apply relationship-building values and the principles of team dynamics to perform effectively in different team roles to plan and deliver patient/population-centered care that is safe, timely, efficient, effective, and equitable.

The Specific Sub-competencies of Teams and Teamwork

TT1. Describe the process of team development and the roles and practices of effective teams.

TT2. Develop consensus on the ethical principles to guide all aspects of patient care and teamwork.

TT3. Engage health and other professionals in shared patient-centered and population-focused problem-solving.

TT4. Integrate the knowledge and experience of health and other professions to inform health and care decisions, while respecting patient and community values and priorities/preferences for care.

TT5. Apply leadership practices that support collaborative practice and team effectiveness.

TT6. Engage self and others to constructively manage disagreements about values, roles, goals, and actions that arise among health and other professionals and with patients, families, and community members.

TT7. Share accountability with other professions, patients, and communities for outcomes relevant to prevention and health care.

TT8. Reflect on individual and team performance for individual, as well as team, performance improvement.

TT9. Use process improvement strategies to increase the effectiveness of interprofessional teamwork and team-based services, programs, and policies.

TT10. Use available evidence to inform effective teamwork and team-based practices.

TT11. Perform effectively on teams and in different team roles in a variety of settings.

---

events to develop in the way they did, some of the specific competencies must have been worked out beforehand.

2. Identify any potential ethical issue(s) in the case study, even if it does not arise to the level of an ethical dilemma. Which Values/Ethics Sub-competencies could help avoid or mitigate the ethical issue?

3. Identify potential gaps or overlaps in the Roles/Responsibilities of the people involved in the case; remember to include patients and family members to the healthcare team. Next, determine which Roles/Responsibilities Sub-competencies could help to close the gaps or clarify the overlaps.

4. Identify examples of interprofessional communication in the case study, and determine which Interprofessional Communication Sub-competencies could have improved those communications.

5. Identify all the individuals involved in the case study. Determine which Teams and Teamwork Sub-competencies could have improved the actions and interactions of the team in the case study. Identify any un-named health professional who, if present, may have improved the performance of the team.

CASE STUDY: EMERGENCY IN A RURAL CLINIC

Frontier Medical Services is a small rural clinic, staffed with a doctor, an experienced nurse, and a receptionist who is responsible for several tasks, including making appointments, stocking supplies, and getting and filing the medical charts. Ms. Miller is a 21-year-old patient who is 7 months pregnant. She has a history of intravenous (IV) drug use and exchanging sex for drugs or money. She is HIV-positive, but she is inconsistent with her HIV treatment and with her prenatal care. Ms. Miller came to Frontier Medical Services complaining of severe abdominal pain and vaginal bleeding. Upon examination, the nurse determined that the young woman was in an advanced stage of labor, but she could not hear a fetal heartbeat. The nurse ran out of the examining room and yelled to the receptionist to call an ambulance and then summoned the doctor, who was attending to another patient. The doctor examined the patient and concurred with the nurse; the doctor requested that the patient be prepared for transport. Because of the several complications and the long ride to the nearest hospital, the doctor decides to ride along in the ambulance and continue treating the patient. The clinic staff called the emergency room of the hospital to alert them of the case. Halfway through the ride to the hospital, Ms. Miller gave birth a stillborn baby boy whom the team could not resuscitate. The mother, though she lost a lot of blood, stabilized and survived.

Discussion Questions

1. What are some ethical considerations in this case study, given the patient is (1) a known drug addict, (2) a patient who engages in prostitution, (3) HIV-positive, and (4) not following up with prenatal care or HIV treatment?
2. Because the ambulance is the domain of the paramedic, what are some Roles/Responsibilities issues that may arise with the doctor riding along with the patient in the ambulance? How could these issues be resolved?

a. If you are working on this case independently, describe the communication concerns of the paramedic in this case study.
   b. If you are working in a group, role play the communication concerns of the paramedic and the doctor.
3. What Core Competencies/Sub-competencies does this case study illustrate? Identify the Core Competencies and Sub-competencies that are applicable in these interactions.
   a. How do the Core Competencies and Sub-competencies you identified complement each other?
   b. Do any of the Core Competencies or Sub-competencies conflict in any way? If so, which Core Competencies and Sub-competencies should be prioritized?
4. Identify at least two Core Competencies, and specific Sub-competencies, not illustrated in the case study and describe how their application would result in optimal patient outcomes.

Role Play Activities

Working in pairs, role play the interactions between the doctor and paramedic during the ambulance trip.

1. First, role play at least one of the Core Competencies or Sub-competencies illustrated in this case study that you identified in question 3.
2. Then, role play at least one of the Core Competencies or Sub-competencies not illustrated in this case study that you identified in question 4.

CASE STUDY: EMERGENCY IN THE FACTORY

Thompson Brothers Steel is a medium-sized regional steel manufacturing factory. The factory has a small health clinic staffed with a part-time occupational physician and a full-time master's-level occupational health nurse. The occupational health nurse assists the doctor when he is present, and the rest of the time the nurse runs health and safety programs, performs screenings, and certifies that the employees are up-to-date on their safety training certifications. The doctor diagnoses and treats work-related injuries, educates the employees, and sees anyone not feeling well on the day that he is present. Mr. Jackson is a 29-year-old employee who came to the factory's clinic complaining of abdominal pain. He stated that he has been in pain for the past couple of days, but in the past couple of hours the pain has become intolerable. The findings of the examination were dull pain in the upper abdomen that became sharp as it moved to the lower right abdomen, loss of appetite, nausea, significant abdominal swelling, and a fever of 102° F. The doctor suspects that Mr. Jackson has appendicitis and that his appendix is at high risk of rupturing. The doctor asks the nurse to call for an ambulance, but Mr. Jackson insists he wants to drive himself to the hospital. Because the doctor is concerned Mr. Jackson's pain may impair his driving, he insists the patient should not drive. Mr. Jackson agrees to call his wife to transport him to the hospital. The nurse calls the emergency room to alert them to Mr. Jackson's arrival.

Discussion Questions

1. Identify positive examples of Interprofessional Collaboration in this case study.
2. Identify the Core Competencies or Sub-competencies that you see demonstrated.
3. What specific issues are most apparent to you?
4. Identify the appropriate Core Competency and its corresponding Sub-competencies that would be helpful in resolving this issue.
5. Describe how you would apply the identified Sub-competencies to resolve this issue.

CASE STUDY: TEAMWORK CHALLENGES

Ms. Trivaldi is a 53-year-old patient with uncontrolled diabetes. She is severely underweight and has gastroparesis that interferes with nutritional absorption and metabolism. The bariatric surgeon wanted to put a PICC (peripherally inserted central catheter) line to supplement her nutrition. He referred the patient to a gastroenterologist (GE) for management of the total parenteral nutrition (TPN) solution. However, the GE was concerned with the management of her diabetes, so she contacted the patient's endocrinologist for consultation on the amount of insulin that should be added to the TPN mixture. The bariatric surgeon did not wait for the GE and the endocrinologist to make their recommendation and placed the PICC line. He then told the GE to get the TPN solution prescribed, but she told the bariatric surgeon that she was not comfortable prescribing the nutritional supplement without the endocrinologist recommendation. When the patient asked the bariatric surgeon why she had not been started on the supplement, the surgeon told her it was because the GE did not want to prescribe the supplement. The patient was very upset with the GE and became difficult to work with after talking with the surgeon. Furthermore, once the endocrinologist reviewed the case, he recommended against the TPN because of her uncontrolled diabetes, and the PICC line had to be removed.

Discussion Questions

1. Who are the members of the interprofessional healthcare team?
2. Can you identify positive and negative examples of interprofessional collaboration? Describe at least one of each.
3. What is the main problem in this case study?
4. Which Core Competencies and specific Sub-competencies could have improved care in this situation? Identify at least three and explain your rationale.

CASE STUDY: NEIGHBORHOOD PHARMACY VERSUS MAIL ORDER PHARMACY

Rishi Sardana is an 11-year-old boy who is being switched from regular Ritalin to Ritalin LA, the long-acting version. His father, Mr. Sardana, goes to the pharmacy to pick up the new prescription, but he is told that the insurance company is refusing to pay for the LA preparation. The upset father tells the pharmacy technician that the pharmacy did not do it right and he wanted the pharmacy to fix the problem. The pharmacy technician calls the insurance company to clarify why they do not want to pay for the LA preparation. The representative of the insurance company explains that Ritalin LA is a maintenance drug and the policy of the insurance is that maintenance drugs must be ordered through their mail order pharmacy program. The representative also explains that they sent information to the family about how to make the switch. The insurance company does agree to approve the drug at the pharmacy, but with a much higher copay. The patient decides to buy a 30-day supply at the pharmacy and then transfer the prescription to the mail order pharmacy program, which has a much smaller copay.

Discussion Questions

1. Identify the members of the team mentioned in this case study.

2. Discuss the responsibility of each team member for the failure in communication. Remember the patient is also part of the team.
3. Should the insurance company be part of the healthcare team? Explain your rationale.
4. The insurance company sent information to the Sardana family about changing Rishi's prescription to the mail pharmacy. The communication of the health insurance company was not effective. If the team members involved in this case were working in collaboration, what other measures may they have taken to ensure the communication of this information was successful?

CASE STUDY: TIC, NOT TICK!

Ms. Brown is a 79-year-old patient in a small gastroenterology clinic. The clinic hired a young gastroenterologist (GE), who took over the care of patients from a doctor who had just retired. It is the custom in the clinic for the nurses to put a sticky note on top of the chart with the name of the patient, the examining room where the patient would be placed, and the reason for the visit. In the case of Ms. Brown, the nurse put "TICK" as the reason for the visit. The young GE thought it was strange that she was seeing someone for a tick bite, but she went ahead to the room. During examination, the doctor asked the patient, "Were you given antibiotics?" The patient responded, "For what?" The doctor said, "For the tick bite?" The patient yelled back, "What tick bite? I am here for diverticulitis!" (A common abbreviation for diverticulitis is "TIC.")

Discussion Questions

1. What was the communication problem in this case? At the personal level? At the clinic level?
2. What could have each of the team members involved in this case have done to prevent this communication problem?
3. Besides the specific Sub-competencies for Interprofessional Communication, which other specific Sub-competencies could improve the care in this situation?

CASE STUDY: WHO SHOULD HAVE TOLD HER?

Ms. Thompson is a 48-year-old cigarette smoker with late-onset asthma. Her primary care provider (PCP) was managing the asthma with conventional respiratory treatments (e.g., steroids and rescue inhalers). The respiratory therapist observed changes in Ms. Thompson's breathing pattern. When she asked the patient about these changes, the respiratory therapist uncovered Ms. Thompson was experiencing some pain when taking deep breaths. In consultation with the respiratory therapist, the PCP ordered a chest radiograph and referred Ms. Thompson to a pulmonologist, who found a mass in her lower right lung on the radiographs and confirmed the presence of a tumor with magnetic resonance imaging (MRI). The pulmonologist referred Ms. Thompson to an oncologist, who performed a biopsy and recommended treating the tumor with chemotherapy. From this point on, the lung cancer treatment was managed by the oncologist. In a follow up 6 months later, the PCP thinks the patient's condition is worsening; the respiratory therapist's progress notes seem to reflect the same concern. The PCP asks Ms. Thompson to see the pulmonologist. During her appointment with the pulmonologist, she finds a report in the chart from the oncologist indicating Ms. Thompson's tumor has grown and spread to the liver. The pulmonologist asks Ms. Thompson, "What other treatment is the oncologist recommending for you next?" Ms. Thompson responds, "Why would I need another treatment? I am doing well with the chemotherapy." The pulmonologist responds, "You are not doing well. Your cancer has spread to the liver. The chemotherapy is not working." Ms. Thompson yelled, "Nobody told me that!" The pulmonologist thought to herself, "Someone needs to tell her she is dying."

Discussion Questions

1. Identify the communication problem(s) in this case.
2. Who should be responsible for letting the patient know she is dying? What is the ethical responsibility of everyone in the team?
3. What could have been done differently to improve the outcome in this case?

CASE STUDY: AMPUTATION

Part 1

Mr. Rivera is a 63-year-old obese patient with uncontrolled type 2 diabetes. He has lost significant mobility and uses a wheelchair. He has had a nonhealing wound in his left foot for the past 2 months; the foot is now gangrenous. Mr. Rivera was admitted to the hospital

2 days ago to amputate his foot at the ankle. Although the surgery went reasonably well, 2 days after the surgery, Mr. Rivera developed a fever, and the tissue around the stump became red and warm to the touch. During morning rounds, the hospitalist recommends that the patient be discharged. However, the surgeon fears an infection is developing and recommends the patient remain hospitalized.

Discussion Questions

1. In what ways might interprofessional collaboration be improved in the care of Mr. Rivera?
2. Which interprofessional team members, besides the two mentioned, could have been involved in this decision?
3. What significant roles can Mr. Rivera and his family play on the interprofessional team? Explain.
4. Propose how disagreement might be resolved by using the appropriate Sub-competencies.
5. Which healthcare professional is ultimately responsible for this patient? Provide your rationale.

Part 2

Mr. Rivera was discharged to a rehabilitation hospital a couple of days later, after treatment for his infection was started. At the rehabilitation center, he is assigned to a standard team that consists of a nurse, a physician, a physical therapist, an occupational therapist, a pharmacist, and a social worker. Other healthcare professionals are often included in the team as needed. In the case of Mr. Rivera, an endocrinologist nurse practitioner and a dietician were added to the team to assist with controlling his diabetes and weight. An orthotist-prosthetist will join the team once Mr. Rivera is ready for a prosthetist. When the patient is admitted to the rehabilitation center, the team meets to discuss treatment goals and develop a plan. In the case of Mr. Rivera, the team decides the nurse and physician will take the lead regarding the general health of the patient, including caring for the incision and stump. The physical therapist will work on strengthening the leg that was operated on and improving his balance. Once he is ready to work on the prosthetic foot, the orthotist-prosthetist will make a prosthetic foot for him, and the occupational therapist will teach him to put on, use, and care for the prosthesis. The pharmacist will manage his medications (with the physician and nurse), and the social worker will coordinate several aspects of Mr. Rivera's care, including interacting with

Mr. Rivera's family, health insurance, and referrals to outpatient services once he is ready for discharge. Once the plan is in place, the team operates asynchronously; however, the team meets periodically to review the progress and make course corrections to the plan.

A week after admission, the physician and the nurse agree the incision is not healing as fast and well as expected. A chart review reveals that although his blood sugar level has improved, the insulin coverage order has not fully controlled the diabetes. The nurse noted she has talked with the patient several times about asking his wife to bring him sweets, but he evades the conversation, making a joke of it; he has also been seen getting candy from the vending machines in the rehabilitation center. The physical therapist and occupational therapist reported that Mr. Rivera does not like to move because the stump hurts, and it takes a lot for him to perform the exercises prescribed by the physical therapist. After a quick conference call, the team decides to refer Mr. Rivera to the health psychologist for behavior modification and include his wife and adult daughter to help them better support Mr. Rivera. The psychologist sees Mr. Rivera individually once per week and daily in a support group with other patients in an amputee support group. After a couple of weeks, Mr. Rivera and his family become more compliant with his treatment, and the physical therapist and occupational therapist can proceed with fitting the prosthesis and teaching him to live with it.

Discussion Questions

1. What are some of the advantages and disadvantages of having such a large interprofessional team?
2. Is it better to have a smaller team? Explain your answer.
3. Are all the healthcare professionals on the team necessary? Why or why not?
4. Which strategies worked and which did not work in this case study? Explain in terms of the appropriate Core Competencies and specific Sub-competencies involved in your rationale.
5. How could introducing patient-centered care from the beginning have improved the unfolding of this case?

CASE STUDY: TO TUBE OR NOT TO TUBE

Mr. Cowell is a 72-year-old patient who fell and developed a subdural hematoma in the right side of his skull. The patient had emergency surgery to evacuate the hematoma. He came out of surgery connected to a ventilator, intubated with an endotracheal tube. The standard extubation protocol is 12 hours postoperation, provided the patient meets the necessary criteria. Two days postoperation, the neurosurgeon decides to discontinue the ventilator and extubates the patient, even though the patient has not met the full criteria. After extubation the patient is put on a nasal cannula. Shortly after extubation, Mr. Cowell's oxygen saturations decline, and he complains of difficulty breathing and is unable to cough effectively. The respiratory therapist increases his oxygen, gives him a breathing treatment, and suctions him per hospital protocol. After 2 hours of observation, the nurse and respiratory therapist come to consensus that the patient is not showing significant improvement. The nurse and the respiratory therapist recommend the patient be intubated; however, the neurosurgeon insists that the patient needs to be breathing on his own 5 days after the operation. The patient continues to deteriorate, and 2 hours later the attending anesthesiologist reintubates the patient.

Discussion Questions

1. Who are the members of the interprofessional team in this case?
2. What specific communication problem(s) can you identify and how did it contribute to the poor healthcare outcomes?
3. Which specific Sub-competencies, from all four Core Competencies, could have improved the healthcare outcomes for the patient in this case?
4. Which other healthcare professionals might have joined the interprofessional team to consult during the initial decision-making process regarding tube removal? Provide your rationale.

CASE STUDY: "NONCOMPLIANT"

Mr. Williams is a 63-year-old patient of a neurology practice that is affiliated to a large hospital. A couple of years ago, he was diagnosed with Charcot-Marie-Tooth disease, a hereditary neurologic disorder that tends to start with the feet and affects the peripheral nerves, producing peripheral neuropathy and loss of muscle mass. Years ago, the patient started feeling numbness he described as "having his feet taped," but he did not seek medical help until he started having problem controlling his feet.

The patient often comes late to his appointments or does not show up. When he arrives for his appointments and is waiting in the reception area, he is loud and rude to the receptionists and nurses in his attempt to be seen faster. He constantly insists the doctors contact his health insurance to get approved for things he can buy over the counter. He does not follow up with the referrals the doctors make. For example, the neurologist referred him to a physical therapist for muscle strength training, muscle and ligament stretching, stamina training, and aerobic exercise. The neurologist also referred him to an orthopedic specialist to get ankle braces to improve his ambulation and to an occupational therapist to learn how to put the ankle braces on. Mr. Williams did not follow up with the orthopedic specialist until walking became too difficult. He got the ankle braces but did not followed up with the occupational therapist.

The neurology practice has a "three no show policy" that enables them to discharge patients from the practice. The neurology team continued to work with Mr. Williams until his fifth "no show." Then they notified him that he had been discharged from the practice. He was sent a letter communicating that he had been discharged and was provided a list of neurologists in the area. However, Mr. Williams still calls once in a while to request his prescription be renewed and to ask the doctors to contact his insurance provider to get him approved for things he needs.

Discussion Questions

1. Who are the members of the interprofessional team in this case?
2. Discuss leadership in this team. Who should have been the leader of this team? Explain your rationale.
3. Was communication appropriate and adequate between all team members? Use the Interprofessional Communication Sub-competencies to explain your answer.
4. Did the neurology practice meet their ethical obligations in this case? Why or why not?
5. Which other healthcare professional(s) may have made a difference if they had been included in this interprofessional team?

CASE STUDY: PEDIATRIC PATIENT

Sammy is an 11-year-old child with chronic back pain and behavioral problems. Because Sammy has been acting out at home and at school and showing signs of depression, the school counselor has put the family in contact with the Department of Family Services. The social worker from family services referred the child to a community counselor to address the behavior problems and depressive symptoms. After evaluation, the counselor determines the symptoms are largely related to the back pain and suggests that the family take the child to a pediatric orthopedic surgeon to evaluate the back pain. The surgeon diagnoses the child with a lumbar herniated disk and suggests Sammy have surgery during a school break. In the interim, the doctor prescribes ibuprofen and refers the child to physical therapy to teach him targeted stretching and exercises for rehabilitation. The school counselor helps the family to secure a more comfortable chair for Sammy because sitting all day in his school desk was aggravating the pain.

Discussion Questions

1. Who are the members of the interprofessional team in this case? Would you define this as a collaborative team? Explain.
2. Who should have been the leader of this team?
3. Discuss team communication related to Sammy's issues. Which of the Interprofessional Communication Sub-competencies that apply to this case study were and were not demonstrated?
4. Which of the Teams and Teamwork Sub-competencies that apply to this case study were and were not demonstrated?
5. Do you think it helped or hindered the outcomes of the case that the healthcare professionals worked in different institutions?

CASE STUDY: MISCOMMUNICATION

Mr. Salib is a 35-year-old man who comes to the hospital with severe abdominal pain. He is diagnosed with an incarcerated abdominal hernia that requires surgery. The doctor orders the patient to fast overnight to be ready for surgery in the morning. Mr. Salib is kept in a double room and put on the schedule for surgery next morning. In the morning, the food service worker working the floor fails to confirm the identity of Mr. Salib and gives him his roommate's food tray. The registered nurse sees the tray being delivered to Mr. Salib and asks the food service worker to make sure he is giving the food to the right patient. The food service worker compares the names of the patients on their wristbands with his delivery list

and confirms that Mr. Salib is not the patient in the room who should get the food tray.

Discussion Questions

1. Identify the members of the team mentioned in this case study and state, in terms of interprofessional communication, what each of them could have done to prevent this problem.
2. Which specific Sub-competencies in the Core Competency of Teams and Teamwork apply to this case study, either because they were or were not demonstrated?
3. Which specific Sub-competencies in the Core Competency of Roles/Responsibilities apply to this case study, either because they were or were not demonstrated?
4. Propose a policy that may prevent this problem in the future.

CASE STUDY: PHARMACY SAVES THE DAY

Ms. Kim is a 34-year-old patient who comes to urgent care for an ear infection. The doctor in urgent care prescribes penicillin, even though the patient states that she is allergic to that antibiotic. The doctor transmits the prescription to Ms. Kim's local pharmacy, and before she arrives at the pharmacy, the pharmacy technician begins working on the prescription. When the technician enters the prescription in the patient's record, a flag appears indicating a possible allergy to penicillin. The technician consults with the pharmacist, who agrees there seems to be a potential negative interaction. The pharmacist calls Ms. Kim and explains that she was prescribed penicillin and the system is indicating that she may be allergic to the antibiotic. After she confirms her allergy to penicillin, the pharmacist contacts the doctor in urgent care to provide this information and suggest that a more appropriate antibiotic be prescribed.

Discussion Questions

1. Who are the members of this healthcare team?
2. What Core Competencies and Sub-competencies did the team members demonstrate?
3. Did the team demonstrate interprofessional collaboration? Explain your answer.

Role Play Activities

1. Using four participants, role play the interactions between the pharmacy technician and the pharmacist,

between the pharmacist and the patient, and between the pharmacist and the prescribing physician.
2. Identify and demonstrate the appropriate Sub-competencies of the Roles/Responsibilities Competency in the role play.
3. Identify and demonstrate the appropriate Sub-competencies of the Interprofessional Communication Competency in the role play.

CASE STUDY: LIVER TRANSPLANT INTENSIVE CARE UNIT TEAM

Mr. Taylor is a 57-year-old liver transplant patient. The team that receives the transplant patients in the intensive care unit (ICU) consists of the nurse assigned to the patient, a pharmacist, a surgical resident, a resident from the internal medicine team, a respiratory therapist, and the ICU head nurse; the family is often involved, especially at the beginning when history is being collected and as discharge approaches. The postoperative transplant team meets every morning to discuss the day's plan for the patients. The day after Mr. Taylor's transplant, the team meets, and the nurse assigned to him reports that he seems restless and anxious. After the team reviews the chart, the pharmacist notes that Mr. Taylor had been receiving the immunosuppressant medication intravenously for more than 24 hours and that he should have been switched already to the oral medication. She explains that "shakiness" is a common side effect of the intravenous (IV) version of the medication. The surgical resident suggests a consultation with the psychiatry department for an anxiolytic, but the ICU head nurse recommends switching the patient to the oral immunosuppressant medication and orienting him to lower the "anxiety" before getting the consultation. The assigned nurse offers to engage Mr. Taylor's adult daughter because she is able to calm him and make him feel less uneasy. The team agrees on the plan.

Discussion Questions

1. What actions in this case study demonstrate proficiency in Interprofessional Collaborative Practice? Identify at least two actions and explain your rationale using the Sub-competencies of any of the four Core Competencies.
2. What are some of the advantages of working as an interprofessional collaborative team, as demonstrated in this case study?

3. Who should be the leader of this team, and why?
4. Who should present the case to the group, and why?

CASE STUDY: THE DOCTOR HAS HAD IT WITH THE PAPERWORK

Mr. Dede is a 53-year-old patient with diabetes. His doctor prescribes a new glucometer for his diabetes management that is much easier to use and requires a much smaller blood sample. When he takes his prescription to the pharmacy, the pharmacy technician tells him that his health insurance requires paperwork to be completed by his doctor before they will allow payment for the device. Mr. Dede comes back a couple of days later saying that his doctor said the pharmacy has to complete the paperwork. The pharmacist calls the doctor to explain that the insurance company specifically prohibits the pharmacy from completing that kind of paperwork. The insurance will only accept the paperwork from the doctor who prescribes the device. The doctor responds, "I've had it with the paperwork. I am not doing it," and hangs up.

Discussion Questions

Completing preauthorization forms, referrals, letters, and other paperwork from other entities take time from the doctors and other health professionals; they are not paid for the time they spend completing such paperwork. However, it may still be part of their responsibilities.
1. Does the doctor have the right to refuse completing this paperwork?
2. What are the ethical implications of the doctor refusing to complete the paperwork, for the doctor and for the pharmacist? Explain using the specific Sub-competencies of the Core Competency Values/Ethics.
3. Besides completing or not completing the paperwork, are there other alternatives the doctor has to help Mr. Dede obtain a glucometer?
4. If these individuals where working as a collaborative team, which actions could they take to have a positive outcome for the patient? What could the doctor, pharmacist, patient, and insurance company do?

CASE STUDY: YOUR DENTIST UNTIL DEATH DO US PART

Dr. Hernandez is a dentist in private practice in a small town. The local police contact her because they found a skull by the river that they suspect belongs to a person who was decapitated in a freak accident the year before. They know the body of the victim belongs to a patient of the doctor, so they hope she can identify the skull using dental records. The doctor is able to make the identification by comparing the teeth in the skull with dental records, including radiographs, progress notes, and a mold that was made of the patient's teeth a couple of years before.

Discussion Questions

1. Is identifying the skull inside or outside of the roles and responsibilities of dentistry? Explain your answer.
2. In this case study, the patient is dead. Does it make sense to think about the professionals involved in this case as a healthcare team? Provide argument in favor and against this idea.
3. If we can consider the professionals involved in this case a healthcare team, who should be part of it?

REFERENCES

Canadian Interprofessional Health Collaborative (CIHC). (2010). *A National interprofessional competency framework*. Vancouver, Canada. Retrieved from https://www.cihc.ca/files/CIHC_IPCompetencies_Feb1210.pdf.

Interprofessional Education Collaborative Expert Panel (IPEC). (2011). *Core competencies for interprofessional collaborative practice: Report of an expert panel*. Washington, DC: Interprofessional Education Collaborative.

Interprofessional Education Collaborative Expert Panel (IPEC). (2016). *Core competencies for interprofessional collaborative practice: 2016 update*. Washington, DC: Interprofessional Education Collaborative.

University of Toronto. (2008). Competency framework. *Advancing the Interprofessional Education Curriculum 2009: Curriculum overview*. Toronto: University of Toronto Office of Interprofessional Education.

Roles and Education of Common Healthcare Professions and Related Careers

Audiology

Role
: Audiologists assess, treat, and rehabilitate hearing, balance, and related disorders (ASHA, n.d.c).

Education
: An undergraduate degree, usually in communication sciences and disorders, is required for admission to an audiology doctoral program.

: Audiologist education includes academic coursework and a minimum of 1820 hours of clinical practicum experience supervised by a certified audiologist.

: It generally takes 4 years to earn a practice Doctorate in Audiology (AuD) degree (BLS, 2015; ASHA, n.d.d).

: Programs that offer a PhD have a research component and usually take 6 years postbaccalaureate degree.

Additional Resources
: American Board of Audiology (ABA). (n.d.). *Board certified in audiology*. Retrieved from: http://www.boardofaudiology.org/board-certified-in-audiology/

Related Careers
: *Audiology Assistant*
: Performs tasks delegated by and under the supervision of a licensed audiologist.
: Duties include cleaning and preparing equipment and working with hearing aids.
: Education is usually on-the-job training.
: *Occupational Hearing Conservationist (OHC)*
: OHCs "provide training, consultation, audiometric testing and hearing protection fitting in occupational settings such as manufacturing plants, mobile health testing vans, occupational health clinics and other facilities with exposure to high noise levels."
: Successful completion of a 20-hour course is required (CAOHC, 2015).

Dentistry

Role
: Dentists "diagnose and treat diseases, injuries and malformations of the teeth and mouth; improve a patient's appearance; perform surgical procedures such as implants, tissue grafts and extractions; educate patients on how to better care for their teeth and prevent oral disease; teach future dentists and dental hygienists; and perform research directed to improving oral health and developing new treatment methods" (ADA, n.d., para 2).

: Dentists diagnose and treat problems with "teeth, gums, and related parts of the mouth; provide advice and instruction on taking care of the teeth and gums and on diet choices that affect oral health" (BLS, 2015).

: There are nine recognized dental specialty areas (ADA, n.d.).

Education	Applicants must take the Dental Admissions Test (DAT) at least a year before applying to dental school.
	A minimum of 4 years of postbaccalaureate education results in either a Doctor of Dental Surgery (DDS) or Doctor of Dental Medicine (DMD) degree.
	All dental education includes an extensive clinical component along with classroom instruction; some schools require a 1- to 2-year clinical residency.
	Specialization requires additional education and clinical experience.
Additional Resources	American Dental Association (ADA). (2015). *State licensure for US dentists.* Retrieved from: http://www.ada.org/en/education-careers/licensure/state-dental-licensure-for-us-dentists
	American Dental Association (ADA). (n.d). *What can a career in dentistry offer you?* Retrieved from: http://www.ada.org/~/media/ADA/Education%20and%20Careers/Files/01_caries_in_primary_dentition-caufield_b/dentistry_fact.ashx
	American Dental Hygiene Association (ADHA). (n.d.). *Education and careers.* Retrieved from: http://www.adha.org/professional-roles
	Commission on Dental Accreditation (CODA). (2015). *Program options and descriptions.* Retrieved from: http://www.ada.org/en/coda/find-a-program/program-options-and-descriptions
	Dental Assistant National Board (DANB). (2016). *Exam & certification FAQ's.* Retrieved from: http://www.danb.org/en/Become-Certified/Exam-and-Certification-FAQs.aspx
Related Careers	**Dental Hygienist**
	These professionals "diagnose, plan, implement, evaluate and document treatment for prevention, intervention and control of oral diseases, while practicing in collaboration with other health professionals" (ADHA, n.d., para 3).
	Minimum education is an associate's degree from a Commission on Dental Accreditation (CODA) accredited program (CODA, 2015).
	Some entry-level programs lead to a bachelor's degree.
	Degree advancement programs award bachelor's or master's degrees in dental hygiene.
	Dental Assistant
	Assists dentists, takes dental radiographs, sterilizes and prepares dental instruments and equipment, and communicates instructions to patients.
	Educational requirements vary by state, with some requiring an associate's degree from a CODA-accredited program and others accepting on-the-job training.
	Some states require credential verification by passing one of several Dental Assistant National Board (DANB) certification examinations (DANB, 2016).

Diagnostic Medical Sonographer, Cardiovascular Technician, Vascular Technologist

Role	Operates equipment that creates images or conducts tests used by providers in the diagnosis of medical conditions.
	Some may assist in surgical procedures by providing imaging (BLS, 2015).
Education	To prepare for a sonography program, high school students should take mathematics, anatomy and physiology, and physics (BLS, 2015).
	Most require an associate's degree education with specific training and clinical experience, but some 1-year certificate programs exist.
	Bachelor's degree programs are available.
Additional Resources	American Registry for Diagnostic Medical Sonography (ARDMS). (2015). *Examinations and certifications.* Retrieved from: http://www.ardms.org/Discover-ARDMS/examinations-and-certifications/Pages/default.aspx

Medicine

Role	To diagnose and treat injuries or illnesses.
	Physicians: Examine patients; take medical histories; prescribe medications; order, perform, and interpret diagnostic tests; counsel patients on diet, hygiene, and preventive health care.
	Surgeons: Operate on patients to treat injuries, such as broken bones; diseases, such as cancerous tumors; and deformities, such as cleft palates (BLS, 2015).
	There are 120 medical specialties and subspecialties (AAMC, 2015a).
Education	Medical degree, internship, and residency
	Medical school applicants must take the Medical College Admission Test (MCAT) and undergo an interview process and criminal background check (AACOM, 2015).
	The Medical Doctor (MD) degree is awarded after successful completion of 4 years of medical school and the Doctor of Osteopathy (DO) degree is awarded by schools of Osteopathic Medicine.
	After earning the MD or DO degree, additional schooling is required before a physician is able to practice independently: 3 to 5 years of internship and residency, and 1 to 3 additional years of fellowship, depending on the medical specialty (AMA, 2015; AACOM, 2015).
Additional Resources	American Association of Colleges of Osteopathic Medicine (AACOM). (2015). *Osteopathic medical education information book 2016*. Chevy Chase, MD: Author.
	American Medical Association (AMA). (2015). *Program options and descriptions*. Retrieved from: http://www.ama-assn.org/ama/pub/education-careers/becoming-physician/medical-licensure/state-medical-boards.page
	Association of American Medical Colleges (AAMC). (n.d). *Using MCAT data in medical student selection*. Washington, DC: Author. Retrieved from: https://aamc-orange.global.ssl.fastly.net/production/media/filer_public/7c/fb/7cfb5f43-f9cd-4a5a-bdad-36e735b5844a/mcatstudentselectionguide.pdf
	Association of American Medical Colleges (AAMC). (2015a). *Careers in Medicine*. Retrieved from: https://www.aamc.org/cim/specialty/list/us/
	Association of American Medical Colleges (AAMC). (2015b). *The official guide to medical school admissions (2015 edition)*. Washington, DC: Author.
	United States Medical Licensing Examination (USMLE). (2015). Retrieved from: http://www.usmle.org/

Nursing-Professional (RN)

Role	Nursing is "the protection, promotion, and optimization of health and abilities, prevention of illness and injury, facilitation of healing, alleviation of suffering through the diagnosis and treatment of human response, and advocacy in the care of individuals, families, groups, communities, and populations" (ANA, 2015).
	Nurses provide and coordinate care, educate patients and the public about health, and provide emotional support to patients and their family members (BLS, 2015).

Education	In the United States, there are three educational pathways to becoming a registered nurse (RN). All require a high school diploma or equivalent to apply.

The most common pathway is the associate's degree program, which consists of 2 to 3 years of education at a community college that grants an associate's degree in nursing (ADN).

RN to BSN Completion Programs exist through which ADN nurses can complete their BSN degree in 1 to 3 years.

The 4-year Bachelor of Science in Nursing degree (BSN) is preferred by most employers and is required for entry into master's and doctoral programs in nursing.

Accelerated or second-degree programs are available for students who have completed a bachelor's degree in another discipline and prerequisite physical and social science courses.

The least common path to becoming a registered nurse is through a diploma program. Nursing skills are taught, but college credit is generally not received.

Globally, the BSN degree is the most common educational preparation for nurses.

There are many specialties in nursing, all of which require certification by a specific specialty organization or the American Nurses Credentialing Center (AACN) (ANA, 2015).

Additional Resources   Accreditation Commission for Education in Nursing (ACEN). (2013). Retrieved from: http://www.acenursing.org/mission-purpose-goals/

Related Careers   *Licensed Practical and Licensed Vocational Nurse (LPN and LVN)*

Provide basic nursing care under the supervision of an RN or physician. Requires state licensure.

They receive training in nondegree vocational programs that take 1 to 2 years to build understanding of responsibilities tailored to individual patients (McNaughton et al., 2013).

Assistant and Certified Home Health Aide

Under the supervision of an RN, they provide basic care in healthcare facilities or homes.

These occupations require training in state-approved training programs that take several weeks and do not involve college education (BLS, 2015).

Nursing–Advanced Practice (APN)

Role   There are four types of advanced practice registered nurses (APRNs): nurse practitioner (NP), certified nurse midwife (CNM), certified registered nurse anesthetist (CRNA), and clinical nurse specialist.

APRNs work independently or in collaboration with physicians.

They prescribe medications, order medical tests, and diagnose health problems (BLS, 2015).

They provide primary and preventive care or may specialize in the care of specific populations or in the treatment of certain diseases.

CRNAs administer anesthesia and are responsible for anesthesia-related care before, during, and after a variety of procedures, including surgery.

CNMs specialize in the care of women, focusing on gynecological care, family planning, care during and after pregnancy, and labor (BLS, 2015).

CNSs are expert clinicians in a specialty area of nursing practice related to a population, setting, disease, or medical subspecialty, type of care, or type of problem (NACNS, 2015).

The terminal practice degree is the Doctor of Nursing Practice (DNP), and the terminal research degree in the discipline of nursing is the PhD.

Education	All APRNs require a minimum of a Master of Science in Nursing (MSN) or a Doctor of Nursing Practice (DNP) degree.
	The DNP is a practice doctorate that may eventually replace the MSN degree for clinical APRNs.
	Programs exist for students to earn the BSN through MSN or DNP.
	A BSN and a valid RN license are required to apply for graduate education in nursing.
	To become a CRNA, a nurse must have a BSN and 1 year of acute care experience, and many programs schools require critical care experience and certification for entrance to a CRNA program (AANA, 2015).
	All APRN programs consist of a combination of classroom instruction and supervised clinical experience.
	APRN programs usually take 2 to 3 years to complete after receiving the BSN degree.
Additional Resources	American Nurses Association (ANA). (2015). *What is nursing?* Retrieved from: http://www.bls.gov/ooh/healthcare/nurse-anesthetists-nurse-midwives-and-nurse-practitioners.htm
	American Nurses Association. (n.d.). *NP and CNS certification rulemaking guide.* Retrieved from: http://www.nursingworld.org/rulemakingguide
	American Association of Nurse Anesthetists (AANA). (2015). *Become a CRNA.* Retrieved from: http://www.aana.com/ceandeducation/becomeacrna/Pages/default.aspx
	National Association of Clinical Nurse Specialists (NACNS). (2015). Retrieved from: http://www.nacns.org/html/cns-faqs.php

Nutrition/Dietetics

Role	Registered dietitian nutritionists (RDNs) or registered dietitians (RDs) are experts in food and nutrition (AND, 2015a) and advise people regarding what to eat to manage disease, promote a healthy lifestyle, or achieve specific health-related goals (BLS, 2015).
Education	A bachelor's degree is required from a program accredited by The Accreditation Council for Education in Nutrition and Dietetics (ACEND) of the Academy of Nutrition and Dietetics (AND).
	There are two types of programs.
	One is a coordinated program that combines academic and supervised practical experience and leads to either a bachelor's or master's degree.
	The other is a 4-year baccalaureate program that requires participation in an ACEND-accredited Dietetic Internship Program or Individualized Supervised Practice Pathway (ISPP) after graduation (AND, 2015a).
	The degree earned may be a Bachelor of Arts (BA), Bachelor of Science (BS), or a BA of Public Health, depending on the school and program (BLS, 2015).
	Advanced practice internships are available.
Additional Resources	Academy of Nutrition and Dietetics (AND). (2015a). *Frequently asked questions about careers in dietetics.* Retrieved from: http://www.eatrightacend.org/ACEND/content.aspx?id=6442485476
	Academy of Nutrition and Dietetics (AND). (2015b). *What is a dietetic technician, registered?* Retrieved from: http://www.eatrightpro.org/resources/about-us/what-is-an-rdn-and-dtr/what-is-a-dietetic-technician-registered
	Board for Certification of Nutrition Specialists (BCNS). (2015). *The certified nutrition specialist credential.* Retrieved from: http://www.nutritionspecialists.org/cns/certified-nutrition-specialist®-cns®-credential
	Commission on Dietetic Registration (CDR). (2015). *Who is a registered dietician?* Retrieved from: https://www.cdrnet.org/about/who-is-a-registered-dietitian-rd

Related Careers	*Nutritionist*
	The role and definition of "nutritionist" is variable (BLS, 2015; AND, 2015a).
	A bachelor's degree is usually required, with special training in nutrition (BLS, 2015).
	Many states regulate the practice of nutritionists in some way, such as licensure or state registration or certification, and restrict the usage of certain titles.
	Dietetic Technician
	Dietetic technicians are "trained at the technical level of nutrition and dietetics practice for the delivery of safe, culturally competent, quality food and nutrition services" (AND, 2015b, para. 1) and work under supervision of registered or licensed dieticians.
	Education requires at least an associate's degree and completion of an ACEND-accredited Dietetic Technician Program that includes 450 hours of supervised practice.

Occupational Therapy (OT)

Role	Occupational therapists focus on the therapeutic use of everyday activities to help people function in all of their environments (AOTA, n.d.c).
	Occupational therapists help injured, ill, or disabled people develop, recover, or improve skills needed to perform activities of daily living and work (BLS, 2015).
Education	A master's degree in occupational therapy is required.
	Students who enter with a bachelor's degree can earn their master's degree (MSOT) in 2 to 3 years or a practice doctorate (OTD) in 3 to 5 years depending on the program.
Additional Resources	American Occupational Association (AOTA). (n.d.a). *About physical therapy.* Retrieved from: http://www.aota.org/About-Occupational-Therapy/Professionals.aspx
	American Occupational Association (AOTA). (n.d.b). *FAQ on OT career and planning.* Retrieved from: http://www.aota.org/Education-Careers/Considering-OT-Career/FAQs/Planning.aspx
	American Occupational Association (AOTA). (n.d.c). *How to get a license.* Retrieved from: http://www.aota.org/Practice/Manage/HowTo.aspx
	Bureau of Labor Statistics (BLS). (2015). *Occupational outlook handbook; Healthcare occupations: 2015-16 edition.* Washington, DC: US Department of Labor. Retrieved from: http://www.bls.gov/ooh/healthcare/home.htm
	Council for the Accreditation in Occupational Hearing Conservation (CAOHC). (2015). *About CAOHC.* Retrieved from: http://www.caohc.org/about-caohc
Related Careers	*OT Assistant*
	An OT assistant is a graduate of an accredited OT Assistant program and must pass a national certification examination.
	OT Aide
	OT aides usually receive on-the-job training and are not eligible for certification or licensure (AOTA, n.d.c).

Pharmacy

Role	"Pharmacist responsibilities include a range of care for patients, from dispensing medications to monitoring patient health and progress to optimize their response to medication therapies" (AACP, 2015b, para. 1).
	Pharmacists are medication experts who educate patients on the use of medications and educate and advise health professionals on medication therapy.
	Pharmacists have expertise in the composition of drugs, ensure drug purity and strength, and make sure that drugs do not interact harmfully (AACP, 2015a).

Education	Students may enter pharmacy programs to earn the Doctor of Pharmacy (PharmD) degree after 2 years of specific undergraduate study; some schools require a 4-year bachelor's degree; most students enter after 3 to 4 years of college.
	Some programs accept students directly from high school and prepare them for pharmacy school through undergraduate study.
	Accelerated programs are available for those with bachelor's degrees in the health sciences.
	Applicants may need to take the Pharmacy Admission Test (PCAT). The PharmD takes 4 years to complete after entry to a school of pharmacy.
	Clinical components of pharmacy education differ among programs.
	The American Society of Health-System Pharmacists offers specialty certification in pharmacotherapy, ambulatory care, oncology, pediatric care, and critical care (ASHP, 2014).
	Most specialties require a 1- to 2-year residency. Some states require Health System Pharmacists to complete a postgraduate residency.
	Postgraduate master or PhD programs are available after the PharmD.
Additional Resources	American Association of Colleges of Pharmacy (AACP). (2015a). *Pharm-D curriculum.* Retrieved from: http://www.pharmcas.org/preparing-to-apply/about-pharmacy/pharmd-curriculum/
	American Association of Colleges of Pharmacy (AACP). (2015b). *Table 5 First year PharmD class.* Retrieved from: http://www.aacp.org/resources/student/pharmacyforyou/admissions/admissionrequirements/Documents/Table%205.pdf
	American Association of Colleges of Pharmacy (AACP). *Role of a pharmacist.* Retrieved from: http://www.pharmcas.org/preparing-to-apply/about-pharmacy/role-of-a-pharmacist/
	American Society of Health-System Pharmacists (ASHP). (2014). *Certification resources.* Retrieved from: http://www.ashpcertifications.org/
	American Society of Health-System Pharmacists (ASHP). (2015). *About technicians.* Retrieved from: http://www.ashp.org/menu/PracticePolicy/ResourceCenters/Pharmacy-Technicians/About-Technicians#sthash.dydJz9t8.dpuf
	National Association of Boards of Pharmacy (NABP). (2015). *Technicians.* Retrieved from: http://www.nabp.net/programs/cpe-monitor/cpe-monitor-service/technicians/#ptcb
Related Careers	***Pharmacy Technician***
	A pharmacy technician "works closely with pharmacists in hospitals, drug and grocery stores, and other medical settings to help prepare and distribute medicines to patients" (ASHP, 2015, para. 1).
	There are several paths to become a pharmacy technician, including on-the-job training, vocational or technical schools, and associate's degree programs (BLS, 2015).
	The ASHP accredits pharmacy technician programs that meet certain standards, such as a minimum length of 600 hours extending over at least 15 weeks (ASHP, 2015).
	Most states license, register, or certify technicians in some way.
Physical Therapy (PT)	
Role	Physical therapists diagnose and manage movement dysfunction and enhance physical and functional abilities; restore, maintain, and promote optimal physical function, and optimal wellness and fitness, and optimal quality of life as it relates to movement and health; and prevent the onset, symptoms, and progression of impairments, functional limitations, and disabilities that may result from diseases, disorders, conditions, or injuries (APTA, 2015a, para. 4).
	Board certification is available in eight recognized specialties through the American Board of Physical Therapy Specialties.

Education	A Doctor of Physical Therapy (DPT) degree from a college or university program is required.
	Most DPT programs take 3 years and comprise 80% classroom instruction and 20% clinical experience, with a final clinical experience that averages 27.5 weeks (APTA, 2015b).
	Most DPT programs require a bachelor's degree before admission, although there are some "3 plus 3 programs" in which students complete 3 years of prerequisites and then 3 years of graduate study.
Additional Resources	American Physical Therapy Association (APTA). (2015a). *Licensure*. Retrieved from: http://www.apta.org/Licensure/
	American Physical Therapy Association (APTA). (2015b). *Role of a physical therapist*. Retrieved from: http://www.apta.org/PTCareers/RoleofaPT/
	American Physical Therapy Association (APTA). (2015c). *Role of a physical therapy assistant*. Retrieved from: http://www.apta.org/PTACareers/RoleofaPTA/
	Physical Therapist Centralized Application Service (PTCAS). (2015). *Summary of course prerequisites for programs in PCTAS: 2015-2016*. Retrieved from: http://www.ptcas.org/uploadedFiles/PTCASorg/Directory/Prerequisites/PTCASCoursePreReqsSummary.pdf
	The Federation of State Boards of Physical Therapy. (2015). *Licensees*. Retrieved from: https://www.fsbpt.org/Licensees.aspx
Related Careers	*PT Assistant*
	PT assistants provide physical therapy under the supervision of a licensed physical therapist.
	They must graduate from an accredited associate's degree program in physical therapy, pass a national examination for PT assistants, and be licensed.
	PT Aide
	PT aides and technicians are trained on the job, provide supportive services under supervision of licensed PT personnel, and are not eligible for licensure (APTA, 2015c).

Physician Assistant (PA)

Role	PAs work under the supervision of a physician or surgeon.
	They diagnose and treat illnesses, perform preventive care, prescribe medication, order and interpret diagnostic tests, and assist in surgery (AAPA, n.d.b).
Education	A Master of Science in Physician Assistant Studies (MSPA) degree is required.
	Most PA programs take 2 to 3 years to complete and consist of classroom instruction and 2000 hours of supervised clinical practice.
	Some 5-year programs exist in which students earn both a bachelor's degree and the MSPA.
Additional Resources	American Academy of Physician Assistants. (AAPA). (n.d.a). *Become a PA*. Retrieved from: https://www.aapa.org/become-a-pa/
	American Academy of Physician Assistants. (AAPA). (n.d.b). *What is a PA?* Retrieved from: https://www.aapa.org/what-is-a-pa/
	American Academy of Physician Assistants. (AAPA). (2014). *Statutory and regulatory requirements for licensure and license renewal*. Retrieved from: https://www.aapa.org/WorkArea/DownloadAsset.aspx?id=599

Psychology

Role	In health care, clinical psychologists "provide clinical or counseling services, assess and treat mental, emotional and behavioral disorders. They use the science of psychology to treat complex human problems and promote change. They also promote resilience and help people discover their strengths" (APA, 2015b, para. 1).

Education	Clinical psychology is a recognized specialty within psychology.
	A doctoral degree is required.
	Graduate programs require a bachelor's degree in psychology or accept a minor in psychology or many psychology courses; GRE scores, research experience, and clinically related community service may also be required (APA, 2015a).
	Many doctoral psychology programs require a master's degree in psychology, while some admit students with a bachelor's degree who progress straight through to a doctoral degree (BLS, 2015).
	Most doctoral degrees take 5 to 7 years to complete, and many mandate completion within 10 years.
	To practice clinical, counseling, or school psychology, a 1-year internship is required.
	Some programs offer a Psychology Doctorate (PsyD) degree for clinical psychologists; others award a PhD (APA, 2015b).
Additional Resources	American Board of Professional Psychology. (2015). *Clinical psychology*. Retrieved from: https://www.abpp.org/i4a/pages/index.cfm?pageid=3355
	American Psychological Association (APA). (2015a). *Frequently asked questions about graduate school*. Retrieved from: http://www.apa.org/education/grad/faqs.aspx
	American Psychological Association (APA). (2015b). *Pursuing a career in clinical psychology*. Retrieved from: http://www.apa.org/action/science/clinical/education-training.aspx
	Dittman, M. (2004). What you need to know to get licensed. *gradPSYCH Magazine*. Retrieved from: http://www.apa.org/gradpsych/2004/01/get-licensed.aspx

Public Health

Role	Public health focuses on improving access to health care; health promotion; preventing and controlling infectious disease; and reducing environmental hazards, violence, substance abuse, and injury.
	A variety of professionals who specialize in public health, including epidemiologists, nurses, social workers, biostatisticians, infectious disease specialists, physicians, health educators, field workers, and others.
Education	4 to 8 or more years depending on the profession.
Additional Resources	American Public Health Association (APHA). (2018). *What is public health?* Retrieved from: https://www.apha.org/what-is-public-health.

Radiologic and Magnetic Resonance Imaging (MRI) Technologists

Role	Radiologic technologists (also called radiographers) operate radiographic diagnostic equipment.
	MRI technologists perform MRI scans (BLS, 2015).
Education	An associate's degree is required from a program accredited by a certifying agency approved by the American Association of Radiologic Technology (AART).
	Bachelor's degree programs are available, and some certificate programs exist.
	MRI technicians start as radiographers and take additional training and certification.
	After additional training, certification is available in several specialties (BLS, 2015).
Additional Resources	American Society of Radiological Technologists (n.d.). Retrieved from: https://www.asrt.org/main/careers/careers-in-radiologic-technology/related-organizations.
	American College of Radiology (ACR). Accreditation. Retrieved from: https://www.acr.org/.

Respiratory Therapy (RT)

Role	Respiratory therapists diagnose lung and breathing disorders and recommend treatment; analyze breath, tissue, and blood specimens to determine levels of oxygen and other gases; manage ventilators and artificial airways; and educate patients and families about lung disease (AARC, 2015).
Education	A minimum of an associate's degree from a program accredited by the Commission on Accreditation for Respiratory Care (CoARC) is required.
	Some entry-level programs lead to a bachelor's degree in RT.
	Degree advancement programs exist for those with an associate's degree in RT to attain a bachelor's degree in RT and for those with a bachelor's degree in RT to receive a master's degree in RT.
Additional Resources	American Association for Respiratory Care (AARC). (2015). *What is an RT?* Retrieved from: http://www.aarc.org/careers/what-is-an-rt/
	National Board for Respiratory Care (NBRC). (2015). *The RRT credential.* Retrieved from: https://www.nbrc.org/rrt/pages/default.aspx
Related Careers	*Pulmonary Function Technologist and Advanced Pulmonary Function Technologist*
	The roles and educational preparation are similar to those for an RRT.
	These technologists take the national Pulmonary Function Technologist (PFT) examination.
	The PFT has cut-off scores. Individuals who achieve the lower-cut score earn the Entry-Level Pulmonary Function Technologist (CPFT) credential, whereas those who achieve the higher-cut score receive the Advanced Pulmonary Function Technologist (RPFT) credential.
	RRTs are eligible to take the PFT examination (NBRC, 2015).

Social Work

Role	Social workers help people obtain tangible services; conduct counseling and psychotherapy; help communities or groups provide or improve social and health services; and participate in legislative processes (NASW, 2015)
Education	There are several levels of education in social work.
	All require a degree from a college or university program accredited by the Council on Social Work Education (CSWE).
	All social work education consists of a combination of classroom instruction and supervised fieldwork.
	A Bachelor of Social Work (BSW) degree requires 4 years of education.
	To perform counseling or therapy, a minimum of a Master's degree in Social Work (MSW) is required.
	Practice doctorate degrees in Social Work (DSW) or PhDs are also available (NASW, n.d).
Additional Resources	Association of Social Work Boards (ASWB). (2013). Retrieved from: https://www.aswb.org/licensees/about-licensing-and-regulation/
	National Association of Social Workers (NASW). (n.d). *The Social Work Career Center: Education.* Retrieved from: http://careers.socialworkers.org/explore/education.asp

Speech-Language Pathology (SLP)

Role	Speech-language pathologists "prevent, assess, diagnose, and treat speech, language, social communication, cognitive-communication, and swallowing disorders in children and adults" (ASHA, n.d.c., para. 4).
Education	An undergraduate degree, usually in communication sciences and disorders, is required for admission to an SLP master's degree program.
	The 2 years of graduate education includes 200 to 300 hours of clinical practicum.
	After completion of academic work, an SLP clinical fellowship supervised by an ASHA-certified SLP consisting of a minimum of 35 hours per week for 36 weeks that totals 1260 hours must be completed (ASHA, n.d.d).
	The minimum entry-level degree for a SLP is a master's degree, which takes 3 years to complete.
	Practice doctorate and PhD programs are available in SLP.
Additional Resources	American Speech Language Hearing Association (ASHA). (n.d.a). *Career pathway for assistants*. Retrieved from: http://www.asha.org/associates/career-pathway-for-assistants/
	American Speech Language Hearing Association (ASHA). (n.d.b). *Certification*. Retrieved from: http://www.asha.org/certification/
	American Speech Language Hearing Association (ASHA). (n.d.c). *Learn about the CSD professions*. Retrieved from: http://www.asha.org/Students/Learn-About-the-CSD-Professions/
	American Speech Language Hearing Association (ASHA). (n.d.d). *Planning your education in communication science disorders*. Retrieved from: http://www.asha.org/Students/Planning-Your-Education-in-CSD/
Related Careers	*Speech-Language Pathology Assistant (SLPA)*
	SLPAs perform tasks prescribed, directed, and supervised by ASHA-certified speech-language pathologists.
	They must complete academic coursework in a CAA-accredited program with a minimum of 100 supervised clinical practicum hours, usually at a community college. Bachelor's degree programs are also available.
	Certification and licensure requirements vary, with some states requiring a bachelor's degree to be a licensed SLPA.
	SLP Aide or Technician
	Aides or technicians receive on-the-job training and work under the direct supervision of ASHA-certified SLPs.
	They are not eligible for licensure.

Page numbers followed by "*f*" indicate figures, "*t*" indicate tables,
and "*b*" indicate boxes.

THE CORE COMPETENCIES FOR INTERPROFESSIONAL COLLABORATIVE PRACTICE WITH SPECIFIC SUB-COMPETENCIES (IPEC, 2016, PP. 11-14)

Values/Ethics for Interprofessional Practice
Work with individuals of other professions to maintain a climate of mutual respect and shared values.

Values/Ethics Sub-competencies
VE1.   Place the interests of patients and populations at the center of interprofessional health care delivery and population health programs and policies, with the goal of promoting health and health equity across the lifespan.

VE2.   Respect the dignity and privacy of patients while maintaining confidentiality in the delivery of team-based care.

VE3.   Embrace the cultural diversity and individual differences that characterize patients, populations, and the health team.

VE4.   Respect the unique cultures, values, roles/responsibilities, and expertise of other health professions and the impact these factors can have on health outcomes.

VE5.   Work in cooperation with those who receive care, those who provide care, and others who contribute to or support the delivery of prevention and health services and programs.

VE6.   Develop a trusting relationship with patients, families, and other team members (CIHC, 2010).

VE7.   Demonstrate high standards of ethical conduct and quality of care in contributions to team-based care.

VE8.   Manage ethical dilemmas specific to interprofessional patient/population centered care situations.

VE9.   Act with honesty and integrity in relationships with patients, families, communities and other team members.

VE10. Maintain competence in one's own profession appropriate to scope of practice.

Roles/Responsibilities
Use the knowledge of one's own role and those of other professions to appropriately assess and address the health care needs of patients and to promote and advance the health of populations.

Roles/Responsibilities Sub-competencies
RR1.   Communicate one's roles and responsibilities clearly to patients, families, community members, and other professionals.

RR2.   Recognize one's limitations in skills, knowledge, and abilities.

RR3.   Engage diverse professionals who complement one's own professional expertise, as well as associated resources, to develop strategies to meet specific health and healthcare needs of patients and populations.

RR4.   Explain the roles and responsibilities of other care providers and how the team works together to provide care, promote health, and prevent disease.

RR5.   Use the full scope of knowledge, skills, and abilities of professionals from health and other fields to provide care that is safe, timely, efficient, effective, and equitable.

RR6.   Communicate with team members to clarify each member's responsibility in executing components of a treatment plan or public health intervention.

RR7.   Forge interdependent relationships with other professions within and outside of the health system to improve care and advance learning.

RR8.   Engage in continuous professional and interprofessional development to enhance team performance and collaboration.

RR9.   Use unique and complementary abilities of all members of the team to optimize health and patient care.

RR10. Describe how professionals in health and other fields can collaborate and integrate clinical care and public health interventions to optimize population health.